Practical Developments in Inherited Metabolic Disease

Practical Developments in Inherited Metabolic Disease: DNA Analysis, Phenylketonuria and Screening for Congenital Adrenal Hyperplasia

Proceedings of the 23rd Annual Symposium of the SSIEM, Liverpool, September 1985

The combined supplements of *Journal of Inherited Metabolic Disease* Volume 9 (1986)

edited by G. M. Addison,
R. A. Harkness,
D. M. Isherwood and R. J. Pollitt

MTP PRESS LIMITED
a member of the KLUWER ACADEMIC PUBLISHERS GROUP
LANCASTER / BOSTON / THE HAGUE / DORDRECHT

Published in the UK and Europe by
MTP Press Limited
Falcon House
Lancaster, England

British Library Cataloguing in Publication Data

Practical developments in inherited metabolic disease: DNA analysis, phenylketonuria and screening for congenital adrenal hyperplasia.
1. Metabolism, Inborn errors of
I. Addison, G. M.
616.3'9042 RC627.8

ISBN 0-85200-690-X

Published in the USA by
MTP Press
A division of Kluwer Academic Publishers
101 Philip Drive
Norwell, MA 02061, USA

Library of Congress Cataloging in Publication Data

Practical developments in inherited metabolic disease.

"The combined supplements of Journal of inherited metabolic disease, volume 9 (1986)."
Based on papers presented at the 23rd Annual Symposium of the SSIEM, held in Liverpool in 1985.
Includes bibliographies and index.
1. Metabolism, Inborn errors of—Congresses.
2. Phenylketonuria—Congresses. 3. Adrenogenital syndrome —Diagnosis—Congresses. 4. Deoxribonucleic acid—Analysis —Congresses. I. Addison, G. M. (Gerald Michael)
II. Society for the Study of Inborn Errors of Metabolism. Symposium (23rd : 1985 : Liverpool, Merseyside) III. Journal of inherited metabolic disease. [DNLM: 1. Adrenal Hyperplasia, Congenital—diagnosis—congresses. 2. DNA—analysis—congresses. 3. Metabolism, Inborn Errors—congresses.
4. Phenylketonuria—congresses. W3 SO5915K 23rd 1985 / WD 205 P895 1985]
RC627.8.P73 1986 616.3'9043 86-20860
ISBN 0-85200-690-X

Phototypeset and Printed in Great Britain by Titus Wilson & Son Ltd., Kendal.

Contents

Clinical Symposium – Phenylketonuria

Short Communications

Author Index

Title Index

THE 23RD ANNUAL SYMPOSIUM OF THE SSIEM: LIVERPOOL 1985

J. Inher. Metab. Dis. 9 Suppl. 1 (1986) 1–2

Preface

In 1964 the Society held a Symposium in Liverpool and this year returned there. The aim of the Symposium was to provide an overview of the application of DNA analysis to the study of inborn errors of metabolism. This rapidly developing field of investigation had its beginnings in 1878 when Friedrich Miescher reported the chemical composition of 'nuclein'. By 1970 Francis Crick was able to speculate that 'between now and the year 2000 . . . there will inevitably be . . . significant advances the nature of which we can hardly guess'. From the programme for the 23rd Annual Symposium it is already apparent that many significant advances have already been made and that we can look forward to an increasing application of DNA analysis to the investigation and treatment of metabolic disease. The scientific programme was planned and implemented by Drs Pembrey, Ireland, Leonard and Harkness.

Many participants at the conference were newcomers to the field of DNA analysis. The terminology of DNA methodology is often daunting to the genetic novice. This hurdle was rapidly and effectively overcome by the presentations of Drs Scott, Swallow and Malcolm. Important techniques such as gene tracking and restriction length polymorphism analysis in the field of genetic counselling were stressed by Dr Pembrey. Investigation of metabolic diseases such as ornithine transcarbamylase deficiency and α_1-antitrypsin deficiency were presented by Dr Rosen and Professor Woo. Dr Güttler and Professor Woo described hydroxylase restriction length polymorphism, Dr Mandrup-Poulsen gave new information of DNA analysis applied to diabetes and Professor Mainwaring dealt with mechanism of hormonal regulation of gene transcription. Of great interest in the use of DNA analysis is its application to diseases where the effect of the gene alteration on intermediary metabolism is not clearly defined. These subjects were covered by Dr Arlett in his lecture on DNA repair defects and by Professor Pierson in his lecture on Duchenne muscular dystrophy. Professor Smithies presented the Symposium the challenge of achieving high accuracy and efficiency in altering genes in the human genome with the prospect of treatment of metabolic disease.

In 1964 the meeting was organized by the co-founders of the Society; one of whom was a council member Mr Joe Ireland. In 1985 the SSIEM, in its return to Liverpool, had on this occasion Mr Ireland as its President. In recognition of the long service that Mr Ireland had given to the Society over the 23 years of its existence, he was invited to organize a clinical colloquium on phenylketonuria as part of the annual symposium. The generous sponsorship of this part of the programme by Scientific Hospital Supplies Ltd., Liverpool, enabled Mr Ireland to

Journal of Inherited Metabolic Disease. ISSN 0141–8955.

invite contributors from the United States and Denmark to summarize some of the problems of phenylketonuria that have still to be resolved. The speakers presented their experience of dietary management of maternal phenylketonuria, brain metabolism and treatment of phenylketonuria. The increasing importance of maternal phenylketonuria was emphasized in the free communications presented at the end of this interesting half day seminar which attracted not only members of the Society but also several visiting dietitians.

A Workshop on the pressing current problem of screening for congenital adrenal hyperplasia was organized by Dr Addison.

The administration of the 23rd symposium was in the hands of Drs Davidson, Isherwood, McKendrick, Mr Ireland, Mrs Kerr, Mrs McKendrick, Miss Hall, the SSIEM secretary Mrs Anne Green and the assistant secretary Mr Griffiths. Invaluable secretarial help was forthcoming from Mrs E Green and Mrs B Hoskisson and useful help at the meeting from Ms P Waller and several other staff of Scientific Hospital Supplies Ltd. The expert secretarial help of Julie Crilly and Josephine Jepson in the production of this publication and the editorial assistance of Philip Johnstone and Valerie Baker are gratefully acknowledged. The Society was also grateful for the generous financial support from Scientific Hospital Supplies Ltd., and also for donations from the Wellcome trust and the Mersey Regional Health Authority.

Dr G. M. Addison
Dr R. A Harkness
Dr D. M. Isherwood
Dr R. J. Pollitt

The papers listed below were also presented at the meeting. Scripts were not available by the time of publication. 1. Hormonal short-term regulation of gene transcription, W. I. P. Mainwaring, Leeds. 2. Developments in genetic counselling for Duchenne muscular dystrophy. P. L. Pierson, Leiden.

J. Inher. Metab. Dis. 9 Suppl. 1 (1986) 3–16

Introduction to Recombinant DNA

J. Scott
Molecular Medicine, Clinical Research Centre, Northwick Park Hospital, Watford Road, Harrow, Middlesex, HA1 3UJ, UK

This paper describes the current state of knowledge of methods for analysing gene structure and localization. Illustrations are given of the preparation of complementary DNA libraries and their screening by positive–negative selection, the use of synthetic oligodeoxynucleotides and the use of antibodies. Analysis of the EGF precursor is used as an example to show its close relationship to plasma membrane receptor and its homology with the LDL receptor. Analysis of cloned genome DNA by use of bacteriophage lambda or cosmids gives useful information about gene regulation and evolution. Mutations by frame shift, point or missence mutations are discussed with reference to the LDL receptor and the apolipoproteins. The techniques of gene mapping by rat–human cell hybridization and hybridization *in situ* are illustrated, again with reference to genes coding for enzymes of cholesterol metabolism, the apolipoproteins and insulin-like growth factors. Finally the potential of *in vitro* mutagenesis and the injection of cloned DNA into the fertilized mouse ovum are discussed.

The Crick and Watson model for the structure of DNA consists of a double-stranded beta helix with a deoxyribose sugar-phosphate backbone in which the phosphate group links the 5′ and 3′ carbons of adjacent pentose rings. This 5–3 linkage gives the designations 5′ and 3′ by which we orientate genes (Figure 1) (Watson and Crick, 1953). Attached to the sugar moiety are the purine and pyrimidine bases, adenosine (A) and thymine (T), guanine (G) and cytosine (C) which form complementary strands by hydrogen bonding of AT or GC base pairs throughout the helix. It is this complementary base pairing which is the essence of the modern science of molecular biology. Thus a single strand of DNA is capable of replication, can be transcribed into RNA and indeed RNA can be reverse transcribed into DNA. The radioactive and non-radioactive probes used in molecular biology depend for their usefulness on this property of complementary base pairing.

Comparisons may be made between genomes of increasing size. The bacteriophage lambda is a virus which infects *E. coli*. It has some 50 000 base pairs (bp) of DNA and contains 30 genes. Thus for a lambda gene there are approximately 1500 bp per unit. *E. coli* shows a considerable increase in complexity with some 2000 genes and 2×10^6 bp of DNA. In moving from prokaryotic to eukaryotic organisms, the fruit fly *Drosophila* has approximately 10 000 genes and the genome

Journal of Inherited Metabolic Disease. ISSN 0141–8955.

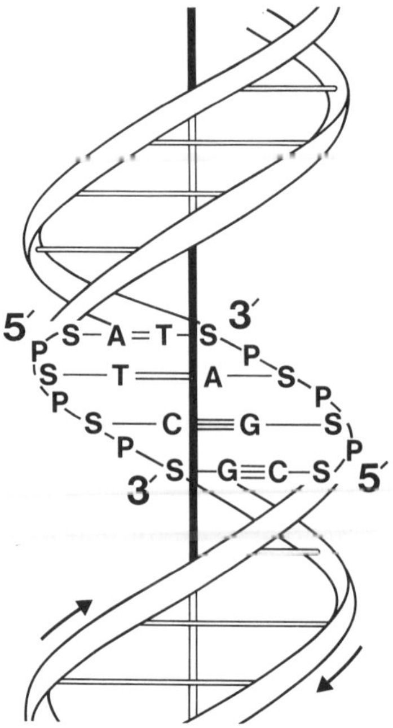

Figure 1 Double-stranded Crick and Watson DNA helix showing hydrogen bonding between complementary base pairs

contains 120×10^6 bp. An enormous leap in complexity takes us to mammals, where there are 50 000–100 000 genes and 5500×10^6 bp of DNA. In mammals approximately 3000 genes have been identified, and it is evident from their structure that mammalian genes are often of similar size to those in the bacteriophage lambda. Therefore much of mammalian DNA is apparently without function and has been called junk or selfish DNA (Orgel *et al.*, 1980).

The structure of an average eukaryotic gene is illustrated in Figure 2. The portions of the gene which code for the protein and untranslated regions at the 5′ and 3′ of the messenger RNA are called exons. These are intersected at various points by intervening sequences of DNA called introns. In the 5′ flanking region of the gene is the promoter region containing the CAT and TATA sequences to which RNA polymerase binds. Also at the 5′ end are sequences which respond to regulatory proteins such as steroid hormone, cholesterol and heavy metal receptors. Frequently at the 5′ end are also so-called enhancer elements which determine the tissue specific expression of a particular gene. These elements may also reside in the 3′ flanking sequences or even in the intervening sequences of the gene. Transcription is initiated by RNA polymerase II at the promoter region. It reads through the exons and introns and beyond the site where polyadenylation will occur in the mRNA. Contained at the 3′ end of the gene and in the mRNA is the polyadenylation signal AATAAA.

Polyadenylation occurs rapidly after transcription. The intervening sequences

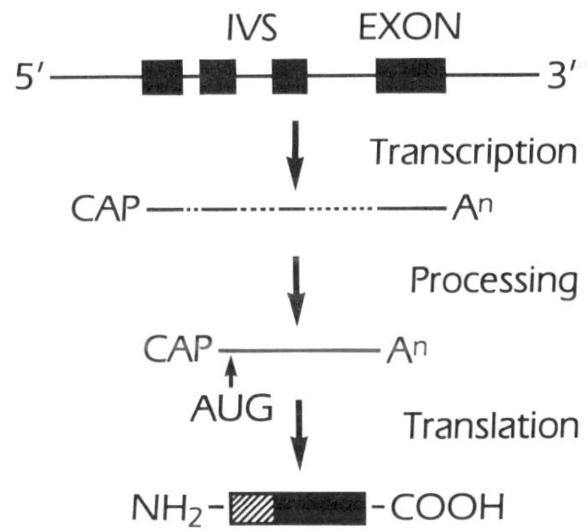

Figure 2 Eukaryotic gene showing transcription and RNA translation

are removed from the pre-mRNA and the site at which transcription begins is modified to form a cap structure. Removal of intervening sequences depends on 5′ splice donor (AGGUAAGU) and 3′ acceptor ($^{U}_{C}$ AGG) sites within the introns. Splicing is mediated by a large ribonucleoprotein complex termed a ‘spliceosome’. Once the mRNA has been capped, polyadenylated and spliced it is transferred from the nucleoplasm to the cytoplasm. Translation is initiated at the first AUG codon which signifies methionine and stops at the first termination codon (UAA, UGA, UAG). Subsequently the precursor protein is processed by removal of the signal peptide for secretory proteins and by other post-translational cleavages and modifications such as glycosylation and phosphorylation.

ANALYSIS OF HUMAN GENOME

How is the complexity of the human genome to be analysed? The structure of DNA has been studied by the techniques of restriction analysis and DNA sequencing. This has been facilitated by the construction of DNA libraries and the identification in them of cloned DNA segments. To identify probes for specific proteins, preparation and screening of complementary DNA (cDNA) libraries is now straightforward. Each cell type contains about 10 000 different messenger mRNAs. Complementary copies of these can be made using reverse transcriptase. The enzyme is primed with an oligo(dT) primer which binds to the poly(A) tail of the mRNA. Thus a single-stranded complement of the mRNA is prepared. Conveniently the transcriptase forms a hairpin at the 3′ end of the cDNA. This hairpin is used to prime second strand synthesis by an enzyme such as DNA polymerase I. Thus a double-stranded Crick and Watson cDNA which represents a copy of the mRNA sequence is formed. The hairpin is cleaved with nuclease SI which cuts single-stranded nucleic acid. The cDNA is tailed with up to 30 dC residues, and annealed with a dG-tailed plasmid which contains antibiotic resistance genes so that recombinant bacteria can be selected. The recombinant plasmid is taken up by *E. coli.* which have been heat shocked to permeabilize their cell walls and plasma membranes. The process of transformation is relatively inefficient but will provide cDNA libraries containing tens of thousands of clones. One problem of this method of preparing cDNA is that SI nuclease tends to remove the 5′ end of cDNA clones. New methods for preparing cDNA avoid this problem so that full-length cDNA clones can be prepared for most proteins (Scott *et al.*, in press; Gubler and Hoffman, 1983). To prepare larger cDNA libraries in which mRNAs represented by only one copy per cell can be cloned, a new vector system has been developed in the bacteriophage lambda (Huynh *et al.*, 1985). After preparing recombinants of cDNA in lambda, this virus is used to infect the *E. coli*. Thus the inefficient process of transformation is replaced by the process of infection. Libraries of up to 10 million clones may be prepared with ease.

SCREENING cDNA LIBRARIES

Three methods are currently fashionable for screening cDNA libraries. The first is positive–negative selection, and it depends on having tissue or cell line sources of RNA between which major differences exist in the level of the mRNA for the product whose cloning is desired. Examples are the identification of T-cell receptor probes by differential screening of cDNAs prepared from T and B lymphocytes (Hedrick *et al.*, 1984): or a cell line which has been induced to express the genes of interest such as the oncogene c-myc after platelet derived growth factor is applied to NIH 3T3 cells (Cochran *et al.*, 1983). Another application of this technique is to the mouse submaxillary gland, where various products of granular convoluted tubule cells respond dramatically to the presence of androgens. These include the kallikrein enzyme system, renin, epidermal growth factor (EGF) and nerve growth factor (NGF). The method may be employed either on filters or in solution. For example, duplicate filters of the cDNA library are prepared, and these are screened separately with ^{32}P-labelled single-stranded cDNA prepared from female and male mouse submaxillary gland mRNA (Figure 3). Screening with male mouse cDNA reveals clones which are not seen on screening with the female mouse cDNA. These represent renin and kallikrein.

The second method of screening, and the most powerful available, is the use of synthetic oligodeoxynucleotides which represent the DNA coding for specific peptides from proteins of known sequence. The genetic code is degenerate, having for example six codons for leucine and serine, but only one for methionine and tryptophan. In the preparation of a short probe of around 20 bases all ambiguities are best filled. Longer probes of more than 35 bases can be designed by choice of frequently used codons and non-destabilizing bases (Scott *et al.*, in press). The probe is labelled with ^{32}P and used for screening of cDNA libraries (Figure 4).

The third method of screening uses antibodies. cDNA may be cloned into restriction sites that reside in COOH terminal portion of the betagalactosidase gene which has been assembled into appropriate plasmids. In the bacterium the betagalactosidase gene is expressed and if the cloned cDNA is in the correct reading frame it will be produced as a fusion product of betagalactosidase and the protein

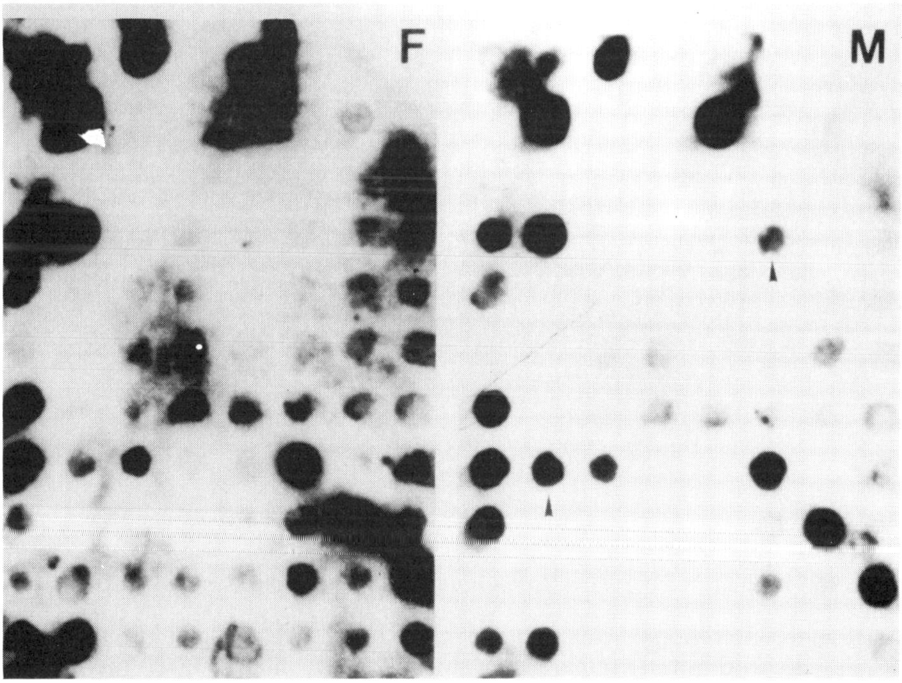

Figure 3 Screening of cDNA clones by positive–negative selection. Screening with single-stranded ^{32}P-labelled cDNA made from male (M) and female (F) submaxillary gland RNA. Male abundant clones are arrowed

for which the cDNA codes. The expressed protein is immobilized on filters which are screened with an antibody and a radiolabelled second antibody or protein A.

cDNA cloning has revealed many interesting aspects of protein structure and biosynthesis. The cDNAs for EGF precursor and for the low density lipoprotein receptor are examples (Scott *et al.*, 1985c). EGF is a potent mitogen of 53 amino acid residues. The precursor for EGF contains 1217 residues. In addition to EGF itself there are seven EGF-like peptides in the precursor and these form two cysteine-rich domains. There is also a membrane spanning domain and several glycosylation sites. EGF precursor therefore closely resembles a plasma membrane receptor. In the middle portion of the molecule a region spanning 400 animo acid residues has a striking homology (30%) to the low density lipoprotein (LDL) receptor. The LDL receptor is in overall structure similar to the EGF precursor having not only the region of homology, but the cysteine-rich domain and the membrane spanning segment.

PREPARATION OF GENOMIC DNA CLONES

To analyse gene structure it is necessary to clone genomic DNA in manageable fragments. Two methods are available for cloning genomic DNA. Firstly it can be

Figure 4 Screening of an ordered cDNA library with ^{32}P-labelled synthetic oligonucleotide

cloned in the bacteriophage lambda (Maniatis *et al.*, 1982). High molecular weight DNA is prepared and cleaved into convenient sized fragments (15–20 kilobase pairs (kbp)) using a sequence specific restriction endonuclease such as *Eco*RI. The *Eco*RI cleaved DNA is ligated between the arms of the bacteriophage. The arms are necessary for the bacteriophage to complete its life cycle but for the purposes of cloning, non-essential DNA has been removed from the bacteriophage. The genomic and bacteriophage DNA are ligated and the recombinant DNA is packaged into a bacteriophage particle which is used to infect *E. coli* and a library is thus established. Cosmids are useful for cloning larger DNA fragments of up to 50 kb. Cosmids contain the antibiotic resistance gene of the plasmid and the cohesive or cos ends of lambda which are necessary for it to circularize during its life cycle. In addition there is an origin for DNA replication. Construction is similar to that of lambda DNA (Maniatis *et al.*, 1982). The virtue of cosmids is their large insert size enabling large genes such as those of EGF precursor (100 kb) and of the LDL receptor (50 kb) to be spanned with relative ease. The analysis of genomic sequence is important to determine how genes are regulated. In addition, surprises about evolution have been revealed. For example, the region of homology that exists between the EGF precursor and the LDL receptor is seen in the genes, where there is remarkable similarity in the intron/exon structure. The LDL receptor also shows homology in its ligand binding domain to the complement C9 protein. Analysis of this gene provides support for the Gilbert hypothesis that introns contribute to the rapid evolution of eukaryotic organisms by intergenic recombination.

RESTRICTION ENDONUCLEASES

Restriction endonuclease digestion and Southern blotting allows the structure of genes to be studied without the necessity for DNA sequencing. There are more

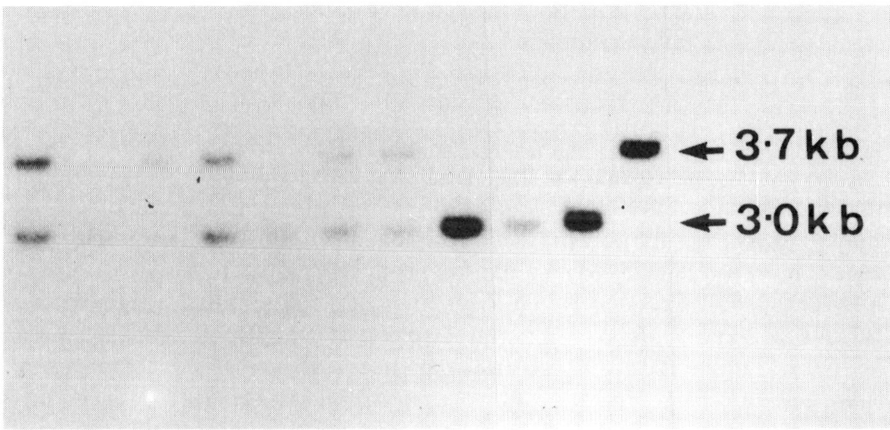

Figure 5 Autoradiograph of Southern blot

than 300 restriction endonucleases which cleave DNA in a sequence specific fashion. Genomic DNA is readily prepared from white blood cells. DNA cleaved with restriction endonuclease is electrophoresed in agarose and, because of its negative charges, it will migrate on the basis of fragment size towards the cathode. The DNA may then be transferred from the gel onto a nitrocellulose or nylon membrane using a high salt solution and capillary action. The DNA is fixed to the membrane by baking and a radioactive probe for the gene of interest is hybridized to the filter. Excess unhybridized probe is removed by washing and the membrane is autoradiographed. Figure 5 shows an autoradiograph of cleavage in the flanking sequences of the apolipoprotein AII gene. Restriction fragment length polymorphism for the enzyme *Msp*I is demonstrated. There is one allele with a fragment of 3 kb and the second allele with a fragment of 3.7 kb. Heterozygotes and homozygotes for each allele are demonstrated. Figure 6 shows the apo AII gene. *Msp*I cleaves in the 5′ flanking region and in an Alu sequence in the 3′ flanking region to create the 3 kb fragment. Deletion of the site in the Alu sequence gives rise to the 3.7 kb allele. This mutation has been associated with increased circulating levels of apo AII (Scott *et al.*, 1985b). The mutation *per se* is unlikely to be the cause of the increase in plasma apo AII as Alu sequences have no function. This mutation is likely to be in linkage disequilibrium with a second mutation that effects either the

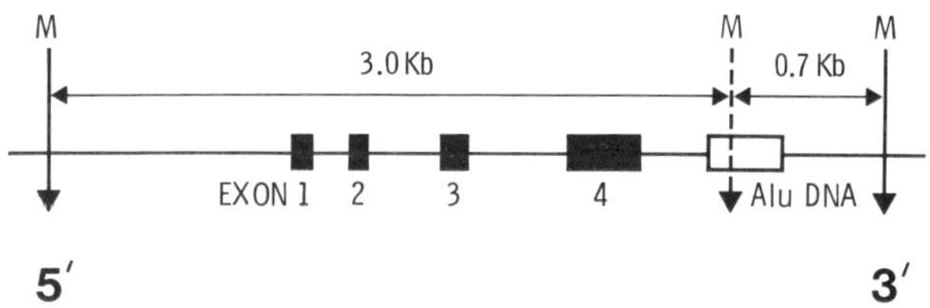

Figure 6 Schematic diagram of apolipoprotein All gene with *Msp*I sites (arrowed black non-polymorphic; dashed polymorphic)

coding sequence and retards apo AII degradation, or the regulatory sequences and increases apo AII gene expression.

MUTATION

Mutation takes three forms, the first two being frame shift and point mutation. In frame shift mutation deletion or insertion of DNA – even of a single base pair – disrupts the reading frame of a gene. This has been illustrated most elegantly in the LDL receptor gene in which mutation produces familial hypercholesterolaemia (Goldstein, 1985). Sequence analysis of this gene has revealed a number of Alu repetitive elements in the 3′ untranslated region of the mRNA. Alu sequences are also to be found in the intervening sequences of the LDL receptor gene. In one variant illegitimate homologous recombination has occurred between an Alu element in an intervening sequence and another in the 3′ untranslated region. This truncates the mRNA and causes the production of a protein which has the LDL binding domain, but lacks the membrane spanning domain. The protein cannot internalize the LDL particle. Point mutations may produce a stop codon in a protein and terminate translation. More commonly point mutation produces a synonymous base change (23%) which does not alter the amino acid because it occurs in the third base which is degenerate.

The third type of protein mutation is called missence (72%). This is illustrated

Apo E polymorphic sites

Position	A.A.(W.T.)	Codon	A.A.(mutants)	Mutation	Receptor binding
142	Arg	CGC	Cys	CGC → TGC	< 20%
145	Arg	CGT	Cys	CGT → TGT	45%
146	Lys	AAG	Gln	AAG → CAG	40%
158	Arg	CGC	Cys	CGC → TGC	2%

Figure 7 Point mutations at this apolipoprotein E receptor binding domain (20)

in relation to apolipoprotein E (Figure 7). Apolipoproteins E and B bind through basic residues to the acidic residues of the LDL receptor. The receptor binding domain of apo E has been identified and there are a number of common mutations which affect this region of the protein. A homologous domain involving apo B has also been identified. Mutation of the arginine codons to cysteine in the receptor binding domain of apo E are surprisingly common, whereas mutation of the lysine in the receptor binding domain has been described on only one occasion. This is because CG base pairs are hot spots for mutation (Barker *et al.*, 1985) and all the arginines in the receptor binding domain of apo E are coded for by the codon CGN (Paik *et al.*, 1985). CG mutates to TG in the germ line because methylated cytidine mutates to thymidine. DNA repair enzymes recognize thymidine as legitimate. Thus, during DNA replication, the codon for arginine (CG$_{T}^{C}$) is mutated to that for cysteine (TG$_{T}^{C}$). In apo B the arginines of the receptor binding domain are coded for by AGN and will not be mutated in the same way as those in apo E (Knott *et al.*, 1985).

GENE MAPPING

Physical methods of gene mapping have allowed the map of the human genome to be established. In somatic cell hybrids of rodent and human cells the rodent chromosomes are maintained, but the human chromosomes are selectively lost. A panel of hybrids can be established and assessed by the assay of constitutive enzymes for the loss of human chromosomes. By use of such a panel of hybrids and Southern

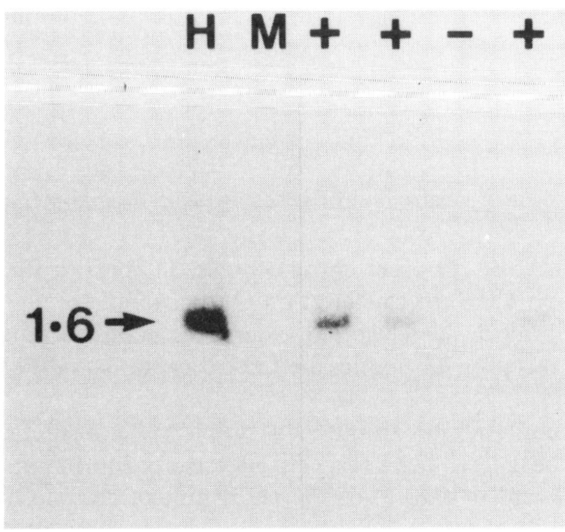

Figure 8 Southern blot of human (H), mouse (M) and somatic cell hybrid DNA cut with *Eco*RI and hybridized with apolipoprotein B cDNA. (+) donates hybrid containing gene. (−) gene lost from hybrid

blotting the chromosomal localization of any gene can be determined (Figure 8). Cell lines with regional chromosome translocations allow local assignment of a gene to be made. Detailed regional analysis may be obtained by *in situ* hybridization of labelled probe to metaphase or prophase chromosome spreads (Zabel *et al.*, 1983). Localization of the silver grains gives the localization of the gene. Examples of the value of gene mapping are given. Figure 9 shows the chromosome localization of genes involved in the metabolism of cholesterol and lipids, variants of which are likely candidates for the generation of dyslipoproteinaemia. In the analysis of this polygenic disorder it is important to know where genes involved in cholesterol metabolism such as apo B, HMGCoA reductase and the LDL receptor are located (HMG8). Similarly genes involved in HDL metabolism such as apo AI, Apo AII

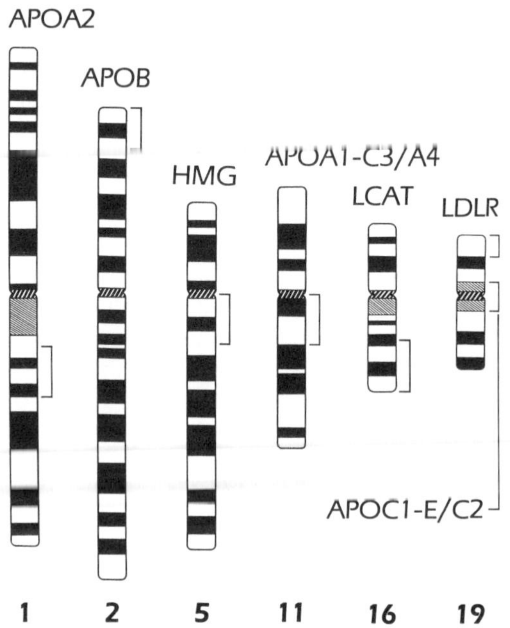

Figure 9 Chromosomal localization of genes involved in lipid metabolism

and apo E are also on different chromosomes. In contrast the genes for apo AI, apo AIV and apo CIII are clustered on chromosome 11, and the genes for apo CI, apo CII and apo E are clustered around the centromere on chromosome 19. In addition the receptor for apo E, the LDL receptor is on the tip of chromosome 19.

A second example relates to the localization of the insulin-like growth factor I and II genes. These have been respectively localized to the tip of the long arm of chromosome 12 and to the tip of the short arm of chromosome 11 respectively (HMG8). These localizations together with the placement of the insulin, Harvey-ras and LDH A genes on chromosome 11 and of the Kirston-ras and LDH B genes on chromosome 12 and the homology in banding structure between chromosomes 11 and 12 suggests an evolutionary relationship between these chromosomes. Chromosomes 11 and 12 may have evolved by duplication and pericentric inversion of an ancestral chromosome. Duplication of the IGF II gene locus on the tip of the short arm of chromosome 11 may be seen in the rare neonatal abnormality, the Beckwith–Wiedemann syndrome (exomphalos, macroglossia and somatomegaly). The disorder is due to amplification of the IGF II gene in some patients (HMG8). Symptomatically, after the first year of life children with Beckwith–Wiedemann syndrome are often normal. However, they have a significant risk of developing the embryonal neoplasms: Wilms' tumour, hepatoblastoma and rhabdomyosarcoma. Intriguingly, Koufos and colleagues (1985) have demonstrated that patients with these tumours develop homozygosity for genes on the short arm of chromosome 11 compared to heterozygosity in non-tumour DNA. The development of homozygosity may allow the expression of a recessive mutation that leads to tumour development. Examination of Northern blots of RNA from Wilms' tumour, rhabdomyosarcoma and from a hepatoblastoma cell line has demonstrated high level IGF II gene expression in these tumours (Scott *et al.*, 1985a). This is far higher than found in the adult tissues, but comparable to the levels in fetal kidney, liver and striated muscle. These are the same tissues from which the embryonal tumours arise that develop homozygosity for 11p markers. Tumours such as Ewing's sarcoma of bone, retinoblastoma, medulloblastoma and neuroblastoma do not develop homozygosity for markers on chromosome 11 and in them the gene for IGF II is not over-expressed. Fetal brain was significantly negative for IGF II gene expression.

Hybridization *in situ* of labelled DNA probes to tissue sections is revealing important results for developmental biology and medicine. In Figure 10 a ^{32}P-labelled cDNA for mouse EGF was hybridized to a longitudinal section of the mouse. EGF mRNA was found in the submaxillary gland, and surprisingly was demonstrated in the kidney and tooth buds. EGF protein had not previously been demonstrated in the kidney. Hybridization of the probe to tissue sections of the kidney showed that the mRNA was mainly in the distal convoluted tubules (Figure 10). Analysis of EGF mRNA size from the submaxillary gland and kidney showed a same-sized mRNA of 4800 bases. Therefore differential splicing of the EGF gene seemed unlikely. This suggested the possibility that there was differential processing of the large EGF precursor. Antibodies were therefore raised against a fusion protein of β-galactosidase and a portion of the EGF precursor, which did not encode EGF. The antibodies against EGF precursor were used in organ culture studies in which submaxillary gland and kidney tissue was labelled *in vitro*. Immunoprecipitation followed by SDS polyacrylamide gel electrophoresis of the samples showed that in the submaxillary gland EGF was precipitated by an antibody raised against the native protein, and portions of the precursor were precipitated by the antibody raised against the precursor fusion protein. In the kidney both antibodies precipitated a high molecular weight protein of the size predicted for the intact EGF precursor. These data presage a new function for an old protein, possibly as a receptor involved in ion transport.

MUTAGENESIS

The technique of *in vitro* mutagenesis allows specific point mutations to be placed within a cloned DNA. The cloned DNA is prepared in the single-stranded M13 bacteriophage. The single-stranded DNA is annealed with a synthetic oligodeoxynucleotide probe which contains the mutation which it is wished to introduce. The oligonucleotide is used to prime the completion of the double-stranded circular DNA. Both wild type and mutant DNAs are prepared, isolated and rendered double-stranded. The mutant DNA can be transfected into a suitable cell line for assay. Gill and colleagues (1985) have recently demonstrated the power of this technique in mutating HMG CoA reductase, the rate-limiting enzyme of cholesterol synthesis. The enzyme has a cytoplasmic domain which contains the active site and

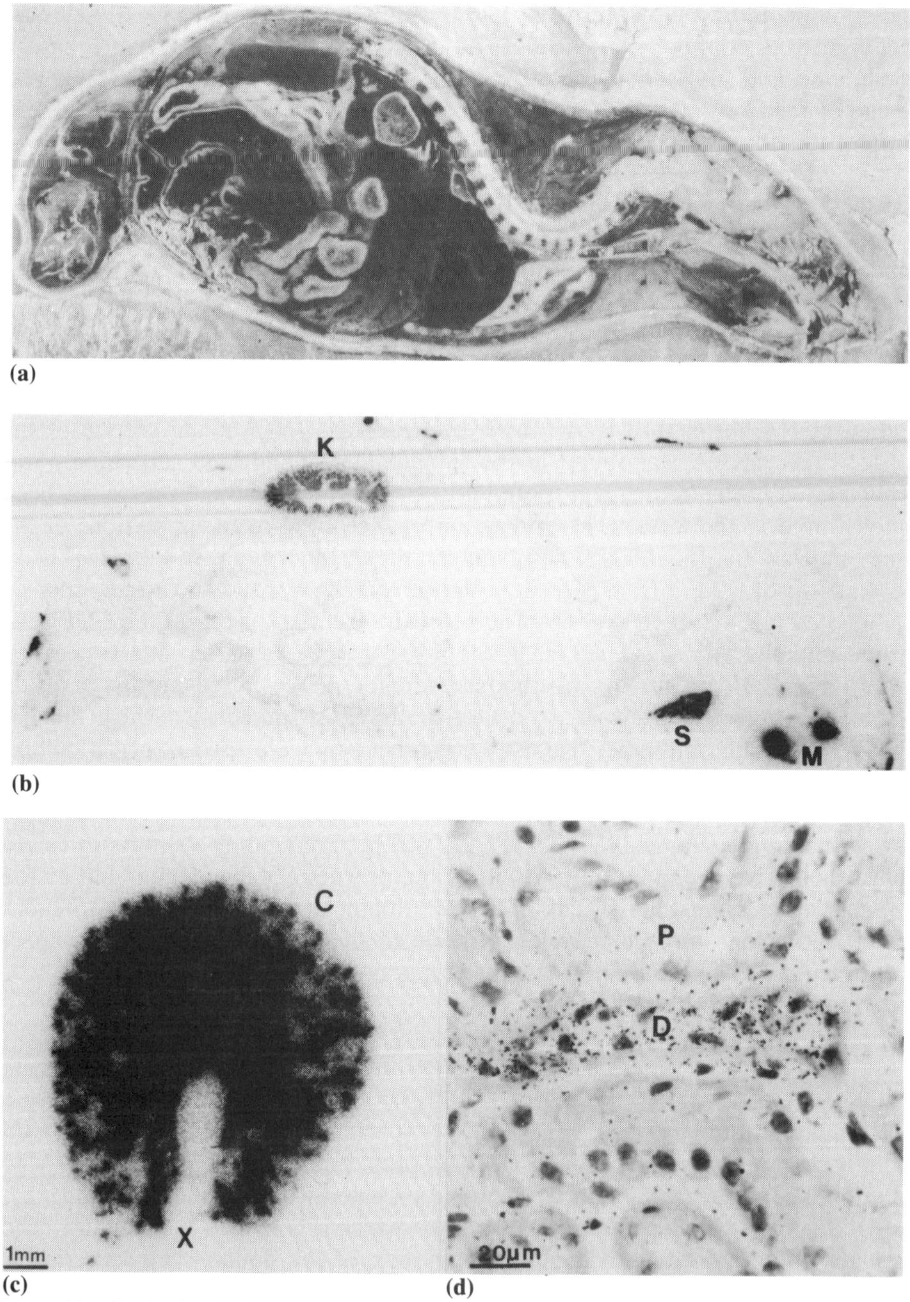

Figure 10 *In situ* hybridization of prepro EGF cDNA to mouse tissues: **(a)** sagittal section of an adult male Swiss–Webster mouse; **(b)** autoradiographs of sections of a whole male mouse; **(c)** transverse section of kidney; and **(d)** male kidney cortex. (S, submaxillary gland; K, kidney; M, mouth region; D, distal tubule; P, proximal tubule; X, renal pelvis; C, kidney cortex. The distal tubules can be distinguished from the proximal kidney tubules by their wider lumen and thinner walls).

a membrane-spanning domain which binds the protein to the smooth endoplasmic reticulum. Degradation of the enzyme is regulated by cholesterol concentration in the cytoplasm. A mutated form of this enzyme was produced in which the amino terminal of the protein which normally resides in the lumen of the smooth endoplasmic reticulum was directly joined to the amino terminal of the cytoplasmic domain and the membrane-spanning domain thereby removed. The mutated enzyme was not degraded in the cytoplasm in the presence of cholesterol. It was concluded that the membrane-spanning domain is essential to regulate the degradation of this enzyme.

IN VIVO STUDIES

One of the most powerful techniques of modern molecular biology is the ability to inject cloned DNA into the male pronucleus of the fertilized mouse ovum. The ovum is implanted in the uterus of the pseudopregnant mouse and the embryo allowed to develop. Palmiter and colleagues performed such studies using a mouse growth hormone gene attached to the metallothionein gene promoter (Palmiter *et al.*, 1983). Metallothionein is a constitutive enzyme in many cells. The metallothionein gene regulated growth hormone was produced in many tissues including the liver, spleen and kidney. Thus the so-called supermouse was created. The same technique has been employed by Hanahan. The SV40 gene coding for the transforming T antigen (Hanahan, 1985) was fused to the 5′ flanking sequence of the insulin gene. T antigen was expressed solely in the B cells of the islets of Langerhans and in no other cell type. The mice developed B cell-specific islet adenomas.

References

Barker, D., Schafer, M and White, R. Restriction sites containing CpG show a higher frequency of polymorphism in human DNA. *Cell* 36 (1984) 131–138

Cochran, B. H., Reffel, A. C. and Stiles, C. D. Molecular cloning of gene sequences regulated by platelet derived growth factor. *Cell* 33 (1983) 939-947

Gill, G., Faust, J. R., Chin, D. J., Goldstein, J. L. and Brown, M. S. Membrane-bound domain of HMGCoA reductase is required for sterol-enhanced degradation of the enzyme. *Cell* 41 (1985) 249-258

Goldstein, J. L. The low density lipoprotein receptor. *J. Cell. Sci.* (1985) Suppl. 3 in press

Gubler, U. and Hoffmann, B. J. A simple and very efficient method for generating cDNA libraries. *Gene* 23 (1983) 263-269

Hanahan, D. Heritable formation of pancreatic B-cell tumours in transgenic mice expressing recombinant insulin/simian virus 40 oncogenes. *Nature* 309 (1985) 115-122

Hedrick, S. M., Cohen, D. I., Nielson, E. A. and Davis, M. M. Isolation of cDNA clones encoding T-cell specific membrane-associated proteins. *Nature* 308 (1984) 149-153

Huynh, T. V., Young, R. A. and Davis, R. W. Constructing and screening cDNA libraries in gt10 and gt11. In Glover, D. M. (ed.) *DNA Cloning Volume 1. A Practical Approach* IRL Press, Oxford and London, 1985

Knott, T. J., Rall, S. C., Innerarity, T. L., Jacobson, S. F., Urdea, M. S., Levy-Wilson, B., Powell, L. M., Pease, R. J., Eddy, R., Nakal, H., Byers, M., Priestly, L. M., Robertson, E., Rall, L. B., Betsholtz, C., Shows, T. B., Mahley, R. W. and Scott, J.

Human apolipoprotein B: structure of carboxyl-terminal domains, sites of gene expression, and chromosomal localization. *Science* 230 (1985) 37-43

Koufos, A., Hansen, M. G., Copeland, N. G., Jenkins, N. A., Lampkin, B. C. and Cavenee, W. K. Loss of heterozygosity in three embryonal tumours suggests a common pathogenic mechanism. *Nature* 316 (1985) 330-334

Mahley, R. W., Innerarity, T. L., Rall, Jr., S. C. and Weisgraber, K. H. Plasma lipoproteins: apoprotein structure and function. *J. Lipid Res.* 25 (1984) 1277-1294

Maniatis, T., Fritsch, E. F. and Sambrook, J. Molecular cloning: a laboratory manual (1982) Cold Spring Harbour

Orgel, L. E., Crick, F. H. C. and Sapienza, C., Selfish DNA. *Nature* 288 (1980) 645-646

Paik, Y. K., Chang, D. J., Reardon, C. A., Davies, G. E., Mahley, R. W. and Taylor, J. M. Nucleotide sequence and structure of the human apolipoprotein E gene. *Proc. Natl. Acad. Sci. (USA)* 82 (1985) 3445-3449

Palmiter, R. D., Norstedt, D., Gelinas, R. E., Hammer, R. E. and Brinster, R. L. Metallothionein-human GH fusion genes stimulate growth of mice. *Science* 222 (1983) 809-814

Scott, J., Cowell, J., Robertson, M. E., Priestley, L. M., Wadey, R., Hopkins, B., Pritchard, J., Bell, G. I., Rall, L. B., Graham, C. F. and Knott, T. J. Insulin-like growth factor II gene expression in Wilms' Tumour and embryonic tissues. *Nature* 317 (1985a) 260-262

Scott, J., Knott, T. J., Priestley, L. M., Robertson, M. E., Mann, D. V., Kostner, G., Miller, G. J. and Miller, N. E. High-density lipoprotein composition is altered by a common DNA polymorphism adjacent to apoprotein AII gene in man. *Lancet* 1 (1985b) 771-773

Scott, J., Patterson, S., Rall, L., Bell, G. I., Crawford, R., Penschow, J., Niall, H. and Coghlan, J. The structure and biosynthesis of epidermal growth factor precursor. *J. Cell Sci.* (1985c) Suppl. 3 (in press)

Scott, J., Selby, M. J. and Bell, G. I. *In* Peptide growth factors (A volume of *Methods in Enzymology*) (in press)

Watson, J. D. and Crick, F. H. C. Molecular structure of nucleic acids: a structure for deoxyribose nucleic acid. *Nature* 171 (1958) 737-738

Zabel, B. N., Naylor, S. L., Sakaguchi, A. Y., Bell, G. I. and Shows, T. B. High-resolution chromosomal localization of human genes for amylase, proopiomelanocortin, somatostatin, and a DNA fragment (D3S2) by *in situ* hybridization. *Proc. Natl. Acad. Sci. (USA)* 80 (1983) 6932-6936

J. Inher. Metab. Dis. 9 Suppl. 1 (1986) 17–31

Human Biochemical Genetics of Enzyme Proteins in the New Age of Molecular Genetics

D. M. SWALLOW and D. A. HOPKINSON
MRC Human Biochemical Genetics, The Galton Laboratory, University College London, Wolfson House, 4 Stephenson Way, London NW1 2HE, UK

Advances in protein biochemistry and immunology have had a major impact on the biochemical and genetical analysis of human proteins and have had applications in the analysis of the primary defects in metabolic disorders, as well as in cDNA cloning. The development and expansion of somatic cell genetic techniques has complemented conventional population and family study genetic methods. A large number of mammalian proteins undergo complex processing to achieve the synthesis of the biologically active protein. Much of this processing is under genetic control. Elucidation of these complexities requires a combination of biochemical, immunological and genetical approaches to determine the nature of the events involved.

Human biochemical genetics emerged as a major area of research in the 1950s and 1960s. Although the concept of the inborn errors of metabolism had been established early in the century by Garrod, and inherited differences in blood groups had been discovered by Landsteiner, it was not until the 1960s that explosive growth occurred in the identification of enzyme defects in inborn errors of metabolism, and that the extent of variation in healthy individuals was fully appreciated. The extensive normal variation, which provided a biochemical and genetical explanation for human individuality, was largely demonstrated by the analysis of enzymes and other proteins by electrophoretic methods and was made possible in the case of enzymes by exploiting their biological function, namely their catalytic activity.

From the initial use of simple synthetic substrates, which when hydrolysed give chromogenic products, the detection procedures used after electrophoresis became increasingly sophisticated making use of enzyme-linked reactions where the products of one reaction act as a substrate for another. Using this kind of approach it was possible to analyse a very large number of enzymes from blood and tissues without their prior purification and to show that about one third of all human enzymes display genetically determined polymorphism – the polymorphism being defined as variation with a population frequency of heterozygotes of more than two per cent. Many rare alleles were also detected. In most cases the allelic variants showed no differences in their functional characteristics, but some were associated with reduced enzymic activity and clinical consequences in homozygous or compound heterozygous states.

Journal of Inherited Metabolic Disease. ISSN 0141–8955.

It also became apparent by the analysis of complex isozyme patterns and their tissue distribution that many enzymes are coded for by more than one gene locus. Indeed this situation obtains for about a third of the human enzymes tested to date. In some cases the multiple isozymes have quite distinctive molecular properties suggesting no simple evolutionary relationship, but in most cases the multiple loci appear to have arisen by gene duplication. Furthermore, multimeric enzymes often exhibit interlocus hybrid isozymes. In addition to these complexities post-translational processing, or secondary modification, is also a common phenomenon.

The aims of this paper are to illustrate the developments in human enzyme genetics during recent years and the interaction between protein chemistry and the current advances in DNA technology, and also to show that the study of protein is not redundant. The first section reviews some of the recent developments in the study of human proteins, in terms of separation techniques, detection procedures and other analytical methods. The second half of the paper reviews, with the use of somewhat idiosyncratic examples, the current picture of the events occurring between translation of the structural gene and the formation of the biologically active enzyme protein.

METHODOLOGY

Separation techniques

By far the most powerful method currently available for uncovering allelic variation due to charge change substitutions is flat bed polyacrylamide gel isoelectric focussing. There are many examples of the demonstration of allelic variation by this method not previously revealed by starch gel electrophoresis. Discrimination of extra alleles in this way clearly has applications in gene mapping studies particularly by linkage analysis, since it increases the number of informative families. Isoelectric focussing may also facilitate the separation of certain human and rodent isozymes in somatic cell hybrid material. Separations on immobilised pH gradients ('Immobilines', L.K.B.) which in principle offer even higher levels of resolution have not as yet lived up to expectations for routine applications.

SDS polyacrylamide gel electrophoresis has also provided a valuable tool for the study of proteins where criteria other than biological activity can be used to identify them. From its initial uses for the analysis of subunit size of proteins and assessment of the purity of protein preparations, its uses have been expanded by the increasing application of immunological techniques as a way of identifying the polypeptides – as described in the following section.

Although SDS gel electrophoresis has not in general been used to search for genetic variation except in two-dimensional separation systems, it is noteworthy that on a number of occasions such variation has been demonstrated by this procedure. In our laboratory we have found a genetically determined polymorphism of a urinary mucin-like glycoprotein which is detected by a number of lectins (Karlsson *et al.*, 1983) and also by a number of different antibodies. Although we do not yet know the basis of this variation there are other examples in the literature where the nature of the difference which leads to separation of the allele products on SDS gels is better understood. A polymorphism of arylsulphatase (EC 3.1.6.1) detected in this way is thought to be due to an alteration in the number of carbohydrate side chains. The data suggests that there is a mutation in the sequence Asn-X-Thr(Ser) which is required for the attachment of asparagine linked oligosaccharide side chains (Waheed *et al.*, 1983). Another example is a rare variant of hypoxanthine phosphoribosyl transferase (EC 2.4.2.8) associated with gout (McKusick 30800), where a neutral to neutral amino acid substitution has been found and the alteration in mobility on SDS gels ascribed to a difference in SDS binding (Wilson *et al.*, 1983).

Detection methods

There have been many new and ingenious ideas exploited for the detection of enzymes and serum proteins which utilise the biological activity of the protein (e.g. Cavalli-Sforza *et al.*, 1977; Naylor *et al.*, 1980). Methods to identify various complement components which involve lysis of red cells in an agar overlay are noteworthy (Whitehouse and Putt, 1983).

Perhaps the most important general method used increasingly in the last ten years is that of immunological detection. It has been possible, for example, to make use of commercial antisera for the detection and genetic analysis of many of the serum proteins (Whitehouse and Putt, 1983). A very effective way of doing this has been to transfer the proteins electrophoretically from the gels on to nitrocellulose, and to incubate the nitrocellulose with antiserum, followed by detection of bound IgG with a second antibody which carries some kind of signal. Examples include the original ELISA detection technique (Voller *et al.*, 1979) and a variety of more recent ultra-sensitive procedures (e.g. Blake *et al.*, 1984; Moeremans *et al.*, 1984). The electrophoretic transfer method, which was originally described by Towbin and colleagues (1979) for SDS gels, also works well for isoelectric focussing gels (Whitehouse and Putt, 1983), and can be used in conjunction with monoclonal antibodies as well as polyclonal antisera, provided the epitope they recognise is exposed after this treatment. The whole procedure has been called immunoblotting, immune replica technique and also Western blotting. Passive transfer, which could perhaps more accurately be described as blotting, also sometimes allows adequate retrieval of the protein under investigation (Gershoni and Palade, 1983; Teige *et al.*, 1985).

Proteins transferred to nitrocellulose can be detected by a variety of other procedures (Towbin and Gordon, 1984). Detection of glycoproteins using biotinylated lectins followed by avidin or streptavidin peroxidase or streptavidin peroxidase complex is very sensitive (Gordon-Weeks and Harding, 1983; Amersham International PLC). ^{125}I-labelled lectins have also been used in this way and also to stain gels directly (Karlsson *et al.*, 1983).

Another approach is to use immunoprecipitation or immunoadsorbant chromatography prior to electrophoresis, followed by an appropriate detection procedure. This might be autoradiography or fluorography if radioactively labelled proteins have been used (the arylsulphatase polymorphism referred to earlier (Waheed *et al.*, 1983) was demonstrated by this technique). The microimmunoadsorbant columns used by Kahn and colleagues (1981) are a very useful adaptation for the identification of low amounts of newly synthesized polypeptides in cell-free translation. Immunological binding assays, both qualitative and quantitative, have also been useful in the genetic analysis of enzymes and can sometimes reveal allelic variations (Harris, 1984).

Antibodies have also been used as a means of identifying specific messenger RNA for cDNA cloning. Such applications include for instance fractionation of mRNA by polysome immunoselection (Konings *et al.*, 1984; Myerowitz and Proia, 1984) and 'hybrid select' procedures (e.g. Lloyd *et al.*, 1985). Antibodies can also be used directly in cDNA cloning for the detection of protein in expression libraries using such vectors as the 'phage λgt11 (Young and Davis, 1983; Fukushima *et al.*, 1985; Ikuta *et al.*, 1985).

All these immunologically based procedures depend on the availability of monospecific antisera. This requires protein both for immunisation and also in some cases for purification of the antiserum (e.g. Reuser *et al.*, 1985). The advantage of monoclonal antibodies is that they can be obtained in unlimited supply without using purified protein, but they are not necessarily monospecific since the small epitopes which they recognise may occur on other proteins. In this context it is perhaps worth emphasizing that the criterion of monospecificity is not absolute. Lack of cross-reactivity by one technique does not necessarily mean that cross-reaction will not be detected by another.

Protein purification

Protein purification has been revolutionized by the advent of affinity methods of separation. Affinity ligands based on substrates and inhibitors have been particularly important (e.g. Geiger *et al.*, 1974; Lange and Vallee, 1976) as have monoclonal antibodies (e.g. Secher and Burke, 1980, Vockley and Harris, 1984; Potter *et al.*, 1985). These newer techniques have enabled the isolation of low abundance proteins previously difficult to purify in sufficient quantity to allow the study of their structural and functional characteristics. Amino acid sequencing has been important for identifying appropriate stretches of sequence for synthesis of oligonucleotide probes for use in cDNA cloning (e.g. Michelson *et al.*, 1983; Ikuta *et al.*, 1985). Although other methods of cDNA cloning do not necessarily require amino acid sequence data it is essential to have some way of confirming the identity of the gene. Direct comparison of DNA sequence and amino acid sequence is the method of choice (e.g. Fukushima *et al.*, 1985; Lloyd *et al.*, 1985).

Somatic cell genetics

Analysis of cultured cells has increased enormously during the last ten years. In particular the somatic cell hybrid technique has been used for mapping the gene loci coding for over 250 human enzymes and proteins (McAlpine *et al.*, 1985). In conjunction with family studies and the use of chromosomal translocations and deletions the human gene map is gradually being refined. Formal genetics by family studies is only possible at the level of the protein if the protein is expressed in accessible tissues such as blood and cultured skin fibroblasts. Likewise somatic cell genetic analysis is usually only possible if the gene is expressed in the parental cell lines. However the availability of cDNA and genomic DNA probes gets around this difficulty. Also it is sometimes possible to exploit tumour cell lines which retain tissue specific functions as one of the parents of somatic cell hybrids. This has been done in our laboratory and others in the analysis of liver specific functions, and it has been possible tentatively to assign the structural genes coding for several such proteins to human chromosomes (e.g. Kielty *et al.*, 1982a, 1982b). A combination of these approaches is even more powerful. Mapping of the structural gene coding for the human class 1 alcohol dehydrogenase (EC 1.1.1.1), to chromosome 4 was done using a cDNA clone (Smith *et al.*, 1983). This was in agreement with the results obtained from the hybrids made with the rat hepatoma line FAZA in which human alcohol dehydrogenase was shown only to be expressed in hybrids which contained chromosome 4, though the presence of chromosome 4 was not sufficient for expression. An advantage of confirming an assignment by analysing the expressed gene product is that possible confusion from pseudogenes is eliminated.

Somatic cell hybrids have also been valuable for dissecting the interactions of genes and their products (Shows *et al.*, 1982). A large variety of somatic cell manipulations involving fusions, transfections and selection procedures are now widely used, and dissection of the regulatory elements as well as the coding regions of genes is now underway.

THE GENETICS OF PROTEIN STRUCTURE AND HETEROGENEITY

Many of the technical advances described above have helped in the cloning of cDNA coding for a number of human enzymes and other proteins. More than 200 such human genes have now been cloned (Willard *et al.*, 1985) of which 50 or more code for enzymes. In many cases this endeavour has been greatly aided by the prior understanding of the biochemical and genetical basis of complex isozyme patterns, which has provided a framework for the purification of the isozymes and preparation of specific antisera. There has also been a steady advance in unravelling the complexities of protein processing and it is particularly in this area that protein biochemical genetics remains so important. It is only now that the full extent of the interaction between products of different genes to generate the final biologically functional protein is being elucidated and the tissue specific differences in structure and processing appreciated.

Relevant events occur at all stages from germ line DNA to the final protein product. An outline of the events that may occur in the processing of a single polypeptide is shown in Figure 1. In this review the processing events which occur prior to translation will not be considered further. Table 1 lists specific examples of many protein processing events that have been described. Many of the steps are under genetic control and mutations at gene loci coding for the processing enzymes as well as mutations affecting the crucial sites of the primary polypeptide can lead

Table 1 Examples of protein processing events

Process		*Examples*	*References*
Proteolytic cleavage	Removal of pre- and pro-sequences	hormones and serum proteins	Zimmerman *et al.* (1980) (review)
		lysosomal enzymes	Proia and Neufeld (1982)
		collagen	Hollister *et al.* (1982) (review)
	Cleavage of polyproteins	hormones	Zimmerman *et al.* (1980) (review)
		sucrase/isomaltase (EC 3.2.1.48)	Hauri *et al.* (1985a)
	Further limited proteolysis	lysosomal enzymes	Hasilik and Neufeld (1980a)
Glycosylation	N-linked via dolichol phosphate pathway	α_1-antiitrypsin	Hercz *et al.* (1978)
		lysosomal enzymes	Hasilik and von Figura (1981)
	O-linked to serine and threonine	red cell membrane sialoglycoproteins	Anstee (1981)
	O-linked to hydroxy lysine and proline	collagen	Hollister *et al.* (1982) (review)
	Modification of outer residues e.g. sialic acid	lysosomal enzymes	Swallow *et al.* (1984)
Chemical modification	Thiol oxidation	adenosine deaminase (EC 3.5.4.4)	Hopkinson and Harris (1969)
	Deamidation	amylase (EC 3.2.1.1)	Keller *et al.* (1971)
	Sulphation	tyrosine residues	Huttner *et al.* (1982)
	Phosphorylation	tyrosine residues	Huttner *et al.* (1982)
		mannose on lysosomal enzymes	Hasilik and Neufeld (1980b)
Ligand binding	Non-catalytic glycoprotein	β-galactosidase (EC 3.2.1.23) protective factor	D'Azzo *et al.* (1982)
		adenosine deaminase (EC 3.5.4.4) binding protein	Swallow *et al.* (1977)
Subunit association and aggregation	Non-identical subunits	β-D-*N*-acetylhexosaminidase (EC 3.2.1.30)	Proia *et al.* (1984)
	Different aggregation states	β-galactosidase (EC 3.2.1.23)	D'Azzo *et al.* (1982)
		alkaline phosphatase (EC 3.1.3.1)	Beratis *et al.* (1971)
		α-fucosidase (EC 3.2.1.51)	Turner (1979)

Table 2 Some examples of variant phenotypes involving processing

Stage	*Effect on protein*	*Site of defect*	*Example*	*References*
Proteolytic cleavage	Extra long protein – failure to cleave pro-sequence	amino acid sequence	Factor IX Chapel Hill McKusick 26490	Noyes *et al* (1983)
		amino acid sequence	Proalbumin Christchurch McKusick 17665	Brennan and Carrell (1978)
		amino acid sequence	Familial hyperproinsulinaemia McKusick 17673	Robbins *et al*. (1981)
		procollagen peptidase	Ehlers–Danlos type VII McKusick 224541	Lichtenstein *et al*. (1973)
		? protease	Familial hyperproinsulinaemia McKusick 17673	Gruppuso *et al*. (1984)
Glycosylation	Variation in number of N-linked side chains	? amino acid sequence	Aryl sulphatase polymorphism	Waheed *et al*. (1983)
Transport	Incomplete complex oligosaccharide side chain processing and serum enzyme deficiency	amino acid sequence	α_1-Antitrypsin ZZ McKusick 10740	Hercz *et al*. (1978)
	Failure to phosphorylate mannose and multiple lysosomal enzyme deficiency	*N*-acetylglucosaminyl phosphotransferase	I-cell disease McKusick 25250	Reitman *et al*. (1981)
	enzyme deficiency	unknown	Sucrase/isomaltase deficiency variant McKusick 22290	Hauri *et al*. (1985b)
Ligand binding/subunit interaction	double enzyme deficiency	deficiency of a 'protective factor'	Combined β-galactosidase/sialidase deficiency McKusick 25654	D'Azzo *et al*. (1982)
	enzyme deficiency	non-associating Hexα chain	Tay-Sachs disease variant McKusick 27277, 27280	D'Azzo *et al*. (1983)

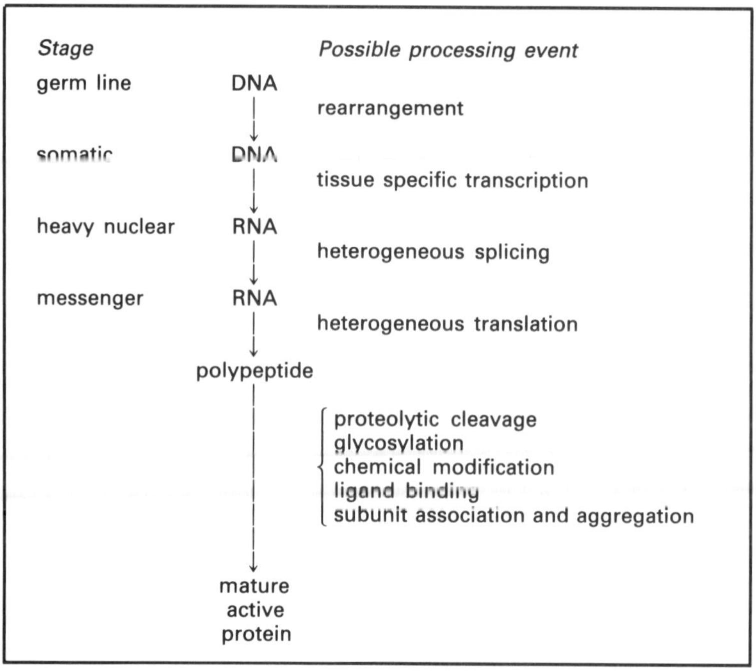

Figure 1 Possible processing steps of DNA, RNA and protein involved in the synthesis of a biologically active polypeptide

to variant proteins, some examples of which are shown in Table 2. One consequence of mutations affecting processing enzymes is that more than one protein may be affected since processing events are often shared by a group of proteins. Lysosomal enzymes provide several examples of this phenomenon. A large number of different enzymes are involved in their processing. These include proteases, glycosidases, glycosyl transferases, a phosphodiesterase and a phosphotransferase. Deficiency of *N*-acetylglucosaminyl phosphotransferase (EC 2.7.8.17) in I-cell disease (McKusick 25250) leads to a generalized secondary deficiency of lysosomal enzymes in many cells of the body. Likewise deficiency of β-galactosidase (EC 3.2.1.23) or sialidase (EC 3.2.1.18) in G_{M1} gangliosidosis (McKusick 23050) or sialidosis (McKusick 25655) respectively causes the other lysosomal enzymes to have extra long carbohydrate side chains.

Lysosomal enzymes, like other proteins, are sometimes comprised of more than one subunit. β-D-*N*-Acetylhexosaminidase A (HEX A) is an interesting example of a protein comprised of polypeptides α and β coded for by distinct genes, *HEXA* and *HEXB*, and has the structure $\alpha\beta_a\beta_b$ where β_a and β_b are proteolytic cleavage products of β (reviews by Neufeld, 1981; Mahuran *et al.*, 1985). HEX A can be considered to be an obligate heteropolymer, and in this respect resembles haemoglobin, since HEX A is the only isozyme that hydrolyses the major natural substrate G_{M2} *in vivo*, although the other polypeptide combinations $(\beta_a\beta_b)_2$ and α_2 occur, as HEX B and HEX S respectively. Mutations at the *HEXA* locus and at the *HEXB* locus both have the same clinical consequences leading to a variety of presentations of G_{M2} gangliosidosis (McKusick 26876, 26880, 27277, 27280) but whose severity is mainly related to the amount of functional HEX A. It is of interest that there is some evidence of an evolutionary relationship between HEX β and HEX α (Geiger *et al.*, 1977). Both subunits carry an active site though these have slightly different substrate specificities (Kytzia and Sandhoff, 1985).

The ability of HEX A to hydrolyse the natural substrate G_{M2} appears to reflect not simply the difference in the active site but a difference in the recognition by yet another glycoprotein, G_{M2} activator protein, coded by a third gene which has the role of presenting the hydrophobic G_{M2} to the enzyme (Conzelmann and Sandhoff, 1978; Conzelmann *et al.*, 1982). This also might be considered a kind of subunit interaction but of a much less stable kind, since it has not proved possible to demonstrate HEX A G_{M2} activator binding experimentally (Conzelmann *et al.*, 1982). It is intriguing but possibly coincidental that the gene coding for the activator protein *GM2A* maps to chromosome 5 – the same chromosome to which *HEXB* has been mapped (Burg *et al.*, 1985). From the genetic point of view it is of interest that deficiency of the G_{M2} activator protein can lead to a failure of G_{M2} hydrolysis and to a clinical presentation similar to deficiency of either the α or β polypeptide (Conzelmann and Sandhoff, 1978; McKusick 27275).

Extensive biochemical heterogeneity within a single clinical condition can also occur where only a single gene codes for the enzyme polypeptide. Since the deficiency of α-glucosidase (EC 3.2.1.20) in Pompe's disease (McKusick 23230) was the first inborn error in a lysosomal storage disorder to be elucidated it seems appropriate to use this example to illustrate the increase in complexity revealed in the last twenty years.

Deficiency of α-glucosidase leads to a wide spectrum of clinical presentations, particularly in terms of age of onset. While there is thought to be some correlation between the clinical severity and residual enzyme activity, it is clear that some of even the mildly affected adult patients have very profound deficiencies (Beratis *et al.*, 1983). Although it can be shown from simple consideration of enzyme kinetics (Conzelmann and Sandhoff, 1983/4) that very low levels of enzyme are often sufficient to prevent significant accumulation of substrate, the dramatic differences in clinical presentation and of the major organs affected still require explanation.

Table 3 lists the allelic variants of acid α-glucosidase (GAA) that have been identified in healthy individuals and in patients with Pompe's disease. Using two different separation methods four alleles *GAA*1–4* have been found in healthy individuals. By metabolic labelling and immunoprecipitation at least as many different phenotypes, due to homozygosity or heterozygosity of *GAA*0* alleles, have been identified in patients (Table 3). There seems to be a crude correlation between the amount of mature enzyme present in fibroblasts and clinical severity (Reuser *et al.*, 1985). Since many of the mutations appear to affect enzyme turnover and since this might be expected to vary in different tissues, the effective level of enzyme activity will also vary. This might account for the relative differences in involvement of different tissues, in particular the heart and skeletal muscle, as a consequence of the different mutations.

Table 3 Acid α-glucosidase (EC 3.2.1.20) GAA alleles

Allele	*Description*	*Method of separation*	*Frequency*	*References*
Normal activity				
*GAA*1*		starch gel electrophoresis isoelectric focussing	0.91 (Caucasians)	Swallow *et al.* (1975) Nickel and McAlpine (1982)
*GAA*2*		starch gel electrophoresis isoelectric focussing	0.03 (Caucasians)	Swallow *et al.* (1975) Nickel and McAlpine (1982)
*GAA*3*		starch gel electrophoresis	0.01 (Indians) 0.002 (Malays)	Teng and Tan (1979)
*GAA*4*		isoelectric focussing	0.06 (Caucasians)	Nickel and McAlpine (1982)
Low activity				
*GAA*0*	1. no protein (infant)	metabolic labelling immunoprecipitation and SDS electrophoresis (methods 1–4)	rare	Reuser *et al.* (1985)
	2. normal precursor – no phosphorylation no mature form (infant & adult)		rare	
	3. normal precursor – phosphorylation no mature form (juvenile)		rare	
	4. all forms reduced (juvenile, adult)		rare	

A feature of α-glucosidase that has interested us over the years is the significance of the *GAA*2* allele, since there is evidence of altered catalytic activity (Beratis *et al.*, 1983). Furthermore the only GAA 2 adult we have encountered presented with muscle problems. This however was thought to be a consequence of his alcoholism, the condition which led to his death before family studies were possible. We have so far looked at the α-glucosidase of twelve adult patients with Pompe's disease by starch gel electrophoresis but found no evidence of the presence of the *GAA*2* allele.

The elucidation of the substitutions involved in the various *GAA* alleles will no doubt await the cloning of these genes, but the biology of the enzymes and their clinical consequences cannot be elucidated simply by analysis of the DNA.

CONCLUDING REMARKS

It is clear that a very broad range of techniques is necessary for the full analysis of enzymes and other proteins in the contexts both of the healthy population and of clinical genetics. These range from the relatively simple quantitative and qualitative analysis to establish the protein deficiency or variant phenotype, to specialized procedures involving protein purification, raising antisera, amino acid sequencing and the recombinant DNA techniques involving isolation of cDNA and genomic clones and their sequencing and analysis. Although some of these approaches are too laborious to be used for population or family studies, both specific antibody and DNA probes can be used in this way. Furthermore the use of somatic cells in culture, particularly of the somatic cell hybrid technique, has supplemented the population and family study method of genetic analysis. The combined approaches are powerful in finding out the number of genes involved in determining the final structure of a protein and elucidating which gene product carries the primary defect or alteration. The study of the functional characteristics of the protein complements the investigations on the patient and is helpful in revealing the way in which a particular defect generates the pathological syndrome, in some cases providing a rationale for treatment.

REFERENCES

Anstee, D. J. The blood group MNSs-active sialoglycoproteins. *Semin. haematol.* 18 (1981) 13–31

D'Azzo, A., Hoogeveen, A., Reuser, A. J. J., Robinson, D. and Galjaard, H. Molecular defect in combined β-galactosidase and neuraminidase deficiency in man. *Proc. Natl. Acad. Sci. USA* 79 (1982) 4535–4539

D'Azzo, A., Proia, R. L., Kolodny, E. H., Kaback, M. M. and Neufeld, E. F. Biosynthesis assembly and maturation of β-hexosaminidase in variants of Tay-Sachs disease. *Am. J. Hum. Genet.* 35 (1983) 40A

Beratis, N. G., LaBadie, G. U. and Hirschhorn, K. Acid α glucosidase: kinetic and immunologic properties of enzyme variants in health and disease. In Rattazzi, M. C., Scandalios, J. G. and Whitt, G. S. (eds.) *Isozymes: Current Topics in Biological and Medical Research, Vol. 11: Medical and Other Applications*, Alan R. Liss, New York, 1983, pp. 25–36

Beratis, N. G., Seegers, W. and Hirschhorn, K. Properties of placental alkaline phosphatase II. Interactions of fast- and slow-migrating components. *Biochem. Genet.* 5 (1971) 367–377

Blake, M. S., Johnston, K. H., Russell-Jones, G. J. and Gotschlich, E. C. A rapid sensitive method for detection of alkaline phosphatase-conjugated antibody on Western blots. *Anal. Biochem.* 136 (1984) 175–179

Brennan, S. O. and Carrell, R. W. A circulating variant of human pro-albumin. *Nature* 274 (1978) 908–909

Burg, J., Conzelmann, E., Sandhoff, K., Solomon, E. and Swallow, D. M. Mapping of the gene coding for the human G_{M2} activator protein to chromosome 5. *Ann. Hum. Genet.* 49 (1985) 41–45

Cavalli-Sforza, L. L., Daiger, S. P. and Rummel, D. P. Detection of genetic variation with radioactive ligands. I. Electrophoretic screening of plasma proteins with a selected panel of compounds. *Am. J. Hum. Genet.* 29 (1977) 581–592

Conzelmann, E., Burg, J., Stephan, G. and Sandhoff, K. Complexing of glycolipids and their transfer between membranes by the activator protein for degradation of lysosomal ganglioside G_{M2}. *Eur. J. Biochem.* 123 (1982) 455–464

Conzelmann, E. and Sandhoff, K. AB variant of infantile G_{M2} gangliosidosis: deficiency of a factor necessary for stimulation of hexosaminidase A-catalyzed degradation of ganglioside G_{M2} and glycolipid G_{A2}. *Proc. Natl. Acad. Sci. USA* 75 (1978) 3979–3983

Conzelmann, E. and Sandhoff, K. Partial enzyme deficiencies: residual activities and the development of neurological disorders. *Dev. Neurosci.* 6 (1983/84) 58–71

Fukushima, H., de Wet, J. R. and O'Brien, J. S. Molecular cloning of a cDNA for human α-L-fucosidase. *Proc. Natl. Acad. Sci. USA* 82 (1985) 1262–1265

Geiger, B., Arnon, R. and Sandhoff K. Immunochemical and biochemical investigation of hexosaminidase S. *Am. J. Hum. Genet.* 29 (1977) 508–522

Geiger, B., Ben-Yoseph, Y. and Arnon, R. Purification of human hexosaminidases A and B affinity chromatography *FEBS Lett.* 45 (1974) 276–281

Gershoni, J. M. and Palade, G. E. Protein blotting: principles and applications. *Anal. Biochem.* 131 (1983) 1–15

Gordon-Weeks, P. R. and Harding, S. Major differences in the concanavalin A binding glycoproteins of post-synaptic densities from rat forebrain and cerebellum. *Brain Res.* 277 (1983)380–385

Gruppuso, P. A., Gorden, P., Kahn, C. R., Cornblath, M., Zeller, W. P. and Schwartz, R. Familial hyperproinsulinemia due to a proposed defect in conversion of proinsulin to insulin. *N. Engl. J. Med.* 311 (1984) 629–634

Harris, H. Monoclonal antibodies to enzymes. In Kennett, R. H., Bechtol, K. B. and McKearn, T. J. (eds.) *Monoclonal Antibodies and Functional Cell Lines*, Plenary, New York, 1984, pp. 36–65

Hasilik, A. and von Figura, K. Oligosaccharides in lysosomal enzymes. *Eur. J. Biochem.* 121 (1981) 125–129

Hasilik, A. and Neufeld, E. F. Biosynthesis of lysosomal enzymes in fibroblasts: synthesis as precursors of higher molecular weight. *J. Biol. Chem.* 255 (1980a) 4937–4945

Hasilik, A. and Neufeld, E. F. Biosynthesis of lysosomal enzymes in fibroblasts: phosphorylation of mannose residues. *J. Biol. Chem.* 255 (1980b) 4946–4950

Hauri, H.-P., Roth, J., Sterchi, E. and Lentze, M. Transport to cell surface of intestinal sucrase–isomaltase is blocked in the Golgi apparatus in a patient with congenital sucrase–isomaltase deficiency. *Proc. Natl. Acad. Sci. USA* 82 (1985b) 4423–4427

Hauri, H.-P., Sterchi, E. E., Bienz, D., Fransen, J. A. M. and Marxer, A. Expression and intracellular transport of microvillus membrane hydrolases in human intestinal epithelial cells. *J. Cell Biol.* 101 (1985a) 838–851

Hercz, A., Katona, E., Cutz, E., Wilson, J. R. and Barton, M. α_1-Antitrypsin: the presence of excess mannose in the Z variant isolated from liver. *Science* 201 (1978) 1229–1232

Hollister, D. W., Byers, P. H. and Holbrook, K. A. Genetic disorders of collagen metabolism. In Harris, H. and Hirschhorn, K. (eds.) *Advances in Human Genetics, Vol. 12*, Plenum, New York and London, 1982, pp. 1–87

Hopkinson, D. A. and Harris, H. The investigation of reactive sulphydryls in enzymes and their variants by starch gel electrophoresis. Studies on red cell adenosine deaminase. *Ann. Hum. Genet.* 33 (1969) 81–87

Huttner, W. B. Sulphation of tyrosine residues – a widespread modification of proteins. *Nature* 299 (1982) 273–276

Ikuta, T., Fujiyoshi, T., Kurachi, K. and Yoshida, A. Molecular cloning of a full-length cDNA for human alcohol dehydrogenase. *Proc. Natl. Acad. Sci. USA* 82 (1985) 2703–2707

Kahn, A., Cottreau, D., Daegelen, D. and Dreyfus, J-C. Cell-free translation of messenger RNAs from adult and fetal human muscle: characterization of neosynthesized glycogen phosphorylase, phosphofructokinase and glucose phosphate isomerase. *Eur. J. Biochem.* 116 (1981) 7–12

Karlsson, S., Swallow, D. M., Griffiths, B., Corney, G., Hopkinson, D. A., Dawnay, A. and Cartron, J. P. A genetic polymorphism of a human urinary mucin. *Ann. Hum. Genet.* 47 (1983) 263–269

Keller, P. J., Kauffman, D. L., Allan, B. J. and Williams, B. L. Further studies on the structural differences between the isoenzymes of human parotid amylase. *Biochemistry* 10 (1971) 4867–4874

Kielty, C. M., Povey, S. and Hopkinson, D. A. Regulation of expression of liver-specific enzymes. II. Activation and chromosomal localization of soluble glutamate-pyruvate transaminase. *Ann. Hum. Genet.* 46 (1982a) 135–143

Kielty, C. M., Povey, S. and Hopkinson, D. A. Regulation of expression of liver-specific enzymes. III. Further analysis of a series of rat hepatoma × human somatic cell hybrids. *Ann. Hum. Genet.* 46 (1982b) 307–327

Konings, A., Hupkes, P., Versteeg, R., Grosveld, G., Reuser, A. and Galjaard, H. Cloning a cDNA for the lysosomal α-glucosidase. *Biochem. Biophys. Res. Comm.* 119 (1984) 252–258

Kytzia, H.-J. and Sandhoff, K. Evidence for two different active sites on human β-hexosaminidase A: interaction of G_{M2} activator protein with β-hexosaminidase A. *J. Biol. Chem.* 260 (1985) 7568–7572

Lange, L. G. and Vallee, B. L. Double ternary complex affinity chromatography: preparation of alcohol dehydrogenase. *Biochemistry* 15 (1976) 4681–4686

Lichtenstein, J. R., Martin, G. R., Kohn, L. D., Byers, P. H. and McKusick, V. A. Defect in conversion of procollagen to collagen in a form of the Ehlers–Danlos syndrome. *Science* 182 (1973) 298–300

Lloyd, J. C., Isenberg, H., Hopkinson, D. A. and Edwards, Y. H. Isolation of a cDNA clone for the human muscle specific carbonic anhydrase, CAIII. *Ann. Hum. Genet.* 49 (1985) 241–251

McAlpine, P. J., Shows, T. B., Miller, R. L. and Pakstis, A. J. The 1985 catalogue of mapped human genetic markers and report of the nomenclature committee. Human Gene Mapping VIII, Helsinki Conference (1985). Reprinted in *Cytogenet. Cell Genet.* 40 (1985) 8–66

Mahuran, D., Novak, A. and Lowden, A. The lysosomal hexosaminidase isozymes. In Rattazzi, M. C., Scandalios, J. G. and Whitt, G. S. (eds.) *Isozymes: Current Topics in Biological and Medical Research, Vol. 12* Alan R. Liss, New York, 1984, pp. 229–288

Michelson, A. M., Markham, A. F. and Orkin, S. H. Isolation and DNA sequence of full-length cDNA clone for human X chromosome-encoded phosphoglycerate kinase. *Proc. Natl. Acad. Sci.* 80 (1983) 472–476

Moeremans, M., Daneels, G., Van Dijck, A., Langanger, G. and De Mey, J. Sensitive visualization of antigen–antibody reactions in dot and blot immune overlay assays with Immunogold and Immunogold silver staining. *J. Immunol. Meth.* 74 (1984) 353–360

Myerowitz, R. and Proia, R. L. cDNA clone for the α-chain of human β-hexosaminidase:

deficiency of α-chain mRNA in Ashkenazi Tay-Sachs fibroblasts. *Proc. Natl. Acad. Sci. USA* 81 (1984) 5394–5398

Naylor, S. L. Bioautographic visualization of enzymes. In Rattazzi, M. C., Scandalios, J. G. and Whitt, G. S. (eds.) *Isozymes: Current Topics in Biological and Medical Research, Vol. 4*, Alan R. Liss, New York, 1980, pp. 69–106

Neufeld, E. F. Recognition and processing of lysosomal enzymes in cultured fibroblasts. In Callahan, J. W. and Lowden, J. A. (eds.) *Lysosomes and Lysosomal Diseases*, Raven Press, New York, 1981, pp. 115–129

Nickel, B. E. and McAlpine, P. J. Extension of human acid α-glucosidase polymorphism by isoelectric focusing in polyacrylamide gel. *Ann. Hum. Genet.* 46 (1982) 97–103

Noyes, C. M., Griffith, M. J., Roberts, H. R. and Lundblad, R. L. Identification of the molecular defect in factor IX Chapel Hill: substitution of histidine for arginine at position 145. *Proc. Natl. Acad. Sci. USA* 80 (1983) 4200–4202

Potter, J., Ho, M.-W., Bolton, H., Furth, A. J., Swallow, D. M. and Griffiths, B. Human lactase and the molecular basis of lactase persistence. *Biochem. Genet.* 23 (1985) 423–439

Proia, R. L., D'Azzo, A. and Neufeld, E. F. Association of α- and β- subunits during the biosynthesis of β-hexosaminidase in cultured human fibroblasts. *J. Biol. Chem.* 259 (1984) 3350–3354

Proia, R. L. and Neufeld, E. F. Synthesis of β-hexosaminidase in cell-free translation and in intact fibroblasts: an insoluble precursor α chain in a rare form of Tay-Sachs disease. *Proc. Natl. Acad. Sci. USA* 79 (1982) 6360–6364

Reitman, M. L., Varki, A. and Kornfeld, S. Fibroblasts from a patient with I-cell disease and pseudo-Hurler polydystrophy are deficient in uridine 5′-diphosphate-*N*-acetylglucosamine: glycoprotein *N*-acetyl-glucosaminylphosphotransferase activity. *J. Clin. Invest.* 67 (1981) 1574–1579

Reuser, A. J. J., Kroos, M., Oude Elferink, R. P. J. and Tager, J. M. Defects in synthesis, phosphorylation and maturation of acid α-glucosidase in glycogenosis type II. *J. Biol. Chem.* 260 (1985) 8336–8342

Robbins, D. C., Blix, P. M., Rubenstein, A. H., Kanazawa, Y., Kosaka, K. and Tager, H. S. A human proinsulin variant at arginine 65. *Nature* 291 (1981) 679–681

Secher, D. S. and Burke, D. C. A monoclonal antibody for large-scale purification of human leukocyte interferon. *Nature* 285 (1980) 446–450

Shows, T. B., Sakaguchi, A. Y. and Naylor, S. L. Mapping the human genome, cloned genes, DNA polymorphisms and inherited disease. In Harris, H. and Hirschhorn, K. (eds.) *Advances in Human Genetics, Vol. 12*, Plenum Press, New York and London, 1982, pp. 341–452

Smith, M., Povey, S., Arredondo-Vega, F. X., Duester, G., Kielty, C., Jeremiah, S. and Hopkinson, D. A. Mapping of human class 1 alcohol dehydrogenase (*ADH*). Human Gene Mapping VII, Los Angeles Conference (1983). Reprinted in *Cytogenet. Cell Genet.* 37 (1984) 586

Swallow, D. M., Corney, G. and Harris, H. Acid α-glucosidase: a new polymorphism in man demonstrable by 'affinity' electrophoresis. *Ann. Hum. Genet. (London)* 38 (1975) 391–406

Swallow, D. M., Evans, L. and Hopkinson, D. A. Several of the adenosine deaminase isozymes are glycoproteins. *Nature* 269 (1977) 261–262

Swallow, D. M., West, L. F. and Van Elsen, A. The role of lysosomal sialidase and β-galactosidase in processing the complex carbohydrate chains on lysosomal enzymes and possibly other glycoproteins. *Ann. Hum. Genet.* 48 (1984) 215–221

Teige, B., Olaisen, B. and Pedersen, L. Subtyping of haptoglobin – presentation of a new method. *Hum. Genet.* 70 (1985) 163–167

Teng, Y. S. and Tan, S. G. Acid α-glucosidase in Malaysians: population studies and the occurrence of a new variant. *Hum. Hered.* 29 (1979) 2–4

Towbin, H. and Gordon, J. Immunoblotting and dot immunobinding – current status and outlook. *J. Immunol. Meth.* 72 (1984) 313–340

Towbin, H., Staehelin, T. and Gordon, J. Electrophoretic transfer of proteins from polyacrylamide gels to nitrocellulose sheets: procedure and some applications. *Proc. Natl. Acad. Sci. USA* 76 (1979) 4350–4354

Turner, B. M. Purification and characterisation of α-L-fucosidase from human placenta. *Biochem. Biophys. Acta* 578 (1979) 325–336

Vockley, J. and Harris, H. Purification of human adult and foetal intestinal alkaline phosphatases by monoclonal antibody immuno-affinity chromatography. *Biochem. J.* 217 (1984) 535–541

Voller, A., Bidwell, D. E. and Bartlett, A. The enzyme linked immunosorbent assay (ELISA). Guernsey: Dynatech Europe (1979)

Waheed, A., Steckel, F., Hasilik, A. and von Figura, K. Two allelic forms of human arylsufatase A with different numbers of asparagine-linked oligosaccharides. *Am. J. Hum. Genet.* 35 (1983) 228–233

Whitehouse, D. B. and Putt, W. Immunological detection of the sixth complement component (C6) following flat bed polyacrylamide gel isoelectric focusing and electrophoretic transfer to nitrocellulose filters. *Ann. Hum. Genet.* 47 (1983) 1–8

Willard, H. F., Skolnick, M., Pearson, P. L. and Mandel, J. L. Human gene mapping by recombinant DNA techniques. Human Gene Mapping VIII, Helsinki Conference (1985). Reprinted in *Cytogenet. Cell Genet.* 40 (1985) 360–489

Wilson, J. M., Tarr, G. E. and Kelley, W. N. Human hypoxanthine (guanine) phosphoribosyltransferase: an amino acid substitution in a mutant form of the enzyme isolated from a patient with gout. *Proc. Natl. Acad. Sci. USA* 80 (1983) 870–873

Young, R. A. and Davis, R. W. Yeast RNA polymerase II genes: isolation with antibody probes. *Science* 222 (1983) 778–782

Zimmerman, M., Mumford, R. A. and Steiner, D. F. (eds.) Precursor processing in the biosynthesis of proteins. *Ann. NY Acad. Sci.* 343 (1980) 1–449

J. Inher. Metab. Dis. 9 Suppl. 1 (1986) 32–37

Direct DNA Analysis in Family Studies

S. Malcolm
Mothercare Unit of Paediatric Genetics, Institute of Child Health, 30 Guilford Street, London, WC1N 1EH, UK

Restriction fragment length polymorphisms can be followed through families to track the incidence of genetic disease. Either cloned genes or anonymous DNA fragments, closely linked to the disease locus, may be used. 10 mL of blood collected into EDTA provide an excellent source of DNA and the blood is suitable for up to 3 days. In addition to gene tracking, the gene mutation itself may be studied to determine whether there is a DNA deletion.

Over the last 5 or 6 years the genes for many human enzymes of significance in metabolism have been cloned even though their mRNAs are present in cells in very low abundance. These include several lysosomal enzymes such as β-glucocerebrosidase (EC 3.2.1.21), fucosidase (EC 3.2.1.51) and hexosaminidase (EC 3.2.1.52), enzymes of glycolysis such as phosphoglycerate kinase (EC 2.7.2.10), and a whole range of clotting factors including factors VIII and IX and von Willebrand's factor.

Once the clones have been isolated the questions of genome organization, sequence, regulation of expression and changes in disease states can be tackled.

TECHNIQUES

Whether a protein forms a major part of the cells' output (such as the muscle proteins or the immunoglobulins in B cells) or a very minor part (such as adenosine deaminase or alcohol dehydrogenase) the number of genes which code for it among the cells' entire DNA content is likely to be very similar. Most proteins are coded for by a single gene or at the most a small family of closely related genes. Thus there will be a similar number of genes for the highly abundant globins or the much rarer red cell membrane proteins such as glycophorin or spectrin. As the total amount of DNA in the human haploid genome is 3×10^9 bp, a single gene containing 3000 bp will make up only one millionth of the total genome. Analysis of a single copy gene therefore requires extremely sensitive methods of analysis. The universal technique used to study the organization of genes within the chromosome was developed by Professor E. Southern and is referred to as DNA transfer or blotting (Southern, 1975).

With certain exceptions each cell in the body contains the same DNA and therefore the material for analysis can come from any convenient source. The most

Journal of Inherited Metabolic Disease. ISSN 0141–8955.

usual are white cells isolated from whole blood, a lymphoblastoid cell line made

Table 1 DNA preparation

1	Transfer or freeze blood in 50 mL tube (disposable plastic Falcon tube is suitable.) Add 30 mL ice-cold distilled water and mix well to lyse red cells
2	Centrifuge at approximately 3000 *g* for 10–20 minutes at 4°C
3	Tip off supernatant and resuspend thoroughly in 25 mL ice-cold 0.1% NP40 (Nonidet)
4	Spin as in stage 2
5	Tip off supernatant. Resuspend pellet in 2.5 mL of 0.075 mol/L NaCl, 0.025 mol/L EDTA pH 8.0
6	Add 125 μL 10% SDS (final concentration 0.5%) and 1 mg proteinase k. (From stock solution 10 mg/mL made up in distilled water
7	Incubate overnight at 37°C, or 4.5 h at 65°C
8	Add 2.5 mL of 0.075 mol/L NaCl, 0.025 mol/L EDTA pH 8.0
9	Add 5 mL phenol saturated with 50 mol/L Tris-HCl. Mix well
10	Spin as in stage 2
11	Remove upper aqueous layer with Pasteur pipette. Try to disturb the interphase as little as possible
12	Extract aqueous layer with 2.5 mL phenol and 2.5 mL $CHCl_3$. Mix well
13	Spin as in stage 2
14	Remove top aqueous layer
15	Mix aqueous layer with 5 mL $CHCl_3$. Spin as in stage 2. Remove top layer
16	Repeat stage 15
17	Add 0.5 mL 3 mol/L sodium acetate pH 5.2 and 10 mL ice-cold ethanol. Mix gently
18	Spool out precipitated DNA
19	Dissolve in 0.5 10 mmol/L Tris, 1 mmol/L EDTA pH 8.0. Shaking overnight at 4°C will probably be necessary
20	Calculate yield by measuring optical density at 260 μm

from transformed white cells, or a fibroblast cell line. The most straightforward method particularly in family studies is the use of whole blood. 20 mL of blood should provide about 0.5 mg of DNA and the blood is stable at least overnight and so can usually be sent by post, which is particularly useful in family studies.

A simple protocol for preparation of DNA from whole blood is given in Table 1. The basic steps are lysis of red cells (which contain no DNA) and collection of white cells; lysis of white cells with detergent to give nuclei; lysis of nuclei and digestion of protein with sodium dodecyl sulphate (SDS) and proteinase K; phenol/choloroform extractions to remove residual protein; ethanol precipitation of DNA.

Probe preparation

Cloned DNA may be inserted into plasmid, phage, cosmids or M13 single stranded phage. Plasmid DNA is perhaps the most simple to handle in the long term and has tended to be the chosen method of propagation. Stocks are usually maintained as frozen glycerol stocks of bacteria containing the plasmid. To produce suitable DNA for use as a hybridization probe a large scale culture must be grown, bacteria lysed to release chromosomal DNA and plasmid DNA, and the plasmid DNA purified and freed of protein. Most methods of achieving this use the fact that plasmid DNA consists of small circular supercoiled molecules. On alkali treatment linear DNA molecules will denature and fail to reassociate on neutralization, giving an insoluble mass which can be removed by centrifugation, but the supercoiled molecules will snap back together and remain soluble. When DNA molecules are mixed with the fluorescent dye, ethiduim bromide, which intercalates between the bases, supercoiled molecules become slightly less dense and can be separated by caesium chloride/ethiduim bromide isopycnic centrifugation. A detailed protocol was given by Maniatis and colleagues (1982). A single preparation should yield sufficient DNA for many analyses.

If the available stock is purified DNA rather than bacteria, then bacteria must be transformed with a small sample of the DNA, using antibiotic selection to select bacteria which have taken up the plasmid DNA carrying antibiotic resistance markers (Maniatis *et al.*, 1982).

Restriction enzymes

Both cloning and DNA analysis technology rely on the absolute specificity of each restriction enzyme to cut at a particular site. An example illustrating this specificity comes from the analysis of the normal and sickle β-globin genes (Chang and Kan, 1981). The enzyme *Mst*II cuts at the site CCTNAGG. This site exists in normal β-globin at amino acid residues B^5 and B^6 but the mutation of A-G which changes B^6 from glutamic acid to valine in β-sickle also removes the cutting site Thus normal β-globin gene is cut by *Mst*II to give 2 pieces of 1.15 kb and 0.2 kb but β-sickle gives only 1 piece of 1.35 kb. Enzyme specificity means that if DNA from 2 individuals is digested then cuts will occur at exactly the same positions around and within a gene in the 2 individuals, unless there is polymorphic sequence variation between individuals. Such variation does indeed occur in about 1 in 100 bp, and it forms the basis of the genetic analysis to be described in the accompanying article (Pembrey, 1986).

Southern blotting

The technique of Southern blotting is fully described in Sealey and Southern (1982). When total genomic DNA is cut with a restriction enzyme about 10^6 fragments are produced, far too many to resolve on a gel. The fragments are size-separated by electrophoresis through an agarose slab gel and visualized by staining with the fluorescent dye ethiduim bromide. DNA is denatured in the gel by soaking in sodium hydroxide and is then soaked in a neutralizing buffer. The next step is the blotting – the DNA is transferred by capillary action to a filter placed above the gel. Thus an exact replica of the gel is made on the filter. The most widely used filters have been nitrocellulose but other filters based on nylon have several advantages, including a greater mechanical strength and the abilities to bind smaller fragments and to bind them sufficiently tightly that the filters may be reused with different probes. Unfortunately all the membranes presently available are equally expensive. The pieces of DNA to be separated are of high molecular weight (around 3×10^6 u) and the gel system is a low percentage (typically 0.8%) agarose gel with large pores. These are extremely easy to prepare, pour and run.

The next step is to identify the piece of DNA containing the sequence of interest from all the others on the filter. This is done by hybridization with a radioactively labelled probe, washing off unbound DNA and detecting the radiolabelled sequence by autoradiography. Great care is needed to eliminate non-specific binding.

Non-radioactive probes

The isotope usually used in these experiments, ^{32}P, has a short half-life (14 days) and poses some problems of hazard and disposal. Considerable effort has been put into developing systems using colorimetric methods of detection. One such method, now commercially available, is based on incorporation of biotin into the DNA molecule (Langer-Safer *et al.*, 1982). Biotinylated dUTP can substitute for TTP in the labelling reaction and can subsequently be detected by labelling with streptavidin followed by a cross-linked biotin horseradish peroxidase complex or biotin alkaline phosphatase probe. The sequences are then detected by the enzymatic production of a coloured precipitate.

USES OF THE TECHNIQUES

Analysis of a genetic defects

Once a gene has been cloned it may or may not be known whether it is the gene which causes the primary defect in a disease. Genetic analysis should help to answer this question. Gene rearrangement can most simply cause a defect by the gene being wholly or partially deleted. This has been found in a number of types of thalassaemia, particularly α-thalassaemia where the α-globin gene is deleted (Nienhuis *et al.*, 1984). Another example has been found to be due to 21-hydroxylase deficiency in the study of HLA-linked congenital adrenal hyperplasia (White *et al.*, 1984). 21-Hydroxylase deficiency has been found to be frequently associated with a particular HLA haplotype, HLA A3; Bw47; DR7, with a null allele for the C4A (Rodgers) component. A plasmid with a 520 bp insert complementary to the middle third of the cytochrome P450 polypeptide of bovine origin was used as a probe for DNA from normals and a 21-hydroxylase deficient individual homozygous for HLA Bw47. Normal DNA revealed 2 fragments after either *Eco*R1 or *Taq*1 digestion, but the affected individual showed only 1 band. This demonstrated that sometimes the 21-hydroxylase deficiency results from the deficiency of a specific cytochrome P450, with the deletion probably including the nearby C4 gene.

Gene families and evolution of genes

Hybridization of the probe may occur to any closely related sequences. The stringency and thus the selectivity of the hybridization may be changed by altering salt conditions and temperature. Very often a probe may reveal surprisingly complex patterns. An example is the gene for phosphoglycerate kinase which was cloned using a synthetic oligo-nucleotide specific to short portions of the amino acid sequence . The gene was known to be localized in the long arm of the X-chromosome but DNA blotting showed other cross-hybridizing bands which revealed other autosomal sequences (Hutz *et al.*, 1984). A further example has been the unexpected finding that DNA clones from the Y-chromosome hybridize strongly to the X-chromosome (Page *et al.*, 1984), and this discovery led to a model showing that transposition must have occurred between the long arm of the X just below the centromere and the Y-chromosome. On occasion cross-hybridization reveals pseudo-genes which are non-functional gene remnants, and some care is needed to establish that a cross-hybridizing sequence is the genuine functional gene.

Expression of the gene

The DNA blotting technique may easily be adapted to study expression of a sequence (Northern blotting) (Thomas, 1980). Total messenger RNA is size-separated on a denaturing gel and transferred to a filter, and the specific RNA sequence is detected by hybridization. The strength of the signal depends on the abundance of the mRNA and provides a method of studying the tissue distribution of transcription.

Control of transcription

Despite extensive studies rather little is yet known of the factors affecting the regulation of transcription in different tissues or at different stages of development or differentiation. One factor which has a non-simple influence is the state of methylation of the DNA. Most methylation in human DNA occurs as 5 methyl-cytosine in the couplet CpG. When this falls within the recognition site of a restriction enzyme it can sometimes be used to distinguish methylated and non-methylated sequences (Waalwijk and Flavell, 1978). The enzyme MspI will cleave CCGG whether or not the middle C is methylated but HpaII will only cleave a non-methylated sequence. The blotting pattern of a probe using the 2 enzymes will reveal the state of methylation of the sites.

Mutant enzymes

Although gene deletions causing genetic disease have been found they occur in far from the majority of cases. A point mutation is often likely to be the cause of gene dysfunction. Examples have been found among haemophiliacs in the highly complex 180 kb factor VIII gene (Gitschier *et al.*, 1985). In 3 cases a C–T point mutation was found in a TaqI restriction site (TCGA) which was altered to TTGA. This turned out to be a phase such that an arginine (CGA) amino acid was converted to a stop codon (TGA), obviously resulting in non-expression of factor VIII (Gitschier *et al.*, 1985). However, cases which can be analysed simply by restriction enzyme changes will be few, and DNA sequencing of the normal and mutant enzymes will often be necessary. Commercial kits for this are now available.

REFERENCES

Chang, J. C. and Kan, Y. W. Antenatal diagnosis of sickle cell anaemia by direct analysis of the sickle mutation. *Lancet* 2 (1981) 1127–1129

Gitschier, J., Wood, W. I., Tuddenham, E. G., Shuman, M. A., Goralka, T. M., Chen, E. Y. and Lawn, R. M. Detection and sequence of mutations in the factor VIII gene of haemophiliacs. *Nature* 315 (1985) 427–430

Hutz, M. A., Michelson, A. M., Antonarakis, S. C., Orkin, S. H. and Kazazian, H. H. Restriction site polymorphism in the phosphoglycerate kinase gene on the X chromosome. *Hum. Genet.* 66 (1984) 217–219

Langer-Safer, P., Levin, M. and Ward, D. C. Immunological method for mapping genes on Drosophila polytene chromosomes. *Proc. Nat. Acad. Sci. USA* 79 (1982) 4381–4385

Maniatis, T., Fritsch, E. F. and Sambrook, J. Molecular cloning: a laboratory manual. Cold Spring Harbor Laboratory, 1982

Nienhuis, A. W., Anagnou, N. P. and Ley, T. J. Advances in thalassaemia research. *Blood* 63 (1984) 738–758

Page, D. C., Harper, M. E., Love, J. and Botstein, D. Occurrence of a transposition from the X-chromosome long arm to the Y-chromosome short arm during human evolution. *Nature* 311 (1984) 119–123

Pembrey, M. E. Applications and limitations of direct DNA analysis in genetic prediction. *J. Inher. Metab. Dis.* 9 Suppl. 1 (1986) 38-48

Sealey, P. H. and Southern, E. M. Gel electrophoresis of DNA. In Rickwood, D. and Hames, B.D. (eds.) *Gel Electrophoresis of Nucleic Acids,* IRL Press (1982), pp. 39–76

Southern, E. M. Detection of specific sequences among DNA fragments separated by gel electrophoresis. *J. Mol. Biol.* 98 (1975) 503–517

Thomas, P. S. Hybridization of denatured RNA and small DNA fragments transferred to nitro-cellulose. *Proc. Nat. Acad. Sci. USA* 77 (1980) 5201–5205

Waalwijk, C. and Flavell, R. A. DNA methylation at a CCGG sequence in the large intron of the rabbit β-globin gene. *Nucleic Acid Res.* 5 (1978) 4631–4641

White, P. C., New, M. I. and Dupont, B. HLA-linked congenital adrenal hyperplasia results from a defective gene encoding a cytochrome P450 specific for steroid 21-hydroxylation. *Proc. Nat. Acad. Sci. USA* 81 (1984) 7705–7709

J. Inher. Metab. Dis. 9 Suppl. 1 (1986) 38–48

Applications and Limitations of Direct DNA Analysis in Genetic Prediction

M. E. Pembrey
Mothercare Unit of Paediatric Genetics, Institute of Child Health, 30 Guilford Street, London WC1N 1EH, UK

Direct analysis of DNA has enormous potential for improved carrier detection or exclusion and early prenatal diagnosis in monogenic diseases. The strategy adopted in practice is determined by the fact that in most diseases allelic genetic heterogeneity precludes elucidation of the mutation in all families. Gene tracking asks the question – has a relative or fetus inherited the same relevant chromosome region as a previously affected family member? – and requires a gene-specific or closely linked DNA probe that reveals a restriction fragment length polymorphism (RFLP) in order to do a linkage study within the family. Gene tracking is independent of allelic heterogeneity in the disease, but is limited to those families in which key relatives are heterozygous for an RFLP.

The diagnosis of any serious disease has implications for the patient's relatives and those with whom they live, but there is, of course, an added dimension if the disorder is genetically determined. What is the risk that any particular future member of the family will have the disease and, if a fetus is at risk, can the disease be detected prenatally and if so, how early? Genetic prediction, the process of answering these questions within the general setting of genetic counselling, involves pedigree analysis often with particular attention to the probability of mutation or the frequency of the mutant gene in the general population, as well as the use of tests for diagnosis of the heterozygous or homozygous state.

Where the metabolic basis of the disease is understood traditional biochemical tests can often reliably and simply diagnose the disease state prenatally, although detection of carriers may be a rather complicated matter with the results being inconclusive in some individuals. This is particularly true of heterozygote detection in X-linked disorders, where the phenomenon of random X inactivation means that distinction between favourably Lyonised carriers and normal females is unlikely to be possible using biochemical tests. This is the problem with creatine kinase measurement as a test for Duchenne muscular dystrophy carriers (Emery, 1980), coagulation factor levels in Haemophilia A and B (Graham, 1979) and protein loading/orotic acid measurement for carrier detection in ornithine carbamoyl transferase (OCT) deficiency (Becroft *et al.*, 1984). These tests can sometimes establish the heterozygous state for certain but cannot exclude it with equal

Journal of Inherited Metabolic Disease. ISSN 0141–8955.

reliability. As a result they may allow the genetic counsellor to give the bad news but never the good news that a woman is definitely not a carrier. There are a number of inherent limitations in the traditional biochemical approach, the principal one being the need to examine tissue in which the gene is normally expressed. For this reason alone direct analysis of DNA has enormous potential as an approach to genetic diagnosis. DNA can be easily extracted from chorionic villus material so its analysis can form the basis of first trimester prenatal diagnosis. The clinical application of these techniques is in its infancy and limited to a few conditions, but certain general strategies (and problems) are emerging.

GENETIC HETEROGENEITY

The first requirement for genetic prediction is, of course, a precise diagnosis in the affected family member. What may be a satisfactory diagnosis at a clinical level may be inadequate at a genetic level because of genetic heterogeneity. Similar clinical disorders may be due to different mutations at the same gene locus (allelic heterogeneity) or may involve different gene loci (non-allelic heterogeneity). In the latter case direct analysis of DNA cannot be employed in genetic prediction unless one is certain which particular gene locus carries the mutation in the family under study. Clearly, if haemophilia A (factor VIII deficiency) and haemophilia B (factor IX deficiency) were still regarded as one disease as they once were, tracking the inheritance of the haemophilia with a factor VIII gene probe would lead to quite erroneous predictions if in reality the family had haemophilia B.

Within any disease entity the definition of those clinical and biochemical groups that involve the same gene locus is a pre-requisite for genetic prediction by direct DNA analysis. DNA analysis is going to complement, not replace clinical and biochemical investigations.

It is also useful to recognize allelic heterogeneity although this presents less of a problem in genetic prediction than might first be imagined. Allelic heterogeneity within a single genetic disorder should be regarded as the rule rather than the exception. Sickle cell anaemia, so often used to illustrate point mutation and molecular pathology, happens to be a very unusual case. A combination of almost direct observation of the amino acid substitution itself when observing sickled cells and the fact that the sickle mutation has been subjected to positive evolutionary selection by malaria means that all cases of sickle cell carry the same point mutation: GAG (glutamic acid) to GTG (valine) at the 6th codon of the β globin gene. In β-thalassaemia, however, more than 30 different mutations within the β globin gene have been described (Orkin *et al.*, 1983), so that knowledge of the precise mutation in one family tells you nothing about the mutation in another family with β-thalassaemia.

In serious X-linked and autosomal dominant disorders of early onset most families seen in clinical practice will represent quite separate mutational events of a few generations back. There is no reason to suppose that the mutation will be at the same site in the gene in each family and experience so far shows that large easily detected deletions of the gene, so characteristic of α-thalassaemia mutations

(Higgs *et al.*, 1983), are rare in diseases like Haemophilia A (Gitschier *et al.*, 1985), Haemophilia B (Gianelli *et al.*, 1983), OCT deficiency (Rozen *et al.*, 1985) and Lesch-Nyhan syndrome (Yang *et al.*, 1984). Thus for many disorders we can expect great allelic genetic heterogeneity, and therefore detection of the mutation itself in every family would present a formidable task. It is for this reason that a linkage strategy for genetic prediction has been devised.

It is therefore important to draw a distinction between the use of a gene-specific DNA probe to detect the mutation itself which can be referred to as gene detection, and the use of gene-specific or closely linked DNA probes for a linkage study within the family which is termed gene tracking.

DETECTION OF POINT MUTATIONS

In the few conditions where all or the majority of cases have the same single nucleotide base change, there is the opportunity for gene detection. Sometimes, as in sickle cell disease, the mutation alters a restriction enzyme recognition site and simple restriction fragment analysis by Southern blotting can be used to distinguish the mutant gene from the normal one. Figure 1 illustrates the way in which an Mst II digest will produce a 1.15 kb fragment from the normal β globin gene, but a

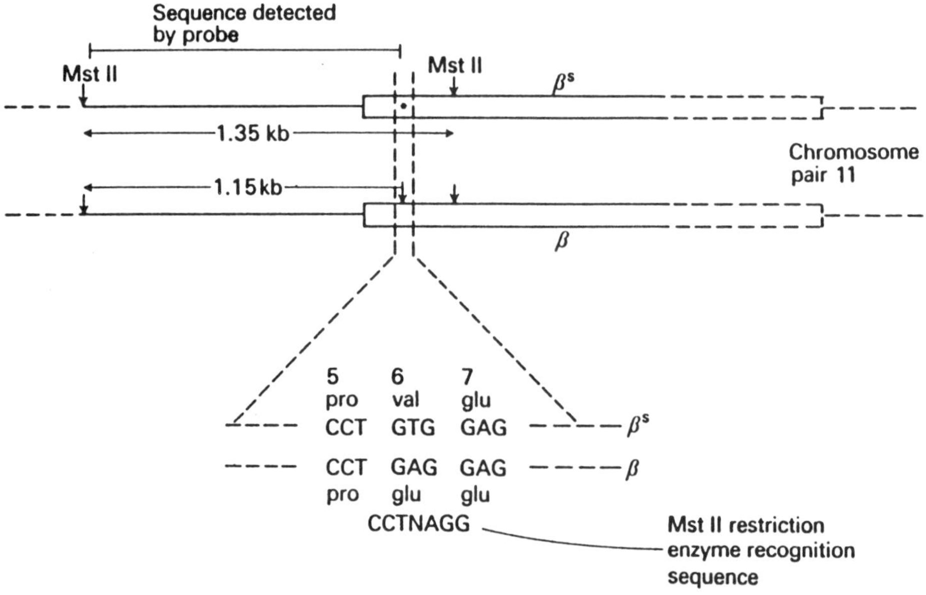

Figure 1 Diagram showing how the nucleotide base change of the sickle mutation GAG→GTG eliminates a cutting site for the restriction enzyme *Mst*II that recognizes the sequence CCTGAGG but not CCTGTGG. Note that the middle base in the *Mst*II site (N in the diagram) can be any nucleotide. The loss of the *Mst*II site on the chromosome carrying the sickle mutation of the β-globin gene results in a larger (1.35 kb) restriction fragment than normal (1.15 kb)

1.35 kb fragment from the β globin gene carrying the sickle mutation (Chang and Kan, 1982).

Point mutations, however, will only occasionally occur at a restriction enzyme recognition sequence and in most cases a different detection technique is required. One approach has been to synthesize an oligonucleotide probe of about 20 nucleotide bases that is complementary to the normal sequence and another that is complementary to the mutant sequence. The stringency of the hybridization conditions can be adjusted so that only a perfect probe/patient DNA match will allow hybridization to occur and therefore produce a signal on the autoradiograph. By carrying out analysis with the normal sequence oligonucleotide probe and then the mutant sequence probe it is possible to detect a specific single nucleotide base difference in total human DNA. Prenatal diagnosis for the ZZ type of α-1-antitrypsin deficiency has been achieved using the oligonucleotide probe technique (Kidd *et al.*, 1983).

DETECTION OF DELETIONS

α-Thalassaemia in the Far East and one not uncommon form of β-thalassaemia in India have substantial deletions of part, or all, of the gene sequence. Such deletions alter the pattern of restriction fragments on Southern blot analysis and are easily detected.

GENE TRACKING

Gene tracking asks the question 'has the fetus or relative inherited the same relevant chromosomal region as a previously affected family member?' There are variations to this question as discussed later, but a small family study is always required. There are 2 requirements for gene tracking: (1) a DNA probe specific for the gene locus involved or a probe for a closely linked DNA sequence, and (2) a common restriction fragment length polymorphism (RFLP) revealed by the DNA probe that can be exploited to distinguish each chromosome of the pair in key family members.

RESTRICTION FRAGMENT LENGTH POLYMORPHISMS

Only a very small percentage of total genomic DNA is actually coding sequence for proteins. The non-coding regions that flank genes, the intergenic DNA, and to some extent the intervening sequences are less conserved during evolution, and point mutations are tolerated and become established in populations. The experience so far suggests that on average 1 in 100–200 nucleotide bases differs between the chromosome pair. A number of these DNA sequence polymorphisms involve the recognition sequence of 4 or 6 bases of a particular restriction enzyme, and this results on digestion in different size restriction fragments from each of the homologous chromosome pair. Thus an RFLP is a relatively common change in

DNA sequence that either destroys or creates a restriction enzyme recognition site, or alters the distance between 2 sites. In any individual who is heterozygous for an RFLP, one restriction band pattern corresponds to one chromosome and the other band pattern to the other chromosome of the pair. This allows one to track the transmission of a single chromosome region through a family and to see if a particular monogenic disease co-inherits with the polymorphic site; in other words, one can perform classical linkage studies (Botstein *et al.*, 1980).

HAEMOPHILIA A AS AN EXAMPLE

The factor VIII gene, the locus at which haemophilia A mutations occur, maps to the Xq28 region of the X-chromosome (Figure 2). By 1983 there were a number

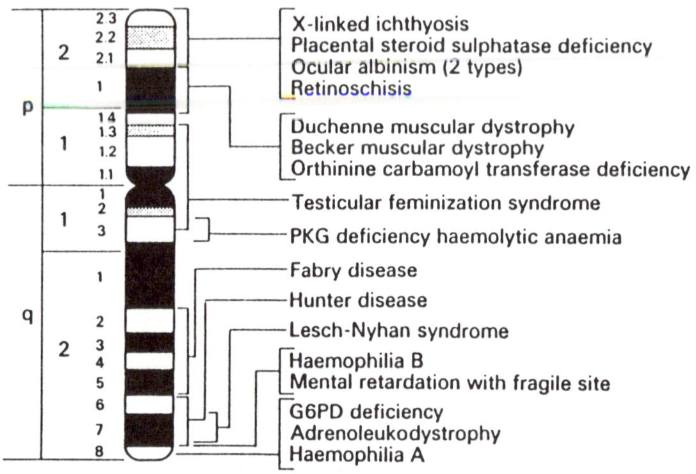

Figure 2 Selected disease gene loci on the X-chromosome

of X-chromosome specific single or low copy random DNA sequences that had been cloned (Davies *et al.*, 1981) and physically mapped to regions of the X (Drayna *et al.*, 1984). One such random sequence probe DX13 (official designation DXS15) mapped to the Xq28 region and was therefore a good candidate to show linkage to haemophilia A in family studies. Whilst the distance along the chromosome between 2 DNA sequences is the factor that primarily determines the closeness of the genetic linkage, it now transpires that certain regions of the X-chromosome are 'hot spots' for recombination. It is therefore essential to establish the recombination frequency between the disease gene locus and the DNA sequence used as a genetic marker by linkage studies in families with the disease in question.

The DX13 probe reveals a common RFLP on digestion of total DNA with the restriction enzyme *Bgl*II, some X-chromosomes revealing a 5.8 kb band (allele 1) and others a 2.8 kb band (allele 2). These alleles occur with equal frequency in the population (and haemophilia A families) and so any female has a half chance of being heterozygous for the RFLP, i.e. showing both bands on restriction fragment analysis. Linkage studies (Harper *et al.*, 1984) in haemophilia A families demonstrated close linkage (recombination frequency less than 5%) and so assessment of carrier status and first trimester prenatal diagnosis by direct DNA analysis became possible in selected families for the first time.

Figure 3 illustrates the pedigree of a woman (II-6) who was the first to seek first

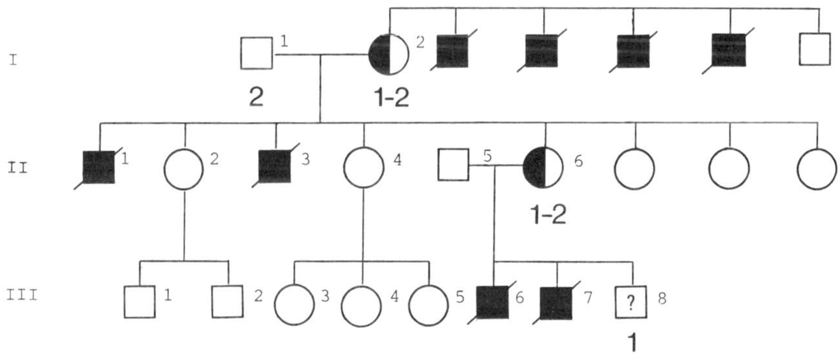

Figure 3 Pedigree of the first woman to seek first trimester prenatal diagnosis for haemophilia A using the linked DNA probe, DX13. The RFLP alleles 1 (5.8 kb band) and 2 (2.8 kb band) are shown for those subjects tested. ■ affected male; ◐ heterozygous female

trimester prenatal diagnosis using DX13 (Winter *et al.*, 1985). She presented with her 3rd pregnancy at 7 weeks gestation. Her 2 previous pregnancies had resulted in males diagnosed as having severe factor VIII deficiency following fetoscopic blood sampling at 18 weeks gestation. In each instance the couple opted for termination of the pregnancy. The pedigree indicates that II-6 had inherited the haemophilia mutation from her mother I-2, who in turn had 4 brothers as well as 2 sons who died from haemophilia. Chorionic villus sampling was performed at 10 weeks gestation and approximately 20 mg of material obtained for DNA analysis. Chorionic villus DNA hybridized strongly with the Y-specific probe pHY2.1, indicating that the fetus was male (Gosden *et al.*, 1982). The segregation of the alleles for the *Bgl*II RFLP using the DX13 probe is shown in Figure 3. The propositus, II-6, and her mother, I-2, were heterozygous, having both the 5.8 kb band (allele 1) and the 2.8 kb band (allele 2). The linkage phase between these alleles and the haemophilia mutation in the propositus could only be established by knowing which allele she received from her non-haemophilic father, I-1. His X-chromosome carried allele 2, so his daughter must have inherited an X-chromosome carrying both the haemophilia mutation and the RFLP allele 1 from her mother. It was this X-chromosome that she transmitted to her fetus, III-8, for chorionic villus DNA analysis revealed only a 5.8 kb band (allele 1). Barring the unlikely events of a cross-over between DX13 and the haemophilia mutation or an erroneous assumption about the paternity of II-6, this result predicted that the fetus was affected. The couple were told the fetus had 'at least a 95% chance' of being affected, and they opted for termination of the pregnancy by vaginal aspiration at 12 weeks gestation. Immediately before this procedure, with the mother's consent, a fetal blood sample was obtained by ultrasound guided cardiac puncture. This revealed no factor VIII activity by the VIII : CAg assay (Rotblat and Tuddenham, 1981) thus confirming the diagnosis.

There is no doubt that the availability of reliable prenatal diagnosis of haemophilia A by fetal blood sampling at 18 weeks gestation (Mibashan *et al.*, 1979) made the introduction of first trimester prenatal diagnosis by gene tracking using the DX13 probe an easier clinical decision.

For some couples the advantage of a genetic prediction in early pregnancy outweighed the slight error rate due to recombination between DX13 and the haemophilia mutation. They accepted the prospect of an occasional false positive result leading to abortion of a normal male fetus, and could if they wished double check the 'good news' on first trimester DNA analysis by fetal blood sampling at 18 weeks to exclude any false negative result. The prospect of fetal blood sampling with a less than 5% chance of a subsequent 2nd trimester abortion is very different from facing a 50% chance of bad news.

A decision to start offering prenatal diagnosis exclusion for conditions like Duchenne muscular dystrophy where there is no 2nd trimester back-up test is a more difficult one. How close a linkage with a DNA marker is close enough and what margin of error on the estimate of the recombination distance from research studies is acceptable? It is not as simple as just deciding to await a completely reliable test based on a gene-specific probe because many women at risk are currently accepting abortion of all males, which is the equivalent of a 50% or greater false positive rate: they may be keen to discuss any improvement on this.

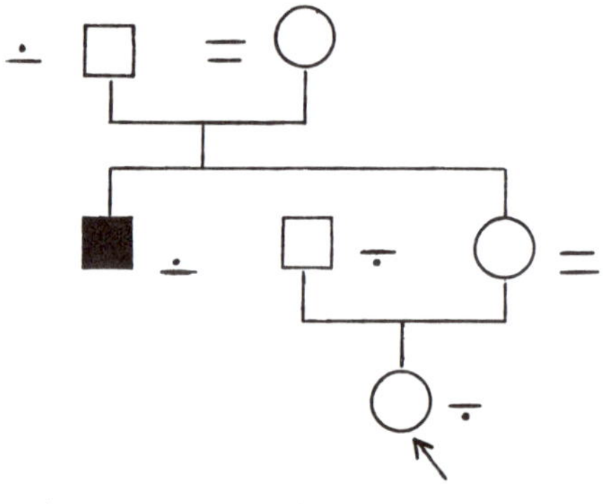

Figure 4 A pedigree showing a woman seeking carrier exclusion and her haemophiliac uncle. The bands of a two allele RFLP are indicated. = heterozygous; ∓ upper band(s) only; ∸ lower band(s) only

These points emphasize one advantage of a gene-specific probe, namely the virtual elimination of errors due to recombination between the mutation and the RFLP used for gene tracking. The second advantage of a gene-specific probe is a consequence of the first. With recombination errors eliminated, the exclusion of heterozygosity for haemophilia A can often be achieved by just examining the DNA of the woman seeking advice and any affected male relative. Figure 4 shows such a situation. There are 3 accumulative opportunities for recombination between a linked DNA probe such as DX13 and the factor VIII locus when passing between the propositus and her affected uncle. This would make any exclusion prediction quite unreliable. However, if analysis with a factor VIII probe RFLP showed that the propositus shared no RFLP allele in common with her uncle, then she could not be a carrier of the haemophilia A mutation. This statement is independent of whether or not the uncle represents a new mutation. If he does, then the propositus is not a carrier; if the grandmother is a carrier, then gene tracking with the gene specific probe also shows the propositus is not a carrier. Gene tracking is therefore very useful in excluding carrier status in X-linked disorders, expecially where new mutations are commonly encountered. Biochemical tests for carrier status do the reverse: they are useful in confirming carrier status in a proportion of cases. If the propositus had indeed inherited the same X-chromosome from her grandmother as her uncle, then a significantly low factor VIIIC : VIIIR.Ag ratio in either the grandmother or mother would confirm carrier status in the propositus.

Soon after the DX13 linkage to the factor VIII locus was demonstrated the factor VIII gene itself was cloned (Gitschier *et al.*, 1984), and a little later a *Bcl*I RFLP was reported (Gitschier *et al.*, 1985a) which has already been used for prenatal

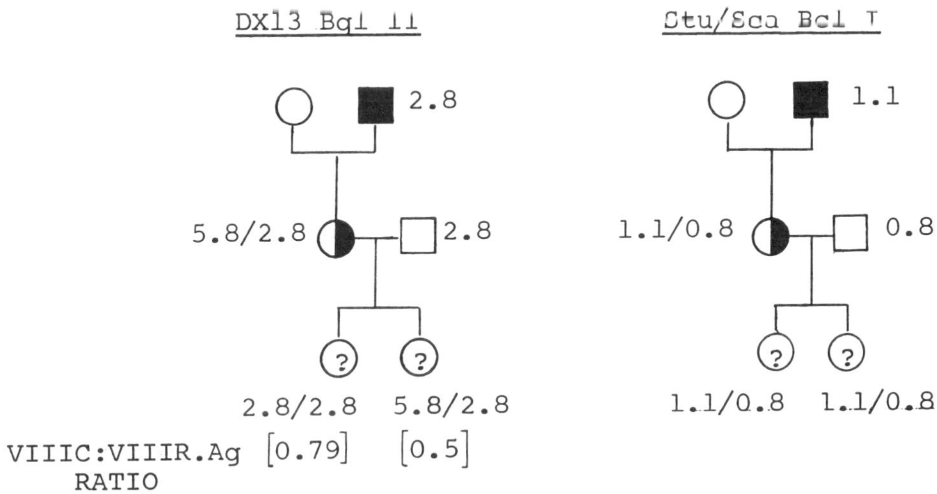

Figure 5 Pedigree showing the results of tracking a haemophilia A mutation from an affected male to his granddaughter using the linked DX13 probe (alleles 5.8 and 2.8 kb bands) and the factor VIII specific probe Stu/Sca (alleles 1.1 and 0.8 kb band). The DX13 probe result in the 2nd granddaughter is inconsistent with her low factor VIIIC : VIIIR. Ag ratio which indicates that she is a carrier. This represents a recombination between DX13 and the haemophilia mutation

diagnosis (Gitschier *et al.*, 1985b). In Europeans, about 50% of women are heterozygous for the *Bcl*I RFLP showing both a 1.1 and 0.8 kb band. Figure 5 shows the only recombination between DX13 and factor VIII observed in our own laboratory. This is one recombination in 43 meioses, which is typical of other people's experience. It will be seen that the low factor VIIIC : VIIIR.Ag ratio in the 2nd daughter alerted us to the recombination with DX13 before we confirmed this using the *Bcl*I RFLP with the factor VIII probe.

A third advantage of a gene-specific probe over a linked DNA probe is, of course, the potential to elucidate the mutation responsible for the haemophilia but, as indicated earlier, the existence of allelic heterogeneity means gene tracking using RFLPs will nearly always be the method of choice in clinical practice.

The current policy in our own unit is to test whether the key female in the family is 'informative', i.e. heterozygous, for the *BclI* RFLP with the factor VIII probe. If not, she is tested with DX13 or with St14 which is another random DNA sequence probe that shows close linkage to the factor VIII locus (Oberle *et al.*, 1985).

PRACTICAL ASPECTS OF GENE TRACKING FOR GENETIC PREDICTION

These have been discussed in detail in relation to carrier status assessment and prenatal diagnosis for haemophilia A using the linked probe DX13 (Winter *et al.*, 1985). There are 4 aspects that apply whether one is using a gene-specific or a linked probe for gene tracking: (1) non-allelic genetic heterogeneity as discussed earlier, (2) non-paternity, (3) assignment of linkage phase in the face of possible new mutation, and (4) the proportion of families in which RFLPs will be 'informative'.

Figure 3 shows that the linkage phase of the haemophilia mutation with the RFLP allele 1 (5.8 kb band) in II-6 is deduced from the knowledge that her father had transmitted allele 2 (2.8 kb band). In other words the prediction is critically dependent on correct paternity. In this instance traditional blood group testing was performed, although it is likely that use of probes for hypervariable 'minisatellite' DNA sequences will allow efficient paternity testing in the future (Jeffreys *et al.*, 1985).

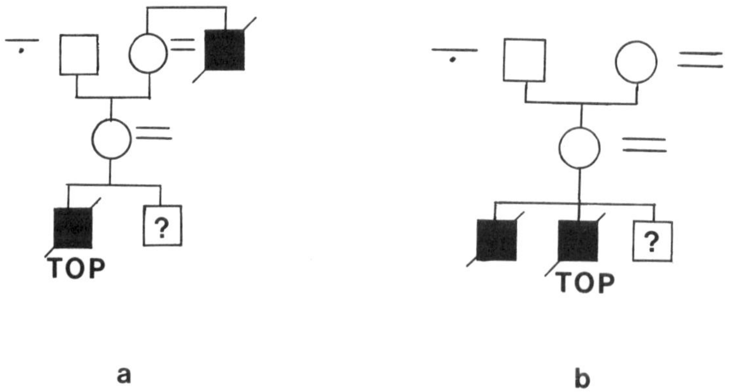

Figure 6 **(a)** Pedigree in which linkage phase between RFLP allele and haemophilia mutation can be deduced, **(b)** Superficially similar pedigree in which linkage phase cannot be deduced

Figure 6 illustrates the sort of pedigrees often encountered in clinical practice. In pedigree (a) the linkage phase in the woman seeking prenatal diagnosis in a male fetus can be deduced from her father's RFLP allele, because we know she inherited the other RFLP allele and the haemophilia mutation from her mother. In pedigree (b), although we know the woman seeking prenatal diagnosis is a carrier and her father was clinically normal, we cannot deduce linkage phase. The woman has close to a half chance of representing a new mutation, and we do not know whether this occurred in the sperm or the ovum that lead to her conception.

With the above points taken into account, gene tracking can be a very efficient approach to genetic prediction, employing the relatively robust technique of restriction fragment analysis by Southern blotting. It is however only available to those families that are 'informative' with one or more RFLPs: this is the major limitation. However, experience over the last few years has shown that as new RFLPs are described the number of families that can be helped rises fairly quickly to 75–80%. DNA from families uninformative for the current RFLPs can be stored and retested on new RFLPs or when better probes become available. DNA from key family members such as a boy with Duchenne muscular dystrophy, a parent with Huntington's chorea or selected elderly relatives must be stored. This commitment to the families is a major undertaking that has to be integrated with regional genetic services. The time has come for health authorities to make such a commitment.

References

Becroft, D. M. O., Barry, D. M. J., Webster, D. R. and Simmonds, H. A. Failure of protein loading tests to identify heterozygosity for ornithine carbamoyl transferase deficiency. *J. Inherit. Metab. Dis*. 7 (1984) 157–159

Botstein, D., White, R. I., Skolnick, M. and Davis, R. W. Construction of a genetic linkage map in man using restriction fragment length polymorphisms. *Am. J. Hum. Genet.* 32 (1980) 314–331

Chang, J. C. and Kan, Y. W. A sensitive new prenatal test for sickle-cell anaemia. *New Engl. J. Med.* 307 (1982) 30–32

Davies, K. E., Young, B. D., Elles, R. G., Hill, M. E. and Williamson, R. Cloning of a representative genomic library of human X chromosome after sorting by flow cytometry. *Nature* 293 (1981) 374–376

Drayna, D., Davies, K. E., Hartley, D., Handel, J. L., Camerino, G., Williamson, R. and White, R. Genetic mapping of the human X chromosome by using restriction fragment length polymorphisms. *Proc. Natl. Acad. Sci. USA* 81 (1984) 2836–2839

Emery, A. E. H. Duchenne muscular dystrophy. Genetic aspects, carrier detection and antenatal diagnosis. *Br. Med. Bull.* 36 (1980) 117–122

Giannelli, F., Choo, K. H., Rees, D. J. G., Boyd, Y., Rizza, C. R. and Brownlee, G. G. Gene deletions in patients with Haemophilia B and anti-factor IX antibodies. *Nature* 303 (1983) 181–182

Gitschier, J., Wood, W. I., Goralka, T. M., Wion, K. L., Chen, E. Y., Eaton, D. H., Vehar, G. A., Capon, D. J. and Lawn, R. M. Characterization of the human factor VIII gene. *Nature* 312 (1984) 326–330

Gitschier, J., Drayna, D., Tuddenham, E. G. D., White, R. L. and Lawn, R. M. Genetic mapping and diagnosis of Haemophilia A achieved through a BcI polymorphism in the factor VIII gene. *Nature* 314 (1985) 738–740

Gitschier, J., Lawn, R. M., Rotblat, F., Goldman, E. and Tuddenham, E. G. D. Antenatal diagnosis and carrier detection of Haemophilia A using factor VIII gene probe. *Lancet* 1 (1985) 1093–1094

Gosden, J. R., Mitchell, A. R., Gosden, C. M., Rodeck, C. H. and Morsman, J. M. Direct vision chorion biopsy and chromosome-specific probes for determination of fetal sex in first trimester prenatal diagnosis. *Lancet* 2 (1982) 1416–1419

Graham, J. B. Genotype assignment (carrier detection) in the haemophilias. *Clin. Haematol.* 8 (1979) 115–145

Harper, K., Winter, R. M., Pembrey, M. E., Hartley, D., Davies, K. E. and Tuddenham, E. G. D. A clinically useful DNA probe closely linked to Haemophilia A. *Lancet* 2 (1984) 6–8

Higgs, D. R. and Weatherall, D. J. Alpha-thalassaemia. *Curr. Top. Hematol.* 4 (1983) 37–97

Jeffreys, A. J., Wilson, V. and Thein, S. L. Hypervariable 'minisatellite' regions in human DNA. *Nature* 314 (1985) 67–73

Kidd, V. J., Wallace, R. B., Itakura, K. and Woo, S. L. C. $Alpha_1$-antitrypsin deficiency detection by direct analysis of the mutation in the gene. *Nature* 304 (1983) 230

Mibashan, R. S., Rodeck, C. H., Thumpston, J. K., Edwards, R. J., Singer, J. D., White, J. M. and Campbell, S. Plasma assay of fetal factor VIIIC and IX for prenatal diagnosis of haemophilia. *Lancet* 1 (1979) 1309

Oberle, I., Camerino, G., Heilig, R., Grunebaum, L., Cazenave, J-P., Crapanzano, C., Mannucci, P. M. and Mandel, J-L. Genetic screening for Hemophilia A (classic hemophilia) with a polymorphic DNA probe. *New Engl. J. Med.* 312 (1985) 682–686

Orkin, S. H., Antonarakis, S. E. and Kazazian, H. H. Jr. Polymorphism and molecular pathology of the human beta-globin gene. *Prog. Hematol.* 13 (1983) 49–73

Rotblat, F. and Tuddenham, E. G. D. Immunologic studies of factor VIII coagulant activity. I: Assays based on a haemophilic and an acquired antibody to VIIIC. *Thromb. Res.* 21 (1981) 431–445

Rozen, R., Fox, J., Fenton, W. A., Horwich, A. L. and Rosenberg, L. E. Gene deletion and restriction fragment length polymorphism at the human ornithine transcarbamylase locus. *Nature* 313 (1985) 815–817

Yang, T. P., Patel, P. I., Chinault, A. C., Stout, J. T., Jackson, L. G. and Hildebrand, B. M. Molecular evidence for new mutation at the *hprt* locus in Lesch-Nyhan patients. *Nature* 310 (1984) 412–414

Winter, R. M., Harper, K., Goldman, E., Mibashan, R. S., Warren, R. C., Rodeck, C. H., Penketh, R. J. A., Ward, R. M. T., Hardisty, R. M. and Pembrey, M. E. First trimester prenatal diagnosis and detection of carriers of Haemophilia A using the linked DNA probe DX13. *Br. Med. J.* 291 (1985) 765–769

J. Inher. Metab. Dis. 9 *Suppl.* 1 (1986) 49–57

DNA Analysis for Ornithine Transcarbamylase Deficiency

R. ROZEN[1], J. E. FOX[2], A. M. HACK[2], W. A. FENTON[2], A. L. HORWICH[2] and L. E. ROSENBERG[2]
[1]*McGill University Center for Human Genetics, 1205 Dr Penfield Avenue, Montreal, Quebec, Canada H3A 1B1*
[2]*Yale University School of Medicine, Department of Human Genetics, 333 Cedar St, PO Box 3333, New Haven, Connecticut, USA 06510*

We have utilized the Southern blotting technique to analyse genomic DNA from males with ornithine transcarbamylase (OTC) deficiency and their families. Using a nearly full length human cDNA probe, we have identified 3 patients with deletions at this locus and have characterized 4 different restriction fragment length polymorphisms that can be used as linkage markers for the OTC mutation. These polymorphisms occur at sufficiently high frequencies so as to enable us to distinguish the two X-chromosomes in approximately 80% of OTC carriers. As a direct consequence of these findings, prenatal diagnosis and carrier assessment can be offered to a large fraction of families at risk for OTC deficiency.

Ornithine transcarbamylase (OTC; EC 2.1.3.3) is a hepatic mitochondrial enzyme that catalyzes the second step of the urea cycle – the condensation of ornithine and carbamyl phosphate to form citrulline (Grisolia, 1976). Deficiency of this enzyme (McKusick 31125), an X-linked disorder (Short *et al.*, 1973; Ricciuti *et al.*, 1976), results in ammonia intoxication and frequent early death of hemizygous male infants (Walser, 1973). Phenotypic expression in heterozygous females is quite variable due to random X-chromosome inactivation (Ricciuti *et al.*, 1976).

Treatment for the disorder involves protein restriction, peritoneal dialysis or haemodialysis, and stimulation of alternate pathways of nitrogen disposal by administration of amino acid acylating agents, such as sodium benzoate and phenylacetate (Brusilow *et al.*, 1984). Prenatal diagnosis by amniocentesis has not been available until recently because the enzyme is not expressed in amniocytes and no unusual metabolites have been detected in amniotic fluid. Prenatal diagnosis by fetal liver biopsy has been performed (Rodeck *et al.*, 1982; Holzgreve and Golbus, 1984), but the general applicability of this approach has not been evaluated.

The frequency of spontaneous mutations in X-linked lethal disorders may be as high as one third of all cases (Haldane, 1935). Consequently, carrier detection for female family members is an important concern. Ammonium chloride (Short *et al.*, 1973) and protein (Brusilow and Valle, 1985) loading tests, with measurement

Journal of Inherited Metabolic Disease. ISSN 0141–8955.

of orotic acid excretion, have been used to identify carrier females, but the sensitivity and specificity of these methods remain to be determined.

The isolation of a nearly full-length human cDNA clone for OTC (Horwich *et al.*, 1984), which maps exclusively to the X-chromosome (Lindgren *et al.*, 1984), has enabled us to perform restriction analysis of DNA on pedigrees with OTC deficiency. In this review, we present some data on the characterization of mutations and on the detection of restriction fragment length polymorphisms (RFLPs) at the OTC locus. The emphasis, however, is on the application of these findings to helping families at risk for OTC deficiency.

GENE DELETIONS AT THE OTC LOCUS

We have performed Southern blot analysis on DNA from at least 25 different OTC-deficient males, using the nick-translated plasmid, pH0731, which contains a nearly full-length human cDNA (1500 bp; Horwich *et al.*, 1984). This approach has

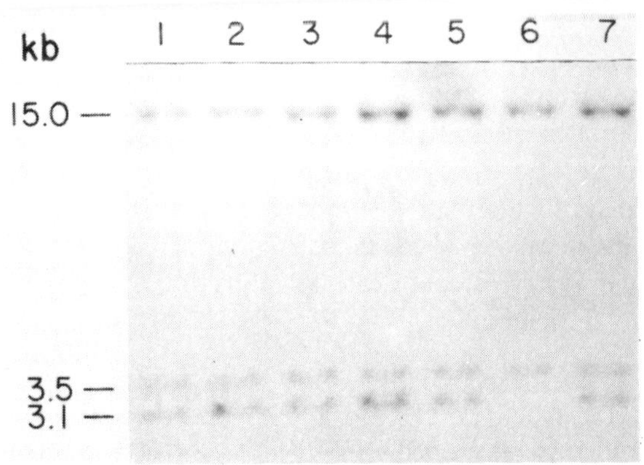

Figure 1 A gene deletion at the OTC locus. Genomic DNA from OTC-deficient males was digested with *Hind*III and subjected to Southern blotting. The nick-translated probe, plasmid pH0731 (Horwich *et al.*, 1984) contained a nearly full-length human cDNA for OTC (1500 bp). Reprinted with permission of the authors and publishers of Rozen *et al.* (1985)

identified 3 patients with partial deletions at this locus. Figure 1 depicts the blot following *Hind*III digestion of DNA from 7 severely affected males. A 3.1 kb band is absent in the digest from the patient in lane 6; this band has been localized to the 3′ end of the gene. Digestion of this patient's DNA with 5 other restriction enzymes has revealed a distinct missing band in each case; no new bands have been detected.

In Figure 2, *Sst*I-digested DNA from another OTC-deficient male (lanes 1, 3 and 5) and from a control female (lanes 2, 4 and 6) was examined by hybridization with the OTC probe (lanes 1 and 2) as well as probes L1.28 (Davies *et al.*, 1984; lanes 3 and 4) and 754 (Hofker *et al.*, 1985; lanes 5 and 6). The last 2 sequences map to the X-chromosome at positions distal and proximal to OTC, respectively (Francke *et al.*, 1985). No hybridizable bands were observed with this enzyme for the proband's DNA using the OTC probe, despite normal hybridization patterns with

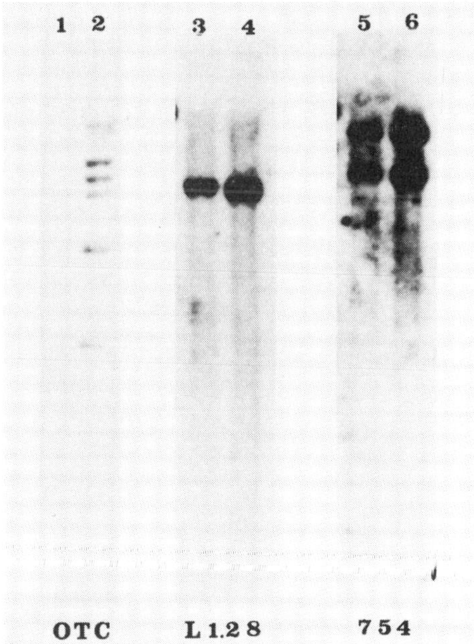

Figure 2 A second gene deletion at the OTC locus. DNA from an OTC-deficient male (lanes 1, 3 and 5) and from a control female (lanes 2, 4 and 6) was digested with *Sst*I, followed by Southern blot analysis. The probes for hybridization were pH0731 in lanes 1 and 2; L1.28 (Davies *et al.*, 1984) in lanes 3 and 4; and 754 (Hofker *et al.*, 1985) in lanes 5 and 6

L1.28 and 754. Subsequent studies have revealed hybridizable bands after digestion with other restriction enzymes. These results indicate that the deletion encompasses a large portion of the OTC gene but does not extend far beyond the locus in either direction along the X-chromosome. A third patient with a partial deletion at the OTC locus has recently been identified (data not shown).

The finding of only 3 deletions in our panel of DNA from OTC-deficient males suggests that most of the clinically significant mutations at the OTC locus are probably single base substitutions or minor deletions/insertions.

RESTRICTION FRAGMENT LENGTH POLYMORPHISMS AT THE OTC LOCUS

We have identified 2 different RFLPs at the OTC locus with the enzyme *Msp*I. A Southern blot of DNA from the 7 affected males discussed in Figure 1 reveals several invariant bands (17.5, 5.4, 3.5, 2.0 and 1.9 kb) (Figure 3a), as well as 2 sets of polymorphic bands (6.6/6.2 kb and 5.1/4.4 kb). Haplotypes have been assigned to the 4 possible combinations: haplotype A shows the 6.6 and 5.1 kb bands; B the 6.6 and 4.4 kb bands; C the 6.2 and 5.1 kb bands; and D the 6.2 and 4.4 kb bands. A hemizygous male can carry only one haplotype; all 4 possible haplotypes are represented in this blot.

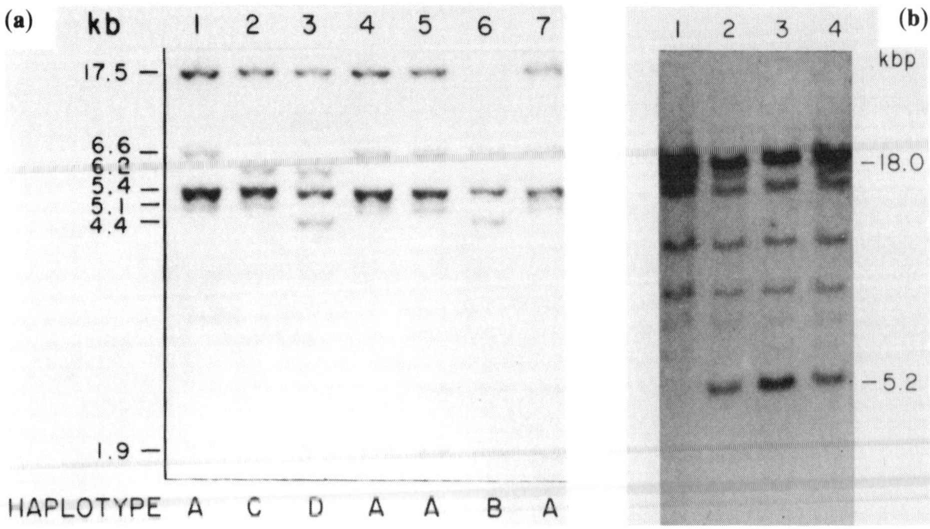

Figure 3 Restriction fragment length polymorphisms at the OTC locus. (**a**) *Msp*I-digested DNA from seven OTC-deficient males was blotted and probed with plasmid pH0731. Haplotypes were assigned as discussed in the text. Reprinted with permission of the authors and publisher of Rozen *et al.* (1985). (**b**) *Bam*HI-digested DNA from 4 control females was analysed as described by Southern blotting with probe pH0731

Females, with 2 X-chromosomes, can be homozygous or heterozygous for these haplotypes. Our analysis of DNA from 35 control women indicates that approximately 69% of females have two different *Msp*I-detectable haplotypes on their X-chromosomes.

Digestion of DNA with *Bam*HI has revealed another RFLP, characterized by polymorphic bands at 18 and 5.2 kb (Figure 3b). Lanes 2 and 4 depict the hybridization pattern of DNA from 2 women who are heterozygous for this RFLP. Lanes 1 and 3 depict the DNA from women who are homozygous for the 18 kb band and the 5.2 kb band, respectively. *Bam*HI digests on 28 control women indicate that 8 (29%) have different *Bam*HI-detectable hybridization patterns on their X-chromosomes.

Another RFLP, distinguished by polymorphic bands at 3.7 and 3.6 kb, has been identified using the enzyme *Taq*I (data not shown). Three women out of 27 controls (11%) are heterozygous for this polymorphism.

The analysis of DNA from OTC carriers has revealed that 80% of this population is heterozygous for at least one of these RFLPs.

RFLP ANALYSIS IN FAMILIES WITH OTC DEFICIENCY

For the small percentage of families in which an OTC gene deletion has been identified, prenatal diagnosis can be performed by qualitative analysis of the DNA from a male fetus i.e. by the absence or presence of specific band(s) in a Southern blot. For the majority of families, however, in which the nature of the mutation has not been characterized, RFLPs must be used as linkage markers.

All women who are obligate carriers of the OTC mutation and who are heterozygous for at least one RFLP are suitable candidates for prenatal diagnosis. Figure 4 shows the blot after *Msp*I digestion of DNA from a proband (lane 1), his mother (lane 2) and his maternal aunt (lane 3). The mother has been designated as an obligate carrier for OTC deficiency, after a protein tolerance test, and is also a heterozygote for the *Msp* polymorphism (haplotypes A and C). The OTC mutation must reside on her X-chromosome with the A haplotype since her affected son inherited that chromosome. For any subsequent pregnancies, all children who inherit the chromosome with the A haplotype will inherit the mutation whereas those who inherit the chromosome with the C haplotype will be unaffected.

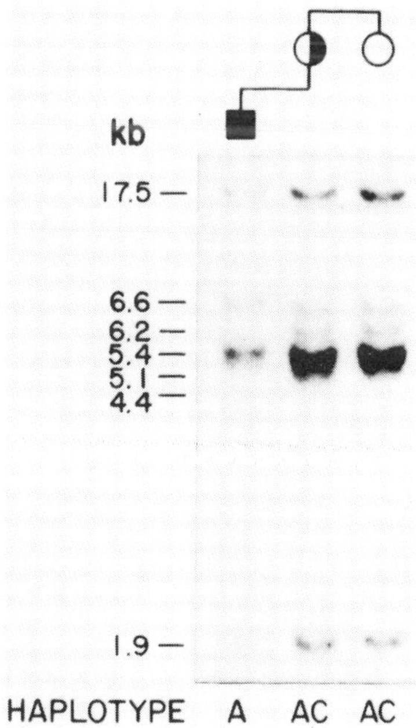

Figure 4 The potential application of RFLPs for prenatal diagnosis of OTC deficiency. DNA from an OTC-deficient male (lane 1), his mother (lane 2) and his maternal aunt (lane 3) was digested with *Msp*I and probed by Southern blotting with plasmid pH 0731. Reprinted with permission of the authors and publisher of Rozen *et al.* (1985)

Haplotype analysis can also be informative even if the female's carrier status has not been determined. The maternal aunt (lane 3) is not necessarily an obligate carrier for OTC deficiency since a spontaneous mutation might have arisen in her sister's chromosome marked by the A haplotype. Nevertheless, one can still predict that all the children of the maternal aunt who inherit her X-chromosome with the C haplotype will be unaffected.

In families with a major gene rearrangement, such as a deletion, carrier detection may be feasible on a qualitative basis, if the rearrangement produces a new hybridizable band(s). If no new bands appear as a result of the deletion, carrier status may be evaluated by quantitative analysis of the intensity of the hybridization

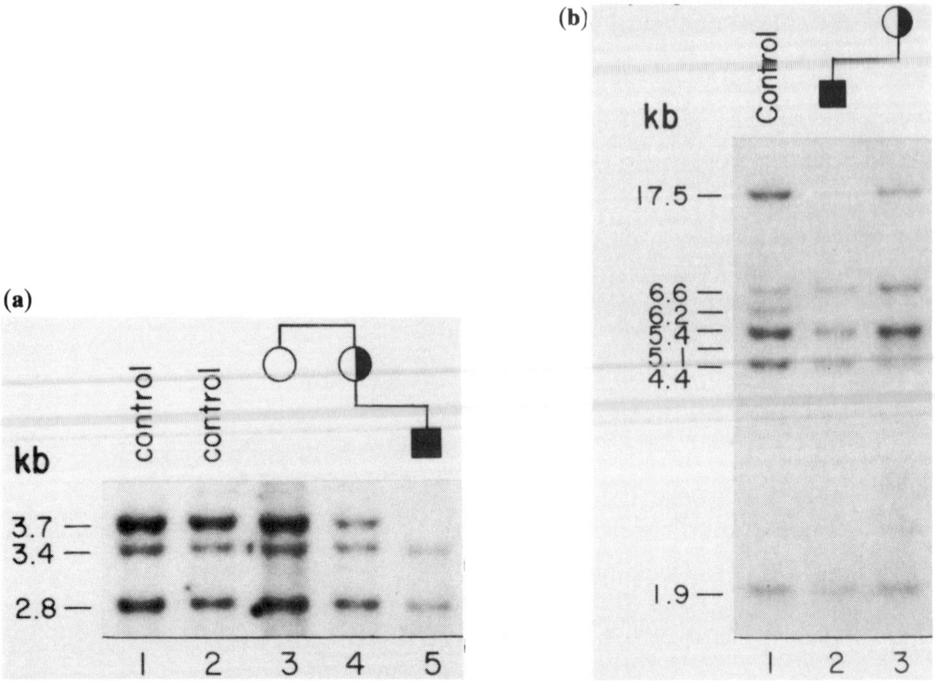

Figure 5 Carrier evaluation in a family with a partial gene deletion at the OTC locus. (**a**) *Eco*RI-digested DNA from two control females (lanes 1 and 2), the maternal aunt (lane 3), the mother (lane 4) and the proband (lane 5) was blotted and probed with pH0731. Only the relevant portion of the blot is shown. (**b**) DNA from a control female (lane 1), the proband (lane 2) and his mother (lane 3) was digested with *Msp*I and analysed as in (**a**). Ethidium bromide staining of the gel indicated that equal amounts of DNA were present in each lane. Reprinted with permission of the authors and publisher of Rozen *et al.* (1985)

signal of the band(s) of interest. For example, Figure 5a depicts a blot following *Eco*RI digestion of DNA from the OTC-deficient male discussed in Figure 1, and from his maternal relatives. The proband (lane 5) is missing a 3.7 kb band. In the DNA of control women (lanes 1 and 2) and of the maternal aunt (lane 3), this band has a stronger hybridization signal than that of the 3.4 kb band, whereas the intensity in the 3.7 kb band of the mother's DNA (lane 2) is virtually equal to that of the 3.4 kb band. Therefore the mother, but not the aunt, can be designated as a carrier for the deletion. Similarly, as seen in Figure 5b with *Msp*I-digested DNA, the intensity of hybridization of the mother's 17.5 kb band (lane 3) is less than that of a control female (lane 1).

For most families, where a specific mutation has not been identified, linkage analysis with RFLPs must be used for carrier assessment as well as for prenatal diagnosis. The inclusion or exclusion of a specific band or haplotype linked to the OTC mutation is the basis for determining carrier status in some families. The

*Bam*HI polymorphism was used to evaluate the family shown in Figure 6a; the probe was a subcloned genomic fragment derived from the 5′ region of the human OTC gene. In this family, the OTC mutation must reside on the X-chromosome characterized by the 5.2 kb band, as determined by the analysis of the proband (lane 2). His mother (lane 1) and one maternal aunt (lane 5) are heterozygous for the RFLP and must also be carriers for the mutation since they inherited the X-

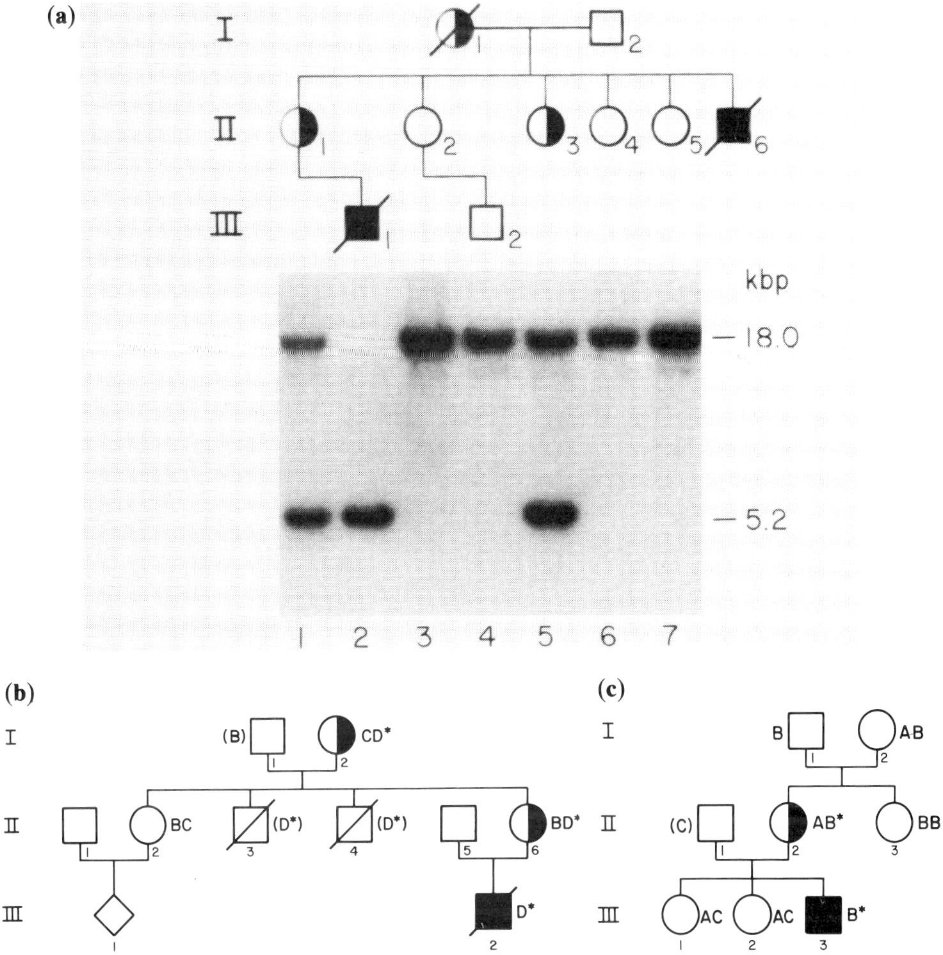

Figure 6 The application of RFLPs for carrier assessment in families at risk for OTC deficiency. (**a**) genomic DNA from family members in generations II and III was digested with *Bam*HI and probed with a subcloned fragment of genomic DNA, derived from the 5′ region of the human OTC gene. Each lane of the blot corresponds to the individual in the pedigree depicted directly above it. (**b**) and (**c**) *Msp*I-digested DNA from pedigrees with OTC deficiency was blotted and probed with pH 0731. Haplotypes were assigned as discussed in the text. Parentheses indicate that the haplotype was inferred from the other haplotypes in the pedigree. * refers to the haplotype of the X-chromosome that presumably carries the OTC mutation. (**b**) and (**c**) were reprinted with permission of the authors and publisher of Rozen *et al.* (1985)

chromosome with the 5.2 kb band. These two women would be suitable candidates for prenatal diagnosis on the basis of this information. On the other hand, the maternal aunts shown in lanes 3, 6 and 7 cannot be carriers since they are homozygous for the 18 kb band.

*Msp*I haplotypes were used for studying the family shown in Figure 6b. The X-chromosome marked by the D haplotype must carry the OTC mutation, since the proband (individual III-2), his mother (individual II-6) and his grandmother (individual I-2) all share this haplotype. The maternal aunt (individual II-2) cannot be a carrier for OTC deficiency since she did not inherit the X-chromosome with the D haplotype from her mother.

Carrier evaluation can also be performed by assigning a spontaneous mutation to a particular individual, as shown in the pedigree in Figure 6c. The mother (individual II-2) of the proband (individual III-3) was designated to be an OTC carrier after a positive protein tolerance test. Since her X-chromosome with haplotype A was inherited from the grandmother, her X-chromosome marked by the B haplotype, which carries the mutation, must have been inherited from the healthy grandfather. Therefore a spontaneous mutation must have occurred in this woman's X-chromosome characterized by the B haplotype. The unlikelihood of a second spontaneous mutation occurring in this pedigree almost certainly designates the maternal aunt (individual II-3) as a non-carrier despite the assignment of B haplotypes to her X-chromosomes.

Interestingly, the proband in this family is the OTC-deficient male with the partial deletion, discussed in Figure 1. His mother and maternal aunt were identified as being a carrier and a non-carrier, respectively, in an independent manner – by dosage analysis of specific bands (Figure 5).

CONCLUSION

With the availability of a human cDNA clone for ornithine transcarbamylase, family planning in pedigrees at risk for OTC deficiency has reached a new dimension. Restriction analysis of DNA from an affected (or unaffected) male family member can link the OTC mutation to a particular RFLP haplotype. Consequently, prenatal diagnosis is a feasible option for obligate carriers of the mutation, provided they are heterozygous for at least one RFLP. Our studies suggest that approximately 80% of all women fall into the latter category.

The issue of carrier status cannot be over-emphasized in this X-linked disorder, where the frequency of spontaneous mutations is quite high. Until now, protein loading studies have been the only resource for information on carrier status in some families, but the results have sometimes been equivocal. Haplotype analysis is a practical alternative for carrier assessment and, at the same time, it is a suitable method for evaluating the efficacy of the protein tolerance tests. Ongoing studies in this regard should prove to be informative.

ACKNOWLEDGEMENTS

We would like to thank Dr P. Pearson for providing probes L1.28 and 754, as well as all the physicians who referred families and supplied cell lines. At the time the study was performed, R. Rozen was the recipient of a postdoctoral fellowship from the MRC of Canada. This work was supported by NIH grant GM 32156.

REFERENCES

Brusilow, S. W., Danney, M., Waber, L. J., Batshaw, M., Burton, B., Levitsky, L., Roth, K., McKeethren, C. and Ward J. Treatment of episodic hyperammonemia in children with inborn errors of urea synthesis. *N. Engl. J. Med.* 310 (1984) 1630–1634

Brusilow, S. W. and Valle, D. L. Identification of heterozygosity for ornithine transcarbamylase deficiency (OTCD). *Pediatr. Res.* 19 (1985) 244A

Davies, K. E., Pearson, P. L., Harper, P. S., Murray, J. M., O'Brien, T. and Williamson, R. Linkage analysis of two cloned DNA sequences flanking the Duchenne muscular dystrophy locus on the short arm of the human X-chromosome. *Nucleic Acids Res.* 11 (1983) 2303–2312

Francke, U., Ochs, H. D., de Martinville, B., Giacalone, J., Lindgren, V., Distèche, C., Pagon, R., Hofker, M. H., van Ommen, G-J. B., Pearson, P. L. and Wedgwood, R. J. Minor Xp21 chromosome deletion in a male associated with expression of Duchenne muscular dystrophy, chronic granulomatous disease, retinitis pigmentosa and McLeod syndrome. *Am. J. Hum. Genet.* 37 (1985) 250–267

Grisolia, S., Baguena, R. and Mayor, F. (eds.) *The Urea Cycle*, Wiley, New York, 1976

Haldane, J. B. S. Rate of spontaneous mutation of the human gene. *J. Genet.* 31 (1935) 317–326

Hofker, M. H., Wapenaar, M., Goor, N., Bakker, E., van Ommen, G-J. B. and Pearson, P. L. Isolation of probes detecting restriction fragment length polymorphisms from chromosome specific libraries: potential use for diagnosis of Duchenne muscular dystrophy. *Hum. Genet.* 70 (1985) 148–156

Holzgreve, W. and Golbus, M. S. Prenatal diagnosis of ornithine transcarbamylase deficiency utilizing fetal liver biopsy. *Am. J. Hum. Genet.* 36 (1984) 320–328

Horwich, A. L., Fenton, W. A., Williams, K. R., Kalousek, F., Kraus, J. P., Doolittle, R. F., Konigsberg, W. and Rosenberg, L. E. Structure and expression of a complementary DNA for the nuclear coded precursor of human mitochondrial ornithine transcarbamylase. *Science* 224 (1984) 1068–1074

Lindgren, V., de Martinville, B., Horwich, A. L., Rosenberg, L. E. and Francke, U. Human ornithine transcarbamylase locus mapped to band Xp21.1 near the Duchenne muscular dystrophy locus. *Science* 226 (1984) 698–700

Ricciuti, F. C., Gelehrter, T. D. and Rosenberg, L. E. X-chromosome inactivation in human liver: confirmation of X-linkage of ornithine transcarbamylase. *Am. J. Hum. Genet.* 28 (1976) 332–338

Rodeck, C. H., Patrick, A. D., Pembrey, M. E., Tzannatos, C. and Whitfield, A. E. Fetal liver biopsy for prenatal diagnosis of ornithine carbamyl transferase deficiency. *Lancet* 1 (1982) 297–299

Rozen, R., Fox, J., Fenton, W. A., Horwich, A. L. and Rosenberg, L. E. Gene deletion and restriction fragment length polymorphisms at the human ornithine transcarbamylase locus. *Nature* 313 (1985) 815–817

Short, E. M., Conn, H. O., Snodgrass, P. J., Campbell, A. G. M. and Rosenberg, L. E. Evidence for X-linked dominant inheritance of ornithine transcarbamylase deficiency. *N. Engl. J. Med.* 288 (1973) 7–12

Walser, M. Urea cycle disorders and other hereditary hyperammonemic syndromes. In Stanbury, J. B., Wyngaarden, J. B., Frederickson, D. S., Goldstein, J. L. and Brown, M. S. (eds.) *The Metabolic Basis of Inherited Disease, 5th edn.* McGraw-Hill, New York, 1983, pp. 402–438

J. Inher. Metab. Dis. 9 Suppl. 1 (1986) 58–68

Molecular Genetics of PKU

F. GÜTTLER[1] and S. L. C. WOO[2]

[1]*The John F. Kennedy Institute, DK-2600 Glostrup, Denmark and* [2]*Howard Hughes Medical Institute, Department of Cell Biology, Baylor College of Medicine, Houston, TX 77030, USA*

This review summarizes the isolation of rat phenylalanine hydroxylase mRNA and its use in the synthesis of its cDNA. As rat cDNA cross-hybridized with human phenylalanine hydroxylase mRNA, the rat cDNA probe was used to screen a human liver cDNA library. A partial length cDNA human phenylalanine hydroxylase probe was obtained which showed restriction fragment length polymorphism (RFLP) with 3 restriction enzymes and was successfully used to trace the transmission of the mutant gene in PKU families with one or more affected children. Recently the partial-length cDNA probe has been used to isolate a full-length cDNA probe for human phenylalanine hydroxylase. Gene transfer experiments with the full-length cDNA have led to expression of human phenylalanine hydroxylase in eukaryotic cultured cells and in recombinant bacteria which normally do not express phenylalanine hydroxylase activity. The full-length cDNA of human phenylalanine hydroxylase has been sequenced, uncovering the nucleic acid sequence of the exons of the human phenylalanine hydroxylase gene, as well as the most likely amino acid structure of the human phenylalanine hydroxylase enzyme. The full-length cDNA probe has 10 identifiable binding sites for restriction enzymes that show RFLP. These additional RFLPs have enabled haplotype analyses of the normal and mutant phenylalanine hydroxylase genes in PKU families. Haplotype analyses in Danish PKU families revealed 12 different haplotypes. However, of 132 chromosomes analysed from 66 obligate heterozygotes, 59 out of 66 PKU genes were associated with only 4 haplotypes. Cosmid cloning and preliminary characterization of the human phenylalanine hydroxylase gene have identified 13 exons distributed across a gene that is more than 190 kb in length. In β-thalassaemia, distinct mutations in the β-globin locus are associated with specific RFLP haplotypes within a given population. As in thalassaemia such an association forms a strategy for cloning and sequence characterization of mutant phenylalanine hydroxylase genes derived from each haplotype. If the PKU genes in the Danish population are the result of mutiple mutations which occurred on chromosomes of the most common haplotypes, the same strategy is potentially applicable for the molecular characterization of the various types of phenylalanine hydroxylase deficiency.

Journal of Inherited Metabolic Disease. ISSN 0141–8955.

Recent advances in recombinant DNA technology have provided a wealth of information about human molecular pathology. An increasing number of inherited metabolic disorders can be diagnosed at the DNA level using appropriate gene probes and restriction endonucleases. When the genetic defect at the DNA level is not yet discovered, as in PKU, but the defective gene product, phenylalanine hydroxylase, is known a complementary DNA (cDNA) gene probe can be cloned. Each gene consists of nucleotide sequences (exons) which are transcribed into messenger RNA (mRNA) and thus into the amino acid sequence of the protein, e.g. phenylalanine hydroxylase, synthesized in the cytoplasm of hepatic cells. The coding DNA sequences are interrupted by intervening sequences or introns. Isolated mRNA can be used as the template to synthesize an exactly complementary cDNA gene probe which is then used to single out its complement in the human genome, rejecting the hundred thousands of other genes.

Restriction endonucleases are enzymes that cleave genomic DNA at precisely defined sequences of 4–6 nucleotide pairs. Recent advances in the study of human DNA suggest that any one individual has a variant but inherited nucleotide for every 100–300 of our 3×10^9 nucleotides. These nucleotide variations will either destroy or create recognition sites for restriction endonucleases. The presence or absence of restriction endonuclease sites are mainly harmless variations in the introns that are inherited in a simple mendelian fashion. The result is individual variations in the size of some of the DNA fragments obtained after digestion with a restriction endonuclease, and a unique pattern of DNA fragments is obtained. Thus, by analysing genomic DNA with a restriction enzyme and an appropriate radioactive cDNA probe, fragments of DNA of differing lengths will appear according to the presence or absence of these recognition sites. The individual restriction fragment length polymorphism (RFLP) obtained provides a source of genetic markers that can be used to trace mutant genes to which they are linked through successive generations of families.

Cloning of a partial-length human phenylalanine hydroxylase cDNA and its use to trace the transmission of PKU genes

Rat liver phenylalanine hydroxylase mRNA was specifically enriched by polysome immunoprecipitation and used for the synthesis of its complementary cDNA (Robson *et al.*, 1982). When it was recognized that the rat phenylalanine hydroxylase cDNA was capable of cross-hybridizing with human liver mRNA, the rat cDNA probe was used to screen a human liver cDNA library. A strong and specific hybridization signal was obtained from a clone with a human phenylalanine hydroxylase cDNA insert of 1.4 kb. Genomic DNAs isolated from leukocytes of random individuals were analysed using a battery of restriction endonucleases and the partial-length human phenylalanine hydroxylase cDNA probe. Three restriction enzymes *Sph*I, *Msp*I and *Hind*III showed polymorphic patterns in the phenylalanine hydroxylase locus (Woo *et al.*, 1983).

An example of the polymorphic bands obtained after digestion of genomic DNA from 3 selected individuals with the enzyme *Msp*I is shown in Figure 1. The

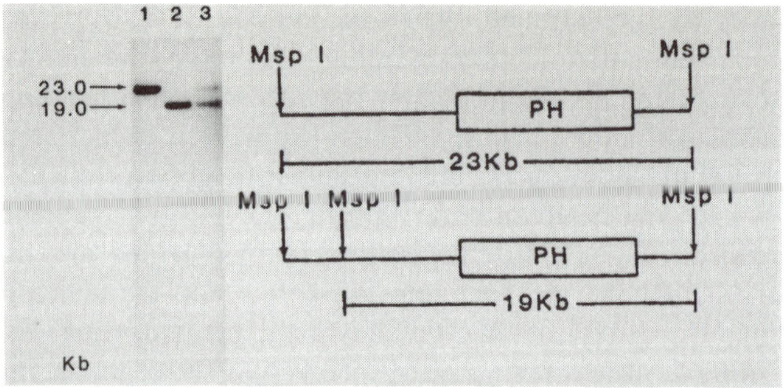

Figure 1 Restriction fragment-length polymorphism in the human phenylalanine hydroxylase gene detected using a partial-length human phenylalanine hydroxylase cDNA probe and the restriction endonuclease *Msp*I for digestion of genomic DNA isolated from leukocytes of 3 normal individuals. The explanation for the restriction fragments obtained is schematically shown on the right hand panel. Individual 2 has the polymorphic 19 kb binding site on both chromosomes, whereas individual 3 has the polymorphic site on one chromosome only. Individual 1 lacks the polymorphic binding site on both chromosomes

explanation for the 3 RFLP patterns is schematically shown on the right hand panel. Suppose that the phenylalanine hydroxylase gene in our genome is flanked by 2 *Msp*I restriction sites that are 23 kb apart. Individuals with 2 chromosomes of the 23 kb type will be homozygous for the 23 kb bands as shown in individual 1. During evolution there has been a mutation contributing an additional *Msp*I site at the 19 kb position.

Individuals with this mutation on both chromosomes are homozygous for the 19 kb band as shown in individual 2. An individual who has one each of the 2 chromosomes will be heterozygous for the 23 kb and 19 kb bands, respectively, as shown in individual 3 (Figure 1).

The polymorphisms found using the restriction enzymes *Msp*I, *Sph*I, and *Hind*III, have been applied to trace the transmission of mutant genes in informative PKU families with one or more affected children. These analyses demonstrated that within individual families, the PKU alleles segregated concordantly with the disease state (Woo *et al*., 1984). An example is given in Figure 2 illustrating a Danish family's DNA after digestion with *Msp*I. Both parents (lanes 1 and 2) are heterozygous with respect to the 23 kb and 19 kb bands. The proband in lane 3 is homozygous for the 19 kb band. Because PKU is an autosomal recessive disorder each parent will normally be an obligate carrier, and they must each contain one copy of the mutant chromosome and one copy of the normal chromosome. By comparing the profiles of the 2 parents and the proband it can be concluded that the proband inherited the 2 copies of the chromosomes of the 19 kb type and therefore that these chromosomes are the mutant chromosomes of the family. By definition the 23 kb bands in the parents must carry the normal phenylalanine hydroxylase gene. These 2 genes have been transmitted to the unaffected sibling (lane 4) who is homozygous for the 23 kb band. This sibling is not only unaffected but free of the PKU trait.

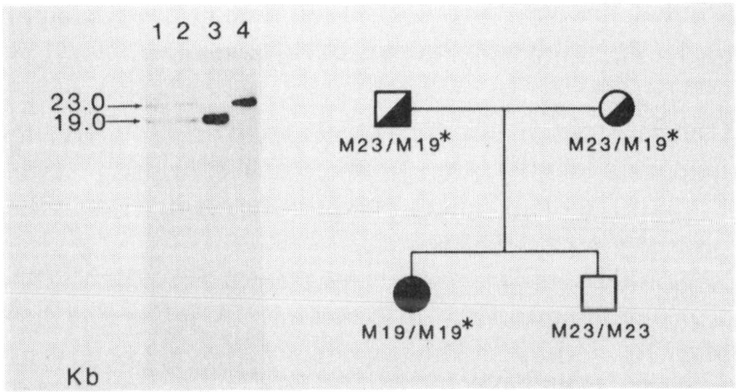

Figure 2 Segregation of the PKU-allele* with the restriction fragments obtained after *Msp*I digestion of DNA isolated from the father (lane 1), the mother (lane 2), the PKU child (lane 3), and an unaffected sibling (lane 4)

Isolation and characterization of a full-length human phenylalanine cDNA clone expressing phenylalanine hydroxylase activity

A second human liver cDNA library was constructed and the partial-length cDNA probe was used to isolate a clone with a human liver phenylalanine hydroxylase cDNA insert of approximately 2.5 kb which is consistent with the size of human phenylalanine hydroxylase mRNA. Further analyses of the cDNA clone revealed a nucleic acid sequence of 2448 base pairs containing a continuous open reading frame of 1353 bases, starting with the first ATG at position 223 and ending with a TAA codon at nucleic acid 1579. Translation of the nucleic acid sequence in the coding region predicted the primary protein structure of human phenylalanine hydroxylase. The deduced amino acid sequence comprises 451 amino acids and constitutes a protein of 51 672 daltons, which is in agreement with the size which has been predicted by biochemical studies of the phenylalanine hydroxylase protein (Kwok *et al.*, 1985).

To determine whether the full-length phenylalanine hydroxylase cDNA clone contained all the genetic information necessary for expression of phenylalanine hydroxylase activity, the full-length cDNA insert was subcloned into an expression vector containing the promotor and the capsite of the human metallothionein gene MT-II. This recombinant clone was transfected into mouse *NIH*3T3 cells which normally do not express phenylalanine hydroxylase activity. The cells containing the phenylalanine hydroxylase recombinant were found to express phenylalanine hydroxylase mRNA and enzymatic activity (Ledley *et al.*, 1985).

Phenylalanine hydroxylase mRNA and enzymatic activity could be induced with cadmium, indicating that the phenylalanine hydroxylase in the transformed cells was derived from the recombinant human phenylalanine hydroxylase gene and the cadmium responsive metallothionein promotor (Ledley *et al.*, 1985). These results indicate that the 2.4 kb cDNA encoding one peptide of 51 900 daltons contains all necessary genetic information for phenylalanine hydroxylase activity and provide evidence that human phenylalanine hydroxylase is encoded for by a single genetic locus.

Extensive restriction site polymorphism at the human phenylalanine hydroxylase locus identified by the full-length human phenylalanine hydroxylase cDNA probe

In addition to the 3 restriction enzymes *Msp*I, *Sph*I, and *Hind*III showing polymorphisms with the partial-length cDNA probe, 5 new restriction enzymes were found that yield restriction fragment length polymorphism: *Bgl*II, *Pvu*II, *Xmn*I, *Eco*RI and *Eco*RV (Lindsky *et al*., 1985a).

As mentioned earlier some individuals have a polymorphic 19 kb binding site for the restriction enzyme *Msp*I. The full-length cDNA probe has detected a second polymorphic *Msp*I site within the 4 kb segment which is obtained when the polymorphic *Msp*I site in the 23 kb segment is cleaved to yield 2 fragments of 19 kb and 4 kb in length. The presence of the new polymorphic site causes the 4 kb fragment to be cleaved into 2 fragments of 2.2 kb and 1.8 kb. The 2 polymorphic restriction sites are designated *Msp*Ia and *Msp*Ib.

Analysis of DNA digested with *Pvu*II shows 4 variant fragments of 19.0, 11.5, 9.1 and 6.0 kb in length, created by 2 polymorphic *Pvu*II restriction sites, designated *a* and *b*. Phenylalanine hydroxylase genes that lack both polymorphic sites would yield 2 bands of 19 kb and 11.5 kb. The presence of site *a* causes cleavage of the 19 kb fragment into a 6 kb fragment, and the presence of site *b* causes cleavage of the 11.5 kb fragment into a 9.1 kb fragment.

Thus, a total of 10 restriction site polymorphisms have been identified at the human phenylalanine hydroxylase locus using the full-length human phenylalanine hydroxylase cDNA probe and 8 restriction enzymes (Lidsky *et al*., 1985a). The size of the different fragments obtained and the frequency of each fragment is shown in Table 1. The estimated frequencies are obtained from analyses of 18 unrelated normal Caucasian individuals. With 18 random individuals the probability of detecting a restriction site polymorphism with a frequency of 10% or greater is 98.5%. The frequencies of the minor fragments exceeded 0.3 for all the enzymes, indicating the existence of a very high degree of polymorphism at the human phenylalanine hydroxylase locus (Lidsky *et al*., 1985a).

Mendelian segregation of the polymorphic sites at the human phenylalanine hydroxylase locus demonstrated by kindred analysis

Mendelian segregation of the *Hind*III, *Sph*I and *Msp*I restriction fragment length polymorphisms in PKU families has previously been demonstrated. Prior to the application of the new restriction enzymes showing polymorphism to tracing the transmission of phenylalanine hydroxylase genes in PKU families, it must be demonstrated conclusively that the RFLPs obtained are indeed authentic and are not the result of artifacts such as partial digestion. Such artifacts are not likely to be transmissable as mendelian traits, and their authenticity can be verified by performing kindred analysis.

Table 2 shows the mendelian segregation of the polymorphic fragments obtained by the restriction enzymes in a Danish PKU family with one affected child and 2 unaffected siblings who happened to be heterozygotes. The PKU proband has

Table 1 Polymorphic restriction sites in the human phenylalanine hydroxylase locus and the calculated frequency of each fragment identified by the full-length cDNA clone

Restriction enzyme	*Fragment size* (kb)	*Frequency*
*Bgl*II	3.6	0.59
	1.7	0.41
*Pvu*IIa	19.0	0.44
	6.0	0.56
*Pvu*IIb	11.5	0.69
	9.1	0.31
*Xmn*I	9.4	0.67
	6.5	0.33
*Eco*RI	17.0	0.59
	11.0	0.41
*Msp*Ia	23.0	0.38
	19.0	0.62
*Msp*Ib	4.0	0.69
	2.2	0.31
*Eco*RV	30.0	0.47
	25.0	0.53
*Hind*III	4.2	0.61
	4.0	0.39
*Sph*I	9.7	0.21
	7.0	0.79

inherited the 17 kb (*Eco*RI), 25 kb (*Eco*RV), 9.4 kb (*Xmn*I), 19 kb (*Msp*I), and 6 kb (*Pvu*IIa) fragments from the father indicating that the mutant allele of the father is associated with this combination of restriction fragments (or this haplotype). The corresponding combination of fragments associated with the normal gene of the father is 17 kb, 30 kb, 6.5 kb, 19 kb and 6 kb, respectively. The PKU proband has inherited the 11 kb (*Eco*RI), 30 kb (*Eco*RV), 6.5 kb (*Xmn*I), 23 kb (*Msp*I), and 19 kb (*Pvu*IIa) fragments from the mother. Thus, this combination of restriction fragments (or haplotype) is associated with the mutant allele of the mother. The corresponding combination of restriction fragments (or haplotype) associated with the normal allele of the mother is: 11 kb, 25 kb, 9.4 kb, 19 kb and 19 kb. Using a similar analysis it can be determined that the 2 unaffected siblings have inherited either a mutant allele from the father or a mutant allele from the mother (Table 2).

Similar analysis of a number of additional kindred has clearly demonstrated mendelian inheritants of these RFLPs. The genotype frequencies are in Hardy–Weinberg equilibrium, and each allelic type has been observed in more than one individual.

RFLP haplotype analysis and genetic counselling

The observation of extensive restriction site polymorphism at the human phenylalanine hydroxylase locus has offered the possibility for haplotype analysis. An

Table 2 RFLP haplotypes of the 4 phenylalanine hydroxylase genes in a Danish PKU family

Genes	RFLP haplotypes						
	*Bgl*II	*Pvu*IIa	*Pvu*IIb	*Eco*RI	*Xmn*I	*Msp*I	*Eco*RV
Father normal	3.6	6	11.5	17	6.5	19	30
mutant	3.6	6	11.5	17	9.4	19	25
Mother normal	1.7	19	9.1	11	9.4	19	25
mutant	1.7	19	11.5	11	6.5	23	30
PKU proband							
mutant F	3.6	6	11.5	17	9.4	19	25
mutant M	1.7	19	11.5	11	6.5	23	30
Heterozygote sibling							
mutant F	3.6	6	11.5	17	9.4	19	25
normal M	1.7	19	9.1	11	9.4	19	25
Heterozygote sibling							
normal F	3.6	6	11.5	17	6.5	19	30
mutant M	1.7	19	11.5	11	6.5	23	30

individual will be either homozygous or heterozygous with respect to the polymorphic fragments obtained after digestion with the restriction enzymes listed in Table 1. The combination of restriction fragments obtained after digestion of an individual's genomic DNA with each of the seven restriction enzymes mentioned in Table 3 forms a haplotype. Thus, a haplotype is the combination of the polymorphic restriction fragments obtained with different restriction enzymes, e.g. the haplotypes of the 4 phenylalanine hydroxylase genes in the family described in Table 2. The RFLP haplotypes of the 4 phenylalanine hydroxylase genes in this family can be readily deduced from the data, and used to trace the transmission of the mutant genes, i.e. permitting determination of affected, carrier, and non-carrier siblings.

To establish the usefulness of haplotype analysis in genetic counselling of PKU the haplotypes have been determined in 38 Danish families, each with one or more affected siblings. Parental haplotypes of 37 families provided information on PKU status and 33 of these families were completely informative, i.e. permitting determination of affected, carrier, and non-carrier siblings. No evidence for recombination was found in any of these families. Theoretically, the observed haplotypes will establish the disease status in 87%.

Association of RFLP haplotypes and PKU genes in the Danish population

Haplotype analysis of 33 Danish PKU families revealed 12 different haplotypes (Table 3). However, of the 132 chromosomes analysed 108 (82%) were associated with only 4 haplotypes (Table 3).

By comparing the haplotype of the mutant phenylalanine hydroxylase genes of the PKU child with the haplotypes of the respective parents, who each have a normal and a mutant gene, it is possible to assign the haplotype associated with

Table 3 **RFLP haplotypes of the phenylalanine hydroxylase gene associated with normal and mutant genes in 33 Danish PKU families**

Haplo-type	*Bgl*II	*Pvu*IIa	*Pvu*IIb	*Xmn*I	*Eco*RI	*Msp*I	*Eco*RV	*Hind*III	*Number of genes*	
									Normal	*PKU*
1	3.6	6.0	11.5	9.4	17.0	19.0	30.0	4.2	23	12
2	3.6	6.0	11.5	9.4	17.0	19.0	25.0	4.0	3	13
3	3.6	6.0	11.5	6.5	11.0	23.0	30.0	4.2	2	25
4	3.6	6.0	11.5	6.5	11.0	23.0	25.0	4.0	21	9
5	1.7	19.0	9.1	9.4	11.0	19.0	25.0	4.2	7	0
6	1.7	19.0	9.1	9.4	11.0	19.0	30.0	4.2	0	2
7	1.7	19.0	11.5	6.5	11.0	23.0	30.0	4.2	7	1
8	3.6	6.0	11.5	9.4	11.0	19.0	25.0	4.2	1	0
9	1.7	6.0	11.5	9.4	11.0	19.0	25.0	4.2	0	1
10	3.6	6.0	11.5	9.4	11.0	19.0	30.0	4.2	1	0
11	1.7	19.0	11.5	9.4	11.0	19.0	25.0	4.2	1	1
12	3.6	6.0	11.5	9.4	17.0	19.0	25.0	4.4	0	2

the normal gene and the haplotype associated with the mutant gene for each patent. Such analyses revealed that a majority of the PKU genes in the Danish PKU families were associated with 2 of the 4 common haplotypes (haplotypes 2 and 3 in Table 3), both of which are different from the predominant haplotypes associated with the normal genes (haplotypes 1 and 4 in Table 3).

The molecular lesions in the phenylalanine hydroxylase gene underlying PKU remain to be established. The observation of different haplotypes associated with β-thalassaemia led to the strategy of sequencing only those mutant genes present in different haplotypes (Orkin *et al.*, 1982). This strategy has produced a high yield of previously undiscovered mutations in β-thalassaemia. The association between haplotype and mutation may be due to a significant lapse of time between the occurrence of mutations and recombinations etc. responsible for the different haplotypes and any subsequent disease producing mutation. Kazazian and colleagues (1984) demonstrated that an average 86% of the mutations responsible for β-thalassaemia within a particular haplotype are identical, while 86% of the occurrence of a particular β-globin is associated with a particular haplotype.

If the PKU genes in the Danish population are the results of multiple mutations which occurred on chromosomes of the most common haplotypes, the same strategy is potentially applicable for the molecular characterization of the various types of phenylalanine hydroxylase deficiency found in Denmark. Preliminary data suggest that children who have inherited the 2 mutant genes associated with haplotypes 2 or 3 (Table 3) are those with classical PKU, whereas children who have inherited one mutant gene associated with haplotypes 1 or 4, and one associated with haplotypes 2 or 3, either have mild PKU or persistent hyperphenylalaninaemia not needing dietary therapy (HPA) (Güttler *et al.*, 1985). If the different phenotypes observed among children with phenylalanine hydroxylase deficiency, i.e. classic PKU, mild PKU and HPA, are due to different mutations and if the haplotypes associated with the mutant genes inherited from the parents can be related to the phenotype of their affected offspring, this preliminary observation suggests that in PKU also there may be a close linkage between haplotypes and specific mutations. As in β-thalassaemia such an association forms a strategy for cloning and sequence characterization of mutant phenylalanine hydroxylase genes derived from each haplotype.

Direct evidence suggesting that different mutations may be responsible for PKU has been obtained by investigating phenylalanine hydroxylase mRNA in PKU patients (DiLella *et al.*, 1985). RNA isolated from needle liver biopsies of individuals with PKU were analysed by Northern hybridization for phenylalanine hydroxylase mRNA. Two phenotypic variations of PKU were observed at the mRNA level. The liver from one PKU individual contained abundant phenylalanine hydroxylase mRNA identical in size to that present in a normal individual, suggesting that PKU in this individual is due to a defective, very unstable enzyme rather than to decreased transcription of the gene into its mRNA. Another PKU individual had negligible amounts of hepatic phenylalanine hydroxylase mRNA. Thus, PKU in this individual could be the result of decreased transcriptional activity of the gene or decreased stability of its mRNA. The studies indicate that phenylalanine hydroxylase mRNA is present in some but not all individuals with PKU suggesting different molecular lesions responsible for PKU.

Cosmid cloning and preliminary characterization of the human phenylalanine hydroxylase gene

The normal chromosomal human phenylalanine hydroxylase gene has been cloned and characterized in structural and sequence details. Studies of genomic DNA using the full-length human phenylalanine hydroxylase cDNA clone as the probe and various restriction enzymes suggested that the chromosomal gene may be 90 kb in length. A cosmid library was therefore constructed from a normal individual and overlapping clones that hydridisized to the full-length cDNA probe were isolated and investigated. The localizations of exons within each of these clones were identified by restriction endonuclease mapping using the full-length cDNA probe (DiLella *et al.*, personal communication).

Thirteen exons have been identified spread over 90 kb of genomic DNA. The

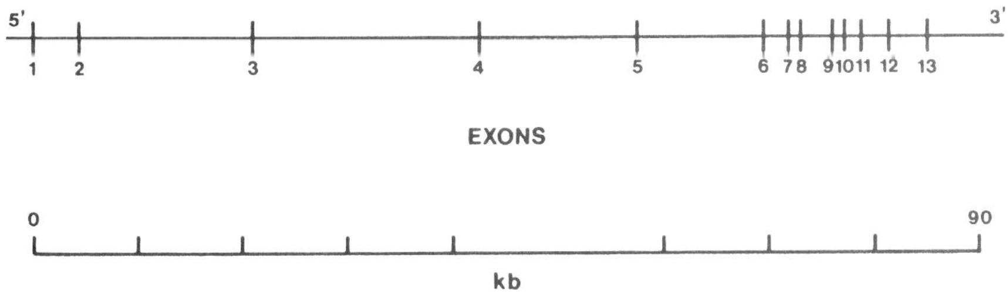

Figure 3 The approximate localization of the exons of the human phenylalanine hydroxylase gene

approximate localization of the exons is shown in Figure 3. Each exon has been subcloned and the exons have been sequenced. The sequences of the exons have been confirmed with the sequence of the full-length human phenylalanine hydroxylase cDNA. The 8 exons (6–13 in Figure 3), comprising approximately 1700 nucleotides are clustered within 15 kb of the 3′ end of the gene, exon 13 being the largest exon of the gene. The remaining 5 exons are scattered throughout a stretch of DNA that is in excess of 90 kb. The cloning and preliminary characterization of the human chromosomal phenylalanine hydroxylase gene has shown that all fragments detected by restriction analysis of genomic DNA arise from a single-copy gene indicating that there are no duplicate genes or pseudogenes in the human genome. Finally, the human phenylalanine hydroxylase gene has been mapped to the region q22–q24.7 on chromosome 12 (Lidsky *et al.*, 1985b).

REFERENCES

DiLella, A. G., Ledley, F. D., Rey, F. Munnich, A. and Woo, S. L. C. Detection of phenylalanine hydroxylase messenger RNA in liver biopsy samples from patients with phenylketonuria. *Lancet* 1 (1985) 160–161

Güttler, F., Woo, S. L. C. and Lidsky, A. Molecular genetics of PKU: prenatal diagnosis and carrier detection by gene analysis. In H. Bickel, ed. *Recent Progress in the Understanding, Recognition and Management of Inherited Diseases of Amino Acid Metabolism*. Georg Thieme Verlag, Stuttgart and New York, 1985, pp. 18–33

Kazazian, H. H. Jr., Orkin, H., Markham, A. F., Chapman, C. R., Youssoufian, H. and Waber, P. G. Quantification of the close association between DNA haplotypes and specific β-thalassaemia mutations in Mediterraneans. *Nature* 310 (1984) 152–154

Ledley, F. D., Grenett, H. E., DiLella, A. G., Kwok, S. C. M. and Woo, S. L. C. Gene transfer and expression of human phenylalanine hydroxylase. *Science* 228 (1985) 77–79

Lidsky, A. S., Ledley, F. D., DiLella, A. G., Kwok, S. C. M., Daiger, S. P., Robson, K. J. H and Woo, S. L. C. Extensive restriction site polymorphism at the human phenylalanine hydroxylase locus and application in prenatal diagnosis of phenylketonuria. *Am. J. Hum. Genet.* 37 (1985a) 324–327

Lidsky, A. S., Law, M. L., Morse, H. G., Kao, F. T. and Woo, S. L. C. Regional mapping of the human phenylalanine hydroxylase gene and the PKU locus on chromosome 12. *Proc. Natl. Acad. Sci. USA* (1985b) (in press)

Kwok, S., Ledley, F. D., DiLella, A. G., Robson, K. J. H. and Woo, S. L. C. Nucleotide sequence of a full-length cDNA clone of human phenylalanine hydroxylase. *Biochemistry* 24 (1985) 556–561

Orkin, S. H., Kazazian, H. H. Jr., Antonarakis, S. E., Goff, S. C., Boehm, C. D., Sexton, J. P., Waber, P. G. and Giardina, P. T. V. Linkage of β-thalassemia mutations and β-globin gene polymorphisms in the human β-globin gene cluster. *Nature* 296 (1982) 627–631

Robson, K. J. H., Chandra, T., MacGillivray, R. T. A. and Woo, S. L. C. Polysome immunoprecipitation of phenylalanine hydroxylase mRNA from rat liver and cloning of its cDNA. *Proc. Natl. Acad. Sci. USA* 79 (1982) 4701–4705

Woo, S. L. C., Lidsky, A. S., Güttler, F., Chandra, T. and Robson, K. J. H. Cloned human phenylalanine hydroxylase gene permits prenatal diagnosis and carrier detection of classical phenylketonuria. *Nature* 306 (1983) 151–155

Woo, S. L. C., Lidsky, A. S., Güttler, F., Chandra, T. and Robson, K. J. H. Prenatal diagnosis of classical phenylketonuria by gene mapping. *JAMA* 251 (1984) 1998–2002

J. Inher. Metab. Dis. 9 Suppl. 1 (1986) 69–84

Human DNA Repair Defects

C. F. ARLETT
MRC Cell Mutation Unit, University of Sussex, Falmer, Brighton, Sussex BN1 9RR, UK

A number of human genetic diseases have come to be described as being defective in DNA repair. The minimum criterion on which this assignment is based is hypersensitivity to the clastogenic or lethal action of specific DNA damaging agents. In one disease, xeroderma pigmentosum, the molecular evidence for a defect in DNA repair is unequivocal. This condition then acts as a model for dissecting others. For the other diseases the formal evidence for defects in repair is less secure or even lacking. The evidence for repair in each disease is assembled together with any methods that have been used to support the differential diagnosis or for prenatal diagnosis. Attempts to clone human DNA repair genes are in hand and may provide the necessary evidence to decide if all the putative DNA repair defective diseases are genuine.

Neoplastic disease and neurological degeneration together with immune defects are frequent clinical features linking this set of diseases, suggesting that effective DNA repair may be important in many aspects of human health.

Our knowledge of the existence and nature of the multiplicity of DNA repair pathways in bacteria is based, in large part, on the study of mutants blocked at various steps in these pathways. In a recent review Friedberg (1985) has listed at least 28 genes in *Escherichia coli* involved in the excision repair of DNA damage. In the light of his more complex organization, man might be anticipated to reveal many more genes similarly engaged. In support of this concept very large numbers of genes are seen to be active in *Saccharomyces cerevisiae* (Lawrence, 1982) and *Drosophilia melangogaster* (Smith *et al*., 1982). In bacteria these repair defective mutants are generally characterized by hypersensitivity to the lethal effects of specific DNA damaging agents; they may also often be hypermutable by these same agents.

Hypersensitivity to sunlight is observed in the sun-sensitive cancer-prone disease xeroderma pigmentosum (McKusick 27870) (Kraemer, 1983). The demonstration by Cleaver (1968) that cells from such individuals are defective in the excision of UV–C photoproducts opened up the prospect that a search for mutagen sensitive individuals would be a rewarding source of human repair defective genes. Some 18 years later a set of putative DNA repair defective syndromes has been assembled by application of this principle. In many instances, however, the evidence for defects in repair is at best equivocal. In this review the evidence for repair will be

Journal of Inherited Metabolic Disease. ISSN 0141–8955. Printed in Great Britain by Titus Wilson & Son Ltd., Kendal.

discussed in a number of these cases, and instances where defects in repair assist in the differential diagnosis will also be noted.

XERODERMA PIGMENTOSUM

The autosomal recessive disease known as xeroderma pigmentosum is the repair defective syndrome which has been studied most. Its frequency has been estimated as 1 in 250 000 in the USA but it is thought to be more common in Japan (Kraemer, 1983). The disease also acts as a model for investigations into other putative repair syndromes.

Affected individuals are unambiguously sun-sensitive and exhibit a distinctive erythemal response; there is also no doubt as to the solar induction of cancer in these patients. The dermatological effects are manifest as pigmented macules, achromic spots and telangiectasia in exposed areas followed ultimately by basal cell carcinoma, squamous cell carcinoma and malignant melanoma. This array of skin changes may be observed in later life in normal Caucasian individuals, especially of Celtic origin, who have occupations or who have lived in regions with high exposure to sunlight. Neurological abnormalities which are seen in their most extreme form in the so-called De Sanctis Cacchione syndrome (McKusick 27880) include microcephaly with progressive mental deterioration, low intelligence, areflexia and ataxia. These symptoms are rarely all present, but many xeroderma pigmentosum patients have one or more of the neurological features. Progressive neurological degeneration is present in 40% of patients.

At the cellular level xeroderma pigmentosum falls into two classes (Cleaver and Bootsma, 1975): those with marked hypersensitivity to the lethal effects of UV light and some chemicals whose action may be regarded as 'UV-like', and those with limited hypersensitivity (Figure 1). The chromosome breakage response to UV light mirrors the lethal response (Marshall and Scott, 1976). Xeroderma pigmentosum cells are also hypersensitive to the induction of sister chromatid exchanges by UV light (de Weerd-Kastelein *et al.*, 1977). The first group of 'classical' xeroderma pigmentosum patients exhibit defects in excision repair of UV-induced pyrimidine dimers or large bulky adducts on DNA (Cleaver and Bootsma, 1975); the second group of 'xeroderma pigmentosum variants' (McKusick 27875) is competent for excision repair (Figure 2) but defective in daughter strand repair (Table 1) (Lehmann *et al.*, 1975).

The defects in excision repair which are usually analysed as unscheduled DNA synthesis have allowed the assignment of at least 9 complementation groups (Fisher *et al.*, 1985) indicating a significant degree of complexity in the genetic control of the disease. The levels of residual unscheduled DNA synthesis overlap between complementation groups so these levels are predictive neither of group nor of the severity of clinical symptoms. Nevertheless the smaller the capacity for unscheduled DNA synthesis the more likely these symptoms are to prove severe. Post-irradiation cell survival measured as colony-forming ability is correlated with complementation group (Andrews *et al.*, 1976), and the residual level of unscheduled DNA synthesis correlates with the hypersensitivity to the lethal effects of UV light (Thielmann *et*

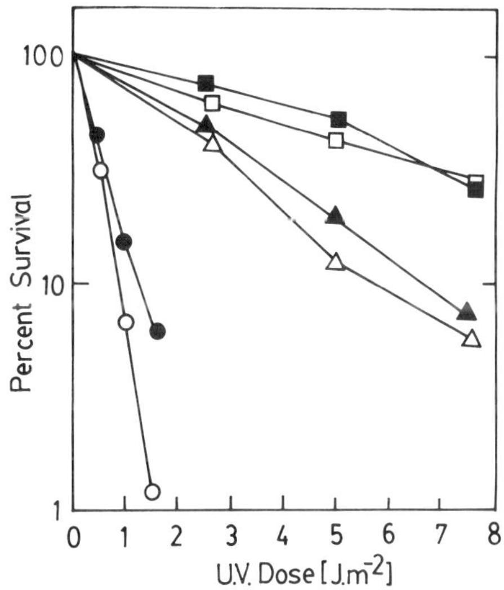

Figure 1 The response of xeroderma pigmentosum and normal fibroblasts to the lethal action of UV light. ■ = 1BR.2, □ = GM730 (normal cell strains); ● = XP2BI, ○ = XP4LO (excision defective xeroderma pigmentosum variants; ▲ = XP3DU, △ = XP7DU (excision competent xeroderma pigmentosum variants). XP3DU and XP7DU were under tests as putative variants from the Department of Dermatology, Ninewells Hospital, Dundee

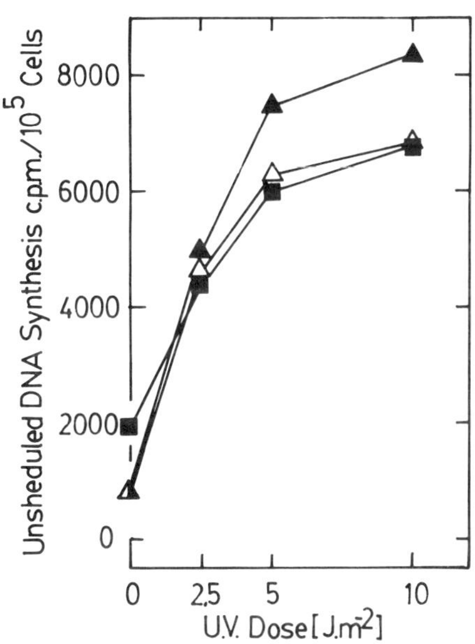

Figure 2 Unscheduled DNA synthesis in xeroderma pigmentosum variant and normal fibroblasts. ■ = 1BR.2 (normal cell strain); ▲ = XP3DU, △ = XP7DU (xeroderma pigmentosum variants)

Table 1 Post-replication repair in UV-irradiated normal and xeroderma pigmentosum variant cell strains

Cell strain	*Pulse*		*Chase*	
	−caffeine	*+caffeine*	*−caffeine*	*+caffeine*
1BR.2 (normal)	109	71	180	153
XP3DU	18	15	135	26
XP7DU	14	10	118	23

The average molecular weights of labelled DNA were calculated from alkaline sucrose gradients following UV irradiation ($8\,J\,m^{-2}$). The values are given in units of 10^6 daltons

al., 1985). It is of some interest to note the correlation between sensitivity to UV and occurrence of neurological abnormalities in the donor (Andrews *et al.*, 1976). Thus post-UV cell survival is highest in fibroblasts from those patients with xeroderma pigmentosum with least or no neurological defects and least in those with severe symptoms. This raises the interesting possibility that those patients with neurological effects may have different or additional cellular defects to those without such symptoms. The number of patients in the different complementation groups reflecting the different molecular forms of xeroderma pigmentosum has been found to differ between Japan and Western Europe/USA (Takebe *et al.*, 1977).

The molecular studies are consistent with the defect in excision repair occurring at the incision or endonuclease step (Lehmann, 1982a). The injection of phage T4 endonuclease (Tanaka *et al.*, 1975) can restore excision repair to some xeroderma pigmentosum cells and reduce the sensitivity to the lethal action of UV. The use of cell-free extracts by Mortelmans and colleagues (1976) showed that such extracts from xeroderma pigmentosum cells were able to excise pyrimidine dimers from DNA but not from DNA complexed with chromatin, indicating that these defects in xeroderma pigmentosum cells are concerned with factors which make the damage accessible to the UV endonuclease. Microinjection of *Micrococcus luteus* UV-endonuclease restored UV-induced unscheduled DNA synthesis to cells from 9 complementation groups (de Jonge *et al.*, 1985).

The cellular identification of xeroderma pigmentosum defective in excision repair both at amniocentesis (Ramsay *et al.*, 1974) or routinely in skin-derived fibroblasts (Arlett *et al.*, 1980) is implied by the ability to demonstrate defects in the levels of unscheduled DNA synthesis following treatment with UV.

The measurement of defects in daughter strand repair manifest in the excision competent xeroderma pigmentosum depends upon experiments which compare the size of newly synthesized DNA in control and irradiated cells. This process does not depend upon excision from parental strands and may thus be regarded as a 'damage tolerance mechanism'. The newly synthesized DNA from UV-irradiated xeroderma pigmentosum variant cells is considerably smaller than from normal cells (Lehmann *et al.*, 1975), and the time taken to achieve the size of DNA strands in unirradiated material is substantially longer. A complementation test based upon this technique has revealed that only one complementation group has been identified so far amongst the xeroderma pigmentosum variants (Jaspers *et al.*, 1981). Fujiwara and Satoh (1981) have provided intriguing evidence that the defect in daughter strand repair can become more severe as the individual ages. Of some relevance to the identification of variants is the observation that caffeine both potentiates the lethal effects of UV–C when applied as a post-irradiation treatment and also magnifies the defects seen in daughter strand repair (Lehmann *et al.*, 1975) (Table 1).

All the xeroderma pigmentosum cells studied to date have shown hypermutability compared with normal cells when exposed to UV-C (Arlett and Harcourt, 1983) or wavelengths simulating sunlight (Patton *et al.*, 1984). The simplest interpretation is that daughter strand repair which is defective in both excision defective and proficient xeroderma pigmentosum is error-prone. The observations of Maher and colleagues (1979) indicate that excision repair may be entirely error-free.

Thus xeroderma pigmentosum provides a satisfying correlation between DNA repair, mutation and cancer, giving strong support for the somatic mutation theory of cancer. The cells of patients with xeroderma pigmentosum are also hypersensitive to and hypermutable by chemical carcinogens such as benzo(a)pyrene (Maher *et al.*, 1977). A survey of epidemiological data (Kraemer *et al.*, 1984) serves to indicate that these individuals are also significantly more prone than normals to some internal cancers where there can be no exposure to UV light. This result supports the contention that competent repair protects against carcinogens.

Real progress in our knowledge of repair mechanisms would follow from cloning of such genes. The successful cloning of a 17 kb human gene which corrects a defect in excision repair from Chinese hamster cells (Westerfield *et al.*, 1984) indicates that this approach should be applicable to human DNA repair defects. Unfortunately, the report by Takano and colleagues (1982) that they had corrected the UV sensitivity of a xeroderma pigmentosum cell line by transfection with DNA from normal cells has not been repeated despite attempts in several other laboratories (Lehmann, 1985). Indeed one difficulty is that revertants may arise frequently during the selection procedure of multiple exposures to UV–C as a consequence of the hypermutability of xeroderma pigmentosum cell lines (Royer-Pokora and Haseltine, 1984).

COCKAYNE SYNDROME

Cockayne syndrome (McKusick 21640) is a second extremely rare autosomal recessive syndrome with severe photosensitivity (Brumback *et al.*, 1978). Associated with dwarfism and mental retardation are skeletal and retinal defects together with a loss of adipose tissue and a progressive neurological degeneration. In contrast to xeroderma pigmentosum there are no reports of an increased incidence of cancer. At the cellular level hypersensitivity to the lethal effects of UV–C is noted (Lehmann, 1982a) although it is not as extreme as seen in excision defective xeroderma pigmentosum. Both excision repair and daughter strand repair are normal in this condition. Cells from patients with Cockayne syndrome may be distinguished from normals by the failure of DNA and RNA synthesis to recover in UV irradiated cells (Lehmann, 1982b). This defect is sufficiently distinctive to permit an assignment to at least 3 complementation groups following an analysis of DNA and RNA synthesis from heterokaryons between cells from different Cockayne syndrome individuals (Tanaka *et al.*, 1981; Lehmann, 1982b).

The differential response between normal and Cockayne syndrome cells for post-UV RNA synthesis has been used by Lehmann and colleagues (1985) in the prenatal diagnosis of Cockayne syndrome. In this example 2 pregnancies were examined and in one Cockayne syndrome was detected and confirmed in the fibroblasts after termination; in the second the fetus was shown to be normal and fibroblast cultures also proved normal when taken after delivery. Cockayne syndrome had previously been diagnosed prenatally by Sugita and colleagues (1982) who used the hypersensitivity to the lethal effects of UV as their diagnostic test. However, this test was considered ambiguous and has now been superceded by a test based upon the rate of DNA synthesis (Kawai *et al.*, 1983). The test procedure using RNA synthesis offers advantages over the DNA synthesis procedure and in addition to its use in prenatal diagnosis it can also be used to confirm a clinical diagnosis (Lehmann, 1982a).

Although there are no reports of cancer in Cockayne syndrome, the extreme photosensitivity and early death in such individuals may mean that there is little opportunity for solar induction of cancer. The data of Arlett and Harcourt (1983) indicates hypermutability in Cockayne syndrome following UV treatment suggesting that it is indeed a cancer prone syndrome.

ATAXIA–TELANGIECTASIA

Ataxia–telangiectasia (McKusick 20890) is an autosomal recessive disorder where sensitivity to ionizing radiation has been recognized (Bridges and Harnden, 1982; Gatti and Swift, 1985). The frequency of ataxia–telangiectasia homozygotes has been variously estimated at 1 in 40 000 to 1 in 100 000 (Bridges *et al.*, 1985), and there is clear evidence of uneven distribution throughout the world. As in xeroderma pigmentosum these patients show neurological defects but are also characterized by defects in the immune system. There is no evidence to suggest that the high frequency of neoplasia, predominantly of the lymphoproliferative tissues, is a consequence of environmental exposure to radiation. Indeed, the classes of tumours differ from those that might be expected to arise from radiation (Waldmann *et al.*, 1983).

An important feature of ataxia–telangiectasia is the elevated level of chromosomal aberrations found in both blood cells and cultured fibroblasts but not in lymphoblastoid lines (Taylor, 1982), causing ataxia–telangiectasia to be described as a chromosome breakage syndrome. A significant feature is the presence in the blood of many patients with ataxia–telangiectasia of clones of cells containing a specific chromosome abnormality. In most instances this is a translocation involving chromosome 14 with the break point at band 14q12. Shahman and colleagues (1980) have shown that ataxia–telangiectasia cells produce a clastogenic factor which produces chromosome aberrations on cocultivation with normal lymphocytes.

Schwartz and colleagues (1985) have discussed a set of tests appropriate to the prenatal diagnosis of ataxia–telangiectasia which included the measurement of amniotic alphafetoprotein levels, the clastogenic potential of amniotic fluid and a cytogenetic evaluation of fetal amniocytes. One affected (Shahman *et al.*, 1982) and 2 normal (Schwartz *et al.*, 1985) fetuses in a single family have been analysed together with normal fetuses in 2 other families. In one the evaluation was based solely on increased sensitivity of amniocytes to X-ray chromosome breakage (Giannelli *et al.*, 1982).

Cellular studies with a considerable number of ataxia–telangiectasia cell strains (Lehmann, 1982c) show a consistent hypersensitivity to the lethal effects of ionizing

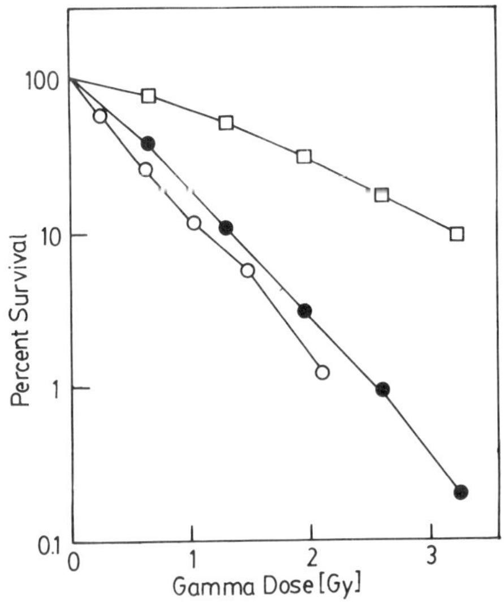

Figure 3 The response to gamma irradiation of normal and ataxia–telangiectasia fibroblasts. □ = GM730 (normal cell strain); ○ = AT5BI (reference ataxia–telangiectasia cell strain), ● = AT1BR putative A–T from Alder-Hey Hospital, Liverpool

radiation suggesting that this may be diagnostic (Figure 3). To this can be added hypersensitivity to bleomycin, neocarzinostatin and, interestingly, the tumour promoting agent phorbol-12-myristate-13 acetate (Shiloh *et al.*, 1985). Defects in the excision of X-ray induced base damage have been reported for some but not all ataxia–telangiectasia cell strains and this led to a preliminary assignment of complementation groups (Paterson *et al.*, 1976). However, the evidence for a specific defect in repair in this syndrome is less secure than for xeroderma pigmentosum. It has been suggested that ataxia–telangiectasia cells are defective in the repair of some form of strand breakage (Lehmann, 1977), but no identification of a specific class of strand break has yet been made (Taylor *et al.*, 1985).

An interesting differential response exhibited by all ataxia–telangiectasia cells tested to date is the lack of inhibition of DNA synthesis by ionizing radiation (Figure 4). De Wit and colleagues (1981) have used this characteristic to assign at

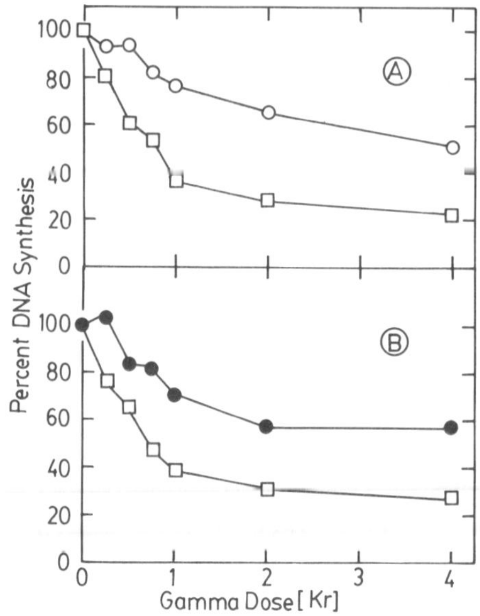

Figure 4 Inhibition of DNA synthesis by gamma-irradiation in normal and ataxia–telangiectasia fibroblasts. (**A**) Experiment 1; □ = 1BR.3 (normal cell strain), ○ = AT5BI (reference ataxia–telangiectasia cell strain). (**B**) Experiment 2; □ = 1BR.3, ● = AT1BR (putative ataxia–telangiectasia from Alder-Hey Hospital, Liverpool)

least 5 complementation groups in ataxia–telangiectasia. The suggestion that this phenomenon is responsible for the hypersensitivity (Painter and Young, 1980) is not tenable because ataxia–telangiectasia cells do not show repair of potentially lethal damage when held in a non-cycling state for some hours after irradiation (Cox, 1982). This cellular characteristic is probably the best evidence, albeit indirect, for a repair defect in ataxia–telangiectasia cells.

The data for mutagenicity in ataxia–telangiectasia is confusing. Our most recent studies (Arlett and Cole, 1985) indicate that untransformed fibroblasts are not mutable by ionizing radiation. However, lymphoblastoid cells and SV40 transformed fibroblast lines are mutable although less so than normals. A formal interpretation of this implies that the untransformed cells lack an error-prone repair process and may thus be analogous to a number of mutations in bacteria (e.g. *recA*, *lexA*, *umuC*, *umuD*) which confer sensitivity to the lethal action whilst abolishing the mutagenic action of ionizing radiation (Walker, 1984). The Epstein–Barr or SV40 viruses may have restored an error-prone repair pathway to these cells.

The suggestion that individuals heterozygous for ataxia–telangiectasia may be more cancer-prone than normals (Swift, 1982) has prompted attempts to devise cellular tests for heterozygotes. To date these have depended on differential sensitivity to the clastogenic or lethal effects of agents such as ionizing radiation (Chen *et al.*, 1978; Arlett and Priestley, 1985) or neocarzinostatin (Shiloh *et al.*, 1982). At present there is no unequivocal test for such individuals although there is a general consensus that they do differ from normals at the cellular level (Bridges *et al.*, 1985). Attempts are in hand to clone the gene for ataxia–telangiectasia (Green *et al.*, 1985) using a DNA-selectable marker cotransfer approach. One radiation resistant clone (clone 67) has been obtained following an extensive series of experiments; it still manifests the ataxia–telangiectasia characteristic of lack of inhibition of DNA synthesis after irradiation. Studies with this clone are continuing in an attempt to resolve whether it represents the product of a genuine transfer of resistant DNA or is a mutant. Clearly, the provision of a cloned fragment containing the ataxia–telangiectasia sequences would assist materially in studies of the molecular defect and also provide a probe to assist in the detection of carriers.

FANCONI'S ANAEMIA

Fanconi's anaemia (McKusick 22765) (Duckworth-Rysiecki *et al.*, 1984) represents a second chromosome breakage syndrome; its frequency is estimated at 1 in 3 000 000 in the USA (Swift, 1976). Early death usually follows from bone marrow failure. Patients who survive longer tend to succumb to cancer, especially leukaemia. However, some caution must be exercised when reviewing the data (German, 1980) since the association between this disease and cancer may be fortuitous. Thus the cancer may be a consequence of the androgen which has been administered to such patients since 1959. Cellular studies indicate a wide-ranging but variable hypersensitivity to the lethal action of an array of DNA damaging agents, but there is a specific hypersensitivity to cross-linking agents such as mitomycin C (Fujiwara *et al.*, 1977). The hypersensitivity to mitomycin C has permitted an assignment to at least 2 complementation groups (Duckworth-Rysiecki *et al.*, 1985).

The chromosome instability seen in Fanconi's anaemia represents a general increase in aberrations observed in lymphocytes and fibroblast cultures (Schroeder and German, 1974). The hypersensitivity to the lethal effects of cross-linking agents is also manifest as chromosome breakage. Duckworth-Rysiecki and colleagues (1985) reported that a combination of spontaneous and induced chromosome breakage is a good aid in differential diagnosis. Prenatal diagnoses in 4 pregnancies at risk have been reported based upon spontaneous and clastogen-induced chromosomal breakage (Auerbach *et al.*, 1981).

DNA repair studies with cells from patients with Fanconi's anaemia have concentrated on 2 areas. First, a demonstration of a defect in the ability to repair cross-links (Fujiwara *et al.*, 1977). Second, the excision of thymine glycols (Remsen and Cerutti, 1976) following treatment with ionizing radiation to which these cells are slightly hypersensitive (Arlett, 1979; Duckworth-Rysiecki and Taylor, 1985). Although the data using mitomycin C is consistent with a defect in the repair of cross-links, when other cross-linking agents are used it is not possible to demonstrate this defect (Duckworth-Rysiecki and Taylor, 1985). Of considerable interest is the report of Kauffman-Hirsch and colleagues (1978) that a defect in DNA ligase activity was present in a single patient with Fanconi's anaemia. The observation of Nagasawa and Little (1983) that superoxide dismutase may alleviate the cytotoxic effects of mitomycin C raises the possibility that the defect in Fanconi's anaemia may be related to impaired radicle scavenging rather than repair *per se*.

As a consequence of the substantial differential in sensitivity to cross-linking agents between cells from patients with Fanconi's anaemia and normals this syndrome is potentially amenable to the selection of resistant clones following transfer of DNA from normal cells.

BLOOM'S SYNDROME

Bloom's syndrome (McKusick 21090) represents a third chromosome breakage syndrome. Associated with chromosome aberrations, especially quadriradials in the circulating lymphocytes (which German regards as diagnostic), are very elevated spontaneous levels of sister chromatid exchanges and increased cancer proneness (German, 1974).

Cellular studies suggest that some cell strains from patients with Bloom's syndrome are hypersensitive to the lethal effects of UV light and mitomycin C (Krepinsky *et al.*, 1980; Ishizaki *et al.*, 1981).

The molecular basis of Bloom's syndrome still requires resolution. The presence of a clastogenic factor is implied in studies where the frequencies of sister chromatid exchanges have been analysed in heterokaryons between cells from Bloom's syndrome patients and normal human or rodent cells, and the partial purification of this clastogenic activity has been achieved (Emerit and Cerutti, 1981). A reduction in its potency is achieved by the addition of superoxide dismutase suggesting that the defects seen in Bloom's syndrome are a consequence of impaired radicle scavenging.

Two important reports have been made on mutation for Bloom's syndrome. Warren and colleagues (1981) reported an elevated spontaneous mutation rate in cultured fibroblasts from 2 Bloom's syndrome individuals. Vijayalaxmi and colleagues (1983) provided data suggesting an elevated mutation frequency *in vivo* when lymphocytes from 7 patients were tested for the frequency of 6-thioguanine resistant mutants. Since HPRT negative mutants may arise frequently from chromosome rearrangements (Cox and Masson, 1978), it may be anticipated that in a syndrome with elevated frequencies of chromosome breakage, increased mutation frequencies should also be observed if they also involve the X-chromosome. Our observations on spontaneous mutation with ataxia–telangiectasia fibroblasts do not support this suggestion (Arlett and Harcourt, 1983).

A HYPOGAMMAGLOBULINAEMIA PATIENT

A hypogammaglobulinaemia patient whose fibroblasts are known to us as 46BR has been subjected to an extensive cellular analysis (Henderson *et al.*, 1985), and of most significance in this discussion is the clinical feature of impaired immune response which may be regarded as analogous to ataxia–telangiectasia (Teo *et al.*, 1983). In this instance a repair defect appears to exist at the level of ligation since the cells are impaired in their ability to rejoin DNA replication intermediates (Okazaki fragments) after treatment with DNA damaging agents such as dimethyl sulphate (Henderson *et al.*, 1985). DNA ligases are involved in DNA replication and amongst their functions is the ligation of these extremely transient intermediates of about 200 nucleotides length which can be detected only with very short pulse-labels of radiosensitivity. The defect in 46BR should be contrasted with xeroderma pigmentosum or ataxia–telangiectasia where the defects are shown or assumed to act at the incision step of repair.

MISCELLANEOUS OBSERVATIONS

A number of other human conditions, some with increased frequency of cancer, have come to be regarded as possible DNA repair diseases on the basis of cellular hypersensitivity to the lethal or clastogenic action of DNA damaging agents (Kraemer, 1983). These include Chediak–Higashi syndrome (McKusick 21450), dyskeratosis congenita (McKusick 30500), Gardner's syndrome (McKusick 17530), basal cell naevus syndrome (McKusick 10940), retinoblastoma (McKusick 18020), tuberous sclerosis (McKusick 19110) and Huntington's disease (McKusick 14310). In many of these there is a lack of concensus between interlaboratories and a singular lack of any evidence at the molecular level for defects in DNA repair.

GENERAL CONCLUSIONS

Hypersensitivity to the clastogenic or lethal effects of physical or chemical DNA damaging agents has been established for a group of heritable diseases. Hypersensitivity at the clinical level is reproduced at the cellular level for sunlight in xeroderma pigmentosum and Cockayne syndrome, and for ionizing radiation in ataxia–telangiectasia. The formal evidence for defective DNA repair is strong for xeroderma pigmentosum but still largely inferential for ataxia–telangiectasia. With Cockayne syndrome no formal evidence for a repair defect is available (Lehmann, 1982a) but the increased sensitivity to the lethal and mutagenic effects of UV-C and induction of sister chromatid exchanges coupled with the post-UV DNA and RNA synthesis defects provides strong presumptive evidence for a DNA repair defect. It must be considered, however, that the DNA and RNA synthesis defect may imply some impairment of the processing of damage rather than in repair.

The demonstration of hypersensitivity in several of these disorders may also assist in the differential diagnosis. Bloom's syndrome, Fanconi's anaemia, xeroderma pigmentosum and ataxia–telangiectasia may all be diagnosed by their chromosome abnormalities. Prenatal diagnosis has been achieved for ataxia–telangiectasia, xeroderma pigmentosum and Cockayne syndrome.

A search for a link between the cellular abnormalities and the clinical features in these conditions may reveal a central role for DNA repair and the maintenance of human health. The progressive neoplastic or neurological degeneration seen in xeroderma pigmentosum, ataxia–telangiectasia and Cockayne syndrome may be a consequence of continued damage and resultant loss of viability in cells damaged by agents acting externally or internally. A similar catalogue of response is seen in dyskeratosis congenita, basal cell naevus syndrome, retinoblastoma, Gardner's syndrome and Huntington's disease, and indeed it has prompted the studies which seek to include them amongst the repair defective syndromes.

Immune deficiency is unambiguous in Bloom's syndrome, ataxia–telangiectasia and the hypogammaglobulinaemia individual. The origin of the immune deficiency is obscure but it is possible to hypothesize on involvement of effective DNA repair mechanisms during the ontogeny of immune diversity and competence. A recent study (Harris *et al.*, 1985) which took as its starting point the fact that immune deficiency is correlated with repair defects has provided evidence for radiation hypersensitivity in lymphocytes from some autoimmune conditions such as systemic lupos erythromatosus.

It would seem that a great deal of work is still required to resolve the contribution of defects in DNA repair for human health.

ACKNOWLEDGEMENTS

This study was supported in part by Euratom contract B10/E/414/81/UK(H). I would like to indicate that the work of S. Harcourt and A. Lehmann is included. I am indebted to Professor B. A. Bridges for many helpful comments.

REFERENCES

Andrews, A. D., Barrett, S. F. and Robbins, J. H. Relation of DNA repair processes to pathological ageing of the nervous system in xeroderma pigmentosum. *Lancet* 1 (1976) 1318–1320

Arlett, C. F. Survival and mutation in gamma-irradiated human cell strains from normal or cancer-prone individuals. In Okada, S., Imamura, M., Terasima, T. and Yamaguchi, H. (eds.) *Proceedings of the Sixth International Congress of Radiation Research*, University of Tokyo Press, Tokyo, 1977, pp. 596–602

Arlett, C. F. and Cole, J. Mutation studies in cells established from human cancer prone syndromes. Proceedings of the IVth Int. Congress Environmental Mutagenesis. Stockholm 1985.

Arlett, C. F. and Harcourt, S. A. Variation in response to mutagens amongst normal and repair-defective human cells. In Lawrence, C. W. (ed.) *Induced Mutagenesis*, Plenum, New York, 1982, pp. 249–270

Arlett, C. F., Harcourt, S. A., Lehmann, A. R., Stevens, S., Ferguson-Smith, M. A. and Morley, W. N. Studies on a new case of xeroderma pigmentosum (XP3BR) from complementation group G with cellular sensitivity to ionizing radiation. *Carcinogenesis* 1 (1980) 745–751

Arlett, C. F. and Priestley, A. An assessment of the radiosensitivity of ataxia–telangiectasia heterozygotes. In Gatti, R. A. and Swift, M. (eds.) *Ataxia–Telangiectasia: Genetics, Neuropathology and Immunopathology of a Degenerative Disease of Childhood,* Liss, New York, 1985, pp. 101–109

Auerbach, A. D., Adler, B. and Chaganti, R. S. K. Prenatal and postnatal diagnosis and carrier detection of Fanconi anemia by a cytogenetic method. *Pediatrics* 67 (1981) 128–135

Bridges, B. A. and Harnden, D. G. *Ataxia–telangiectasia – A Cellular and Molecular Link Between Cancer, Neuropathology, and Immune Deficiency*, Wiley, Chichester, 1982, p. 402

Bridges, B. A., Lenoir, G. and Tomatis, L. Workshop on ataxia–telangiectasia heterozygotes and cancer. *Cancer Res.* 45 (1985) 3979–3980

Brumback, R. A., Yoder, F. W., Andrews, A. D., Peck, G. L. and Robbins, J. H. Normal pressure hydrocephalus. Recognition and relationship to neurological abnormalities in Cockayne Syndrome. *Arch. Neurol.* 35 (1978) 337–345

Chen, P. C., Lavin, M. F. and Kidson, C. Identification of ataxia–telangiectasia heterozygotes, a cancer prone population. *Nature* 274 (1978) 484–486

Cleaver, J. E. Defective repair replication of DNA in xeroderma pigmentosum. *Nature* 218 (1968) 652–656

Cleaver, J. E. and Bootsma, D. Xeroderma pigmentosum – biochemical and genetic characteristics. *Ann. Rev. Genetics* 9 (1975) 19–38

Cox, R. A cellular description of the repair defect in ataxia–telangiectasia. In Bridges, B. A. and Harnden, D. G. (eds.) *Ataxia–telangiectasia – A Cellular and Molecular Link Between Cancer, Neuropathology and Immune Deficiency*, Wiley, Chichester, 1982, pp. 141–153

Cox, R. and Masson, W. K. Do radiation-induced thioguanine-resistant mutants of cultured mammalian cells arise by HGPRT gene mutations or X-chromosome rearrangement? *Nature* 276 (1978) 629–630

Duckworth-Rysiecki, G., Cornish, K., Clarke, C. A. and Buckwald, M. Identification of two complementation groups in Fanconi's anemia. *Somatic Cell and Mol. Genet.* 11 (1985) 35–41

Duckworth-Rysiecki, G., Hulten, M., Mann, J. and Taylor, A. M. R. Clinical and cytogenetic diversity in Fanconi's anaemia. *J. Med. Genet.* 21 (1984) 197–203

Duckworth-Rysiecki, G. and Taylor, A. M. R. Effects of ionising radiation on cells from Fanconi's anaemia patients. *Cancer Res.* 45 (1985) 416–420

Emerit, I. and Cerutti, P. Clastogenic activity from Bloom syndrome fibroblast cultures. *Proc. Natl. Acad. Sci. USA* 78 (1981) 1868–1872

Fischer, E., Keijzer, W., Thielmann, H. W., Popanda, O., Bohner, E., Edler, L., Jung, E. G. and Bootsma, D. A ninth complementation group in xeroderma pigmentosum, XP I. *Mutation Res.* 145 (1985) 217–225

Friedberg, E. C. *DNA Repair*, Freeman, New York, 1985, p. 614

Fujiwara, Y. and Satoh, Y. Age-dependent changes in fibroblast cultures from a xeroderma pigmentosum variant. *J. Invest. Dermatol.* 76 (1981) 215–220

Fujiwara, Y., Tatsumi, M. and Sasaki, M. Cross-link repair in human cells and its possible defect in Fanconi's anemia cells. *J. Mol. Biol.* 113 (1977) 635–649

Gatti, R. and Swift, M. *Ataxia–Telangiectasia: Genetics, Neuropathology and Immunology of a Degenerative Disease of Childhood*, Liss, New York, 1985, p. 407

German, J. Chromosome-breakage syndromes: different genes, different treatments, different cancers. In Generoso, W. M., Shelby, M. D. and de Serres, F. J. (eds.) *DNA Repair and Mutagenesis in Eukaryotes*, Plenum, New York, 1980, 429–439

German, J., Bloom, D. and Passarge, E. Bloom's syndrome. V. Surveillance for cancer in affected families. *Clin. Genet.* 12 (1977) 162–168

Giannelli, F., Avery, J. A., Pembrey, M. E. and Blunt, S. Prenatal exclusion of ataxia–telangiectasia. In Bridges, B. A. and Harnden, D. G. (eds.) *Ataxia–Telangiectasia – A Cellular and Molecular Link Between Cancer, Neuropathology, and Immune Deficiency*, Wiley, Chichester, 1982, pp. 393–400

Green, M. H. L., Lowe, J. E., James, M. R. and Arlett, C. F. An attempt to transfer radiation resistance to an ataxia–telangiectasia cell line. In Gatti, R. A. and Swift, M. (eds.) *Ataxia–Telangiectasia: Genetics, Neuropathology and Immunopathology of a Degenerative Disease of Childhood*, Liss, New York, 1985, pp. 173–179

Harris, G., Cramp, W. A., Edwards, J. C., George, A. M., Sabovljev, S. A., Hart, L., Hughes, G. R. V., Denman, A. M. and Yatvin, M. B. Radiosensitivity of peripheral blood lymphocytes in autoimmune disease. *Int. J. Radiat. Biol.* 47 (1985) 689–699

Henderson, L. M., Arlett, C. F., Harcourt, S. A., Lehmann, A. R. and Broughton, B. C. Cells from an immunodeficient patient (46BR) with a defect in DNA ligation are hypomutable but hypersensitive to the induction of sister chromatid exchanges. *Proc. Natl. Acad. Sci. USA* 82 (1985) 2044–2048

Ishizaki, K., Yagi, T., Inoue, M., Nikaido, O. and Takebe, H. DNA repair in Bloom's syndrome fibroblasts after UV irradiation or treatment with mitomycin C. *Mutation Res.* 80 (1981) 213–219

Jaspers, N. G. J., Jansen van de Kuilen, G. and Bootsma, D. Complementation analysis of xeroderma pigmentosum variants. *Expl. Cell Res.* 136 (1981) 81–90

de Jonge, A. J. R., Vermeulen, W., Keijzer, W., Hoeijmakers, J. H. J. and Bootsma, D. Microinjection of *Micrococcus luteus* UV-endonuclease restores UV-induced unscheduled DNA synthesis in cells of nine xeroderma pigmentosum complementation groups. *Mutation Res.* 150 (1985) 99–105

Kauffman-Hirsch, M., Schweiger, M., Wagner, E. F. and Sperling, K. Deficiency of DNA ligase activity in Fanconi's anemia. *Hum. Genet.* 45 (1978) 25–32

Kawai, K., Ikenaga, M., Ohtani, H., Fukuchi, K. I., Yamamura, K. I. and Kumahara, Y. Rapid procedures for prenatal diagnosis of Cockayne Syndrome. *Jpn. J. Hum. Genet.* 28 (1983) 223–229

Kraemer, K. H. Heritable diseases with increased sensitivity to cellular injury. In Fitzpatrick, T. B., Eisen, A. Z., Wolff, K., Freedberg, I. M. and Austen, K. F. (eds.) *Update: Dermatology in General Medicine*, McGraw-Hill, 1983, pp. 113–144

Kraemer, K. H., Lee, M. M. and Scotto, J. DNA repair protects against cutaneous and internal neoplasia: evidence from xeroderma pigmentosum. *Carcinogenesis* 5 (1984) 511–514

Krepinsky, A. B., Rainbow, A. J., Heddle, J. A. Studies on the ultraviolet light sensitivity of Bloom's syndrome fibroblasts. *Mutation Res.* 69 (1980) 357–368

Lawrence, C. W. Mechanisms of induced mutagenesis in yeast. In Sugimura, T., Kondo, S. and Takebe, H. (eds.) *Environmental Mutagens and Carcinogens*, University of Tokyo Press, Tokyo, 1982, pp. 129–136

Lehmann, A. R. Ataxia–telangiectasia and the lethal lesion produced by ionising radiation. In Nichols, W. N. and Murphy, D. (eds.) *DNA Repair Processes*, Symposia Specialists, Miami, 1977, pp. 167–175

Lehmann, A. R. Xeroderma pigmentosum, Cockayne syndrome and ataxia–telangiectasia: disorders relating DNA repair to carcinogenesis. *Cancer Surveys* 1 (1982a) 93–118

Lehmann, A. R. Three complementation groups in Cockayne syndrome. *Mutation Res.* 106 (1982b) 347–356

Lehmann, A. R. The cellular and molecular responses of ataxia–telangiectasia cells to DNA damage. In Bridges, B. A. and Harnden, D. G. (eds.) *Ataxia–telangiectasia – A Cellular and Molecular Link between Cancer, Neuropathology, and Immune Deficiency*, Wiley, Chichester, 1982c, pp. 83–101

Lehmann, A. R. Use of recombinant DNA techniques in cloning DNA repair genes and in the study of mutagenesis in mammalian cells. *Mutation Res.* 150 (1985) 61–67

Lehmann, A. R., Francis, A. J. and Giannelli, F. Prenatal diagnosis of Cockayne's syndrome. *Lancet* (1985) 486–488

Lehmann, A. R., Kirk-Bell, S., Arlett, C. F., Paterson, M. C., Lohman, P. H. M., de Weerd-Kastelein, E. A. and Bootsma, D. Xeroderma pigmentosum cells with normal levels of excision repair have a defect in DNA synthesis after UV-irradiation. *Proc. Natl. Acad. Sci. USA* 72 (1975) 219–223

Maher, V. M., Dorney, D. J., Mendrala, A. L., Konze-Thomas, B. and McCormick, J. J. DNA excision-repair processes in human cells can eliminate the cytotoxic and mutagenic consequences of ultraviolet irradiation. *Mutation Res.* 62 (1979) 311–323

Maher, V. M., McCormick, J. J., Grover, P. L. and Sims, P. Effect of DNA repair on the cytotoxicity and mutagenicity of polycyclic hydrocarbon derivatives in normal and xeroderma pigmentosum fibroblasts. *Mutation Res.* 43 (1977) 117–138

Marshall, R. R. and Scott, D. The relationship between chromosome damage and cell killing in UV-irradiated normal and xeroderma pigmentosum cells. *Mutation Res.* 36 (1976) 397–400

Mortelmans, K., Friedberg, E. C., Slor, H., Thomas, G. and Cleaver, J. E. Defective thymine dimer excision by cell free extracts of xeroderma pigmentosum cells. *Proc. Natl. Acad. Sci. USA* 73 (1976) 2757–2761

Nagasawa, H. and Little, J. B. Suppression of cytotoxic effect of mitomycin-C by superoxide dismutase in Fanconi's anemia and dyskeratosis congenita fibroblasts. *Carcinogenesis* 4 (1983) 795–798

Painter, R. B. and Young, B. R. Radiosensitivity in ataxia–telangiectasia – a new explanation. *Proc. Natl. Acad. Sci. USA* 77 (1980) 7315–7317

Paterson, M. C., Smith, B. P., Lohman, P. H. M., Anderson, A. K. and Fishman, L. Defective excision repair of gamma-ray-damaged DNA in human (ataxia–telangiectasia) fibroblasts. *Nature* 169 (1976) 444–447

Patton, J. D., Rowan, L. A., Mendrala, A. L., Howell, J. N., Maher, V. M. and McCormick, J. J. Xeroderma pigmentosum fibroblasts including cells from XP variants are abnormally sensitive to the mutagenic and cytotoxic action of broad-spectrum simulated sunlight. *Photochem. Photobiol.* 40 (1984) 37–42

Ramsay, C. A., Coltart, T. M., Blunt, S., Pawsey, S. A. and Giannelli, F. Prenatal diagnosis of xeroderma pigmentosum. *Lancet* 2 (1974) 1109–1112

Remsen, J. F. and Cerutti, P. A. Deficiency of gamma-ray excision repair in skin fibroblasts from patients with Fanconi's anemia. *Proc. Natl. Acad. Sci. USA* 73 (1976) 2419–2423

Royer-Pokora, B. and Haseltine, B. Isolation of UV-resistant revertants from a xeroderma pigmentosum complementation group A cell line. *Nature* 311 (1984) 390–392

Schroeder, T. M. and German, J. Bloom's syndrome and Fanconi's anaemia: demonstration of two distinctive patterns of chromosome disruption and rearrangement. *Humangenetik* 25 (1974) 299–306

Schwartz, S., Flannery, D. B. and Cohen, M. M. Tests appropriate for the prenatal diagnosis of ataxia–telangiectasia. *Prenatal Diag.* 5 (1985) 9–14

Shahman, M., Becker, Y. and Cohen, M. M. A diffusable clastogenic factor in ataxia–telangiectasia. *Cytogenet. Cell Genet.* 27 (1980) 155–161

Shahman, M., Voss, R., Becker, Y., Yarhoni, S., Ornoy, A. and Kohn, G. Prenatal diagnosis of ataxia–telangiectasia. *J. Pediat.* 100 (1982) 134–137

Shiloh, Y., Tabor, E. and Becker, Y. The response of ataxia–telangiectasia homozygous and heterozygous skin fibroblasts to neocarzinostatin. *Carcinogenesis* 3 (1982) 815–820

Shiloh, Y., Tabor, E. and Becker, Y. Cells from patients with ataxia–telangiectasia are abnormally sensitive to the cytotoxic effect of a tumor promoter, phobol-12-myristate-13-acetate. *Mutation Res.* 149 (1985) 283–286

Smith, P. D., Dusenbery, R. L., Cooper, S. H. and Baumen, C. F. Examining the mechanism of mutagenesis in DNA repair-deficient strains of *Drosophila melanogaster*. In Sugimura, T., Kondo, S. and Takebe, H. (eds.) *Environmental Mutagens and Carcinogens*, University of Tokyo Press, Tokyo, 1982, pp. 147–155

Sugita, T., Ikenaga, M., Suehara, N., Kozuka, T., Furuyama, J. I. and Yabuuchi, H. Prenatal diagnosis of Cockayne syndrome using assay of colony-forming ability in ultraviolet-irradiated cells. *Clin. Genet.* 22 (1982) 137–142

Swift, M. Malignant disease heterozygous carriers. *Birth Defects Orig. Antic. Ser.* 12 (1976) 133–144

Swift, M. Disease predisposition of ataxia–telangiectasia heterozygotes. In Bridges, B. A. and Harnden, D. G. (eds.) *Ataxia–telangiectasia – A Cellular and Molecular Link Between Cancer, Neuropathology and Immune Deficiency*, Wiley, Chichester, 1982, pp. 355–361

Takano, T., Noda, M. and Tamura, T. Transfection of cells from a xeroderma pigmentosum patient with normal human DNA confers UV resistance. *Nature* 296 (1982) 269–270

Takebe, H., Miki, Y., Kozuka, T., Furuyama, J. I., Tanaka, K., Sasaki, M. S., Fujiwara, Y. and Akiba, H. DNA repair characteristics and skin cancers of xeroderma pigmentosum patients in Japan. *Cancer Res.* 37 (1977) 490–495

Tanaka, K., Kawai, K., Kumahara, Y., Ikenaga, M. and Okada, Y. Genetic complementation groups in Cockayne syndrome. *Somatic Cell Genet.* 7 (1981) 445–456

Tanaka, K., Sekiguchi, M. and Okada, Y. Restoration of ultraviolet induced unscheduled DNA synthesis of xeroderma pigmentosum cells by the concomitant treatment with bacteriophage T4 endonuclease V and HVJ (Sendai virus). *Proc. Natl. Acad. Sci. USA* 72 (1975) 4071–4075

Taylor, A. M. R. Cytogenetics of ataxia–telangiectasia. In Bridges, B. A. and Harnden, D. G. (eds.) *Ataxia–telangiectasia – a Cellular and Molecular Link Between Cancer, Neuropathology, and Immune Deficiency*, Wiley, Chichester, 1982, pp. 52–81

Taylor, A. M. R., Laker, H. B. and Morgan, G. R. Unscheduled DNA synthesis induced by streptonigrin in ataxia–telangiectasia fibroblasts. *Carcinogenesis* 6 (1985) 945–947

Teo, I. A., Arlett, C. F., Harcourt, S. A., Priestley, A. and Broughton, B. C. Multiple hypersensitivity to mutagens in a cell strain (46BR) derived from a patient with immunodeficiencies. *Mutation Res.* 107 (1983) 371–386

Thielmann, H. W., Edler, L., Popanda, O. and Friemel, S. Xeroderma pigmentosum patients from the Federal Republic of Germany: decrease in post-UV colony-forming ability in 30 xeroderma pigmentosum strains is quantitatively correlated with a decrease in DNA-incising capacity. *J. Cancer Res. Clin. Oncol.* 109 (1985) 227–240

Vijayalaxmi, Evans, H. J., Ray, J. H. and German, J. Bloom's syndrome: evidence for an increased mutation frequency *in vivo*. *Science* 221 (1983) 851–853

Waldmann, T. A., Misiti, J., Nelson, D. L. and Kraemer, K. H. Ataxia–telangiectasia: a multisystem hereditary disease with immunodeficiency, impaired organ maturation, X-ray hypersensitivity, and a high incidence of neoplasia. *Ann. Int. Med.* 99 (1983) 367–379

Walker, G. C. Mutagenesis and inducible responses to deoxyribonucleic acid damage in *Escherichia coli*. *Microbiol. Rev.* 48 (1984) 60–93

Warren, S. T., Schultz, R. A., Chang, C. C., Wade, M. H. and Trosko, J. E. Elevated spontaneous mutation rate in Bloom syndrome fibroblasts. *Proc. Natl. Acad. Sci. USA* 78 (1981) 3133–3137

de Weerd-Kastelein, E. A., Keijzer, W., Rainaldi, G. and Bootsma, D. Induction of sister-chromatid exchanges in xeroderma pigmentosum cells after exposure to ultraviolet light. *Mutation Res.* 45 (1977) 253–261

Westerfield, A., Hoeijmakers, J. H. J., van Duin, M., de Wit, J., Odijk, H., Pastink, A., Wood, R. D. and Bootsma, D. Molecular cloning of a human DNA repair gene. *Nature* 310 (1984) 425–429

de Wit, J., Jaspers, N. G. J. and Bootsma, D. The rate of DNA synthesis in normal human and ataxia–telangiectasia cells after exposure to X-irradiation. *Mutation Res.* 80 (1981) 221–226

J. Inher. Metab. Dis. 9 Suppl. 1 (1986) 85–91

Molecular Basis of α_1-Antitrypsin Deficiency and its Potential Therapy by Gene Transfer

F. D. LEDLEY and S. L. C. WOO
Howard Hughes Medical Institute, Department of Cell Biology, Baylor College of Medicine, Houston, Texas, USA

The gene for α_1-antitrypsin, a serum anti-protease, has been cloned and sequenced. The underlying mutation in the PiZ allele has been identified as a G to A conversion giving rise to the substitution of glu by lys at position 342. Preparation of specific probes has allowed prenatal diagnosis. Recombinant retroviruses containing the normal human α_1-antitrypsin gene have been constructed and used to infect NIH3T3 cells. Analysis of DNA, RNA and protein indicate that successful incorporation of the α_1-antitrypsin was achieved and that the gene was capable of being expressed. The feasibility of genetic replacement therapy has been demonstrated and further experiments justified.

α_1-Antitrypsin accounts for approximately 90% of the total inhibitory capacity of human serum. It is a single polypeptide of molecular weight approximately 50000, with a carbohydrate content of about 12%. It shows affinity to and inhibits a variety of serine proteases such as trypsin, chymotrypsin, thrombin, plasmin, kallikrein, elastase, and collagenase.

Although α_1-antitrypsin is a serum protease inhibitor of hepatic origin, its major site of physiological action is thought to be in the lung (Morse, 1978). The protein is transported by passive diffusion from the blood into the alveolar space of the lung where it protects the lung from destruction by neutrophil elastase. The balance of elastase–anti-elastase activities in the lung can be perturbed genetically in favour of the elastase activity if the individual has an inborn deficiency in α_1-antitrypsin, or by environmental determinants such as cigarette smoke, leading to autodigestion of the alveolar surface by granulocytic proteases and clinical emphysema.

α_1-Antitrypsin is encoded by a single autosomal locus in the human genome (Fagerhol and Laurell, 1970). The α_1-antitrypsin locus has been assigned the term Pi (P for protease and i for inhibitor), and each variant form of α_1-antitrypsin is indicated by a capital letter. Most individuals are homozygotes for PiM, which has a gene frequency of 0.95. The genetic deficiency is inherited through an autosomal recessive trait. The most common mutant is PiZ phenotype which has a frequency in Caucasians of northern European ancestry of 0.02–0.03. Another milder mutant, PiS, is more common in the United States with a gene frequency of 0.03–0.04 (Fagerhol and Laverell, 1970).

Journal of Inherited Metabolic Disease. ISSN 0141–8955. Printed in Great Britain by Titus Wilson & Son Ltd., Kendal.

Although serum α_1-antitrypsin levels in individuals of the ZZ and SZ phenotypes are only 12% and 35% that of the normal MM phenotype, the molecular weight, amino acid composition, carbohydrate content, and specific antiprotease activity are very similar to those of the normal protein. Peptide mapping experiments and analysis of the amino acid composition of tryptic and CNBr fragments of the proteins and their complete amino acid sequence demonstrated the substitution of a glutamic acid in the PiM type protein by a lysine in the PiZ type protein. In the PiS variant there is a substitution of a glutamic acid by valine (Owen and Carrell, 1977).

CLONING AND SEQUENCING OF NORMAL AND MUTANT α_1-ANTITRYPSIN GENES

Our laboratory has reported the cloning of a normal and a mutant α_1-antitrypsin cDNA (Kurachi *et al.*, 1981; Long *et al.*, 1985). The nucleic acid sequence of these clones was determined, and the underlying mutation in the gene coding for the PiZ protein was shown to be a G to A transition in the codon for the glutamate residue (Kidd *et. al.*, 1983). More recently our laboratory has cloned the entire chromosomal gene for both normal and mutant α_1-antitrypsin. Sequence comparison of the exonic regions of the PiM and PiZ α_1-antitrypsin genes has demonstrated complete agreement between the two sequences, with the single exception of a G to A transition in exon V of the PiZ gene. This mutation causes the substitution of a glutamic acid at residue 342 in the PiM protein by a lysine in the PiZ protein, thus confirming previous reports of this substitution as determined by peptide sequencing analysis. Of particular interest is the complete sequence agreement between the PiM and PiZ genes in other regions of the genome which have been sequenced, indicating that the single base substitution is the only significant difference between the PiM and PiZ genes (Sifers *et al.*, unpublished observation).

MOLECULAR GENETIC DIAGNOSIS OF α_1-ANTITRYPSIN GENOTYPES

Knowledge of the exact genetic difference between the normal and mutant α_1-antitrypsin genes has enabled the use of molecular genetic techniques for prenatal diagnosis of α_1-antitrypsin deficiency. The nucleotide substitution in the α_1-antitrypsin gene neither creates nor destroys a restriction endonuclease recognition sequence: the appearance of the normal and mutant α_1-antitrypsin genes are therefore identical when analysed by conventional techniques of restriction endonuclease digestion and Southern hybridization.

Thus, specific oligonucleotides were designed with sequences complementary to the normal PiM or mutant PiZ genomes at the point where these two sequences differ (Figure 1). Experimental conditions were established such that the oligonucleotides would hybridize only with the perfectly homologous sequences. Under conditions of appropriate stringency the ^{32}P-labelled oligonucleotide complementary to the PiM gene will bind only to the PiM gene and not to the PiZ gene, while the ^{32}P-labelled oligonucleotide complementary to the PiZ gene will bind only to

Amino Acid Substitutions Between the Normal and Deficient Phenotypes of Human α1-Antitrypsin Could be the Result of a Point Mutation in the Gene

Phenotype	Condition	Genotype
		342
M	normal	...thr ile asp glu lys gly thr...
		...ACC ATC GAC GAG AAA GGG A.. ...
		↕
Z	deficient	...ACC ATC GAC AAG AAA GGG A......
		...thr ile asp lys lys gly thr...

Figure 1 Oligonucleotide sequences matching the normal and PiZ α_1-antitrypsin sequences used to distinguish the two alleles by differential hybridization

the PiZ gene and not to the PiM gene (Figure 2). These genotype specific probes were then used to analyse genomic DNA of individuals with different genotypes. Individuals who were homozygous for the normal PiM genotype showed hybridization with the PiM probe not with the PiZ probe. Individuals who were heterozygous for the PiM and PiZ alleles showed hybridization with both the PiM and PiZ probes, and individuals who were homozygous for the mutant PiZ genotype showed hybridization with both the PiM and PiZ probes, and individuals who were homozygous for the mutant PiZ genotype showed hybridization to the PiZ probe but not the PiM probe. In this way it is possible to distinguish the genotype of an individual from any DNA sample (Kidd *et al.*, 1983).

This method has been applied to prenatal diagnosis of α_1-antitrypsin deficiency. The initial study involved the prenatal diagnosis in two families at risk. The fetuses were diagnosed to be MZ heterozygotes and the results were verified by Pi typing of the neonates. Thus, the oligonucleotides hybridization method can be used in combination with amniocentesis or chorionic villi sampling as a diagnostic tool to identify ZZ homozygotes prenatally (Kidd *et. al.*, 1984).

Analysis of restriction fragment length polymorphisms (RFLP) at the α_1-antitrypsin locus provides a second method for genetic diagnosis of α_1-antitrypsin deficiency. A very high degree of linkage disequilibrium has been found between RFLPs at the α_1-antitrypsin locus and the PiZ allele (Cox *et al.*, 1985). In particular an *Ava*II RFLP haplotype is associated exclusively with PiZ alleles. 27 PiZ alleles and 47 other alleles were tested with no discordance between the presence of the *Ava*II polymorphisms and the PiZ mutation. This finding suggests that all of the PiZ alleles have a common origin roughly coincident with the appearance of the *Ava*II polymorphic site, and that the occurrence of these two point mutations within the human genome is sufficiently recent for little or no recombination to have taken place between these two loci.

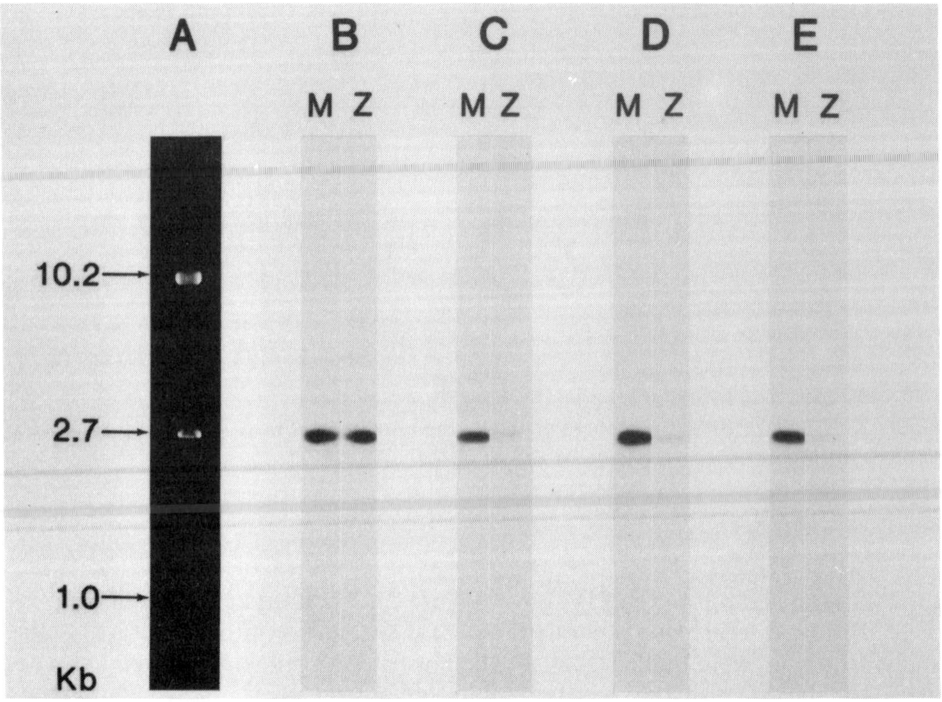

Figure 2 Specificity of oligonucleotide probe for the cloned normal M and mutant Z genotype. DNA was digested with *Hind*III, and stained with ethidium bromide (**A**). Lanes B–E show hybridization under different conditions of stringency: (**B**) hybridization 45°C, wash 4°C; (**C**) hybridization 45°C, wash 55°C; (**D**) hybridization 55°C, wash 4°C; (**E**) hybridization 55°C, wash 55°C; thus showing specific hybridization to normal and not mutant DNA

RATIONALE FOR GENETIC THERAPY OF α_1-ANTITRYPSIN DEFICIENCY

We and others have performed gene transfer experiments in which cloned normal human α_1-antitrypsin was introduced into cultured cells which do not normally produce α_1-antitrypsin. Cells transformed with the human α_1-antitrypsin gene expressed α_1-antitrypsin mRNA and immunoreactive protein. These experiments demonstrated the feasibility of synthesizing authentic α_1-antitrypsin from the cloned gene and raised the possibility that gene transfer into somatic cells might represent a potential therapy for the deficiency syndrome. Introduction of the functional human α_1-antitrypsin gene into somatic cells of deficient individuals by DNA-mediated gene transfer could provide a population of cells capable of synthesizing and secreting normal α_1-antitrypsin into the circulatory system. The recombinant protein, like the normal protein, should diffuse into the alveolar spaces of the lung and provide the necessary antiprotease function to prevent tissue destruction by neutrophil elastase. Although it would be optimal to be able to replace the normal α_1-antitrypsin gene in hepatocytes, it might not be necessary to target the α_1-antitrypsin gene specifically to hepatocytes as long as the recipient cells were capable of secreting significant quantities of the recombinant protein into blood. It is important to note that this form of genetic therapy could only be effective in ameliorating the pulmonary manifestations of α_1-antitrypsin deficiency, and would not be expected to have any efficacy against the hepatic disease which might be caused by excessive accumulation of the mutant protein in the liver.

The methods of DNA-mediated gene transfer used in experiments in cultured cells are, however, poorly suited for genetic transfer into primary cell cultures or live animals due to low efficiency. Viral-mediated genetic transfer using recombinant retroviruses offers many advantages for gene transfer experiments. Retroviral vectors can be engineered to carry a variety of recombinant genes and will efficiently infect a variety of host cells and cause stable integration of the chimeric retroviral genome in the chromosome of the infected cell. Most importantly, it is possible to remove entirely all of the genes coding for viral proteins, and to replace these sequences with a recombinant gene of interest without affecting the ability of the virus to infect cells and integrate stably into the host genome (Cepko *et al.*, 1984). Such viruses, termed 'defective retroviruses', can carry a recombinant gene such as α_1-antitrypsin. They are capable of infecting and transforming somatic cells, yet they are incapable of producing any viral proteins and cannot form infectious viral particles for subsequent propagation.

RETROVIRAL-MEDIATED GENE TRANSFER OF α_1-ANTITRYPSIN

Human α_1-antitrypsin

Recombinant retroviruses containing the normal human α_1-antitrypsin were constructed using the retroviral vector pZIPNEO-SV(X) provided for us by Dr R. Mulligan (Cepko *et al.*, 1984). This vector contains the retroviral promotors and packaging sequences along with the bacterial *neo* resistance gene (which carries resistance to the eukaryotic poison G418), but is devoid of the genes coding for viral proteins. Retroviruses were produced by introducing this DNA into a cell line (ψ2) which contains a different recombinant retroviral gene missing from the packaging sequences required for packing the retroviral nucleic acid genome into a retroviral capsid (Mann *et al.*, 1983). The packaging defective recombinant contained genes for all of the essential viral proteins and directed the synthesis of an intact but empty viral capsid. The retroviral vector containing the α_1-antitrypsin gene, *neo* gene, and packaging sequences was then packaged into the empty viral capsids producing a 'defective' retrovirus. The entire open reading frame for α_1-antitrypsin as well as short 5′ and 3′ untranslated sequences were inserted into the retroviral vector pZIPNEO-SV(X) producing a recombinant designated pZα1AT(+) (Figure 3).

The pZα1AT(+) plasmid DNA was transfected into the ψ2 cell line and G418 resistant colonies containing stably integrated plasmid DNA were isolated, subcloned, and tested for their ability to produce recombinant retroviruses. Supernatants from these cells were harvested and used to infect NIH3T3 cells. The number of G418 resistant colonies arising by infection of NIH3T3 cells represented the titer of retroviral particles.

NIH3T3 cells infected with the α_1-antitrypsin containing retrovirus and selected

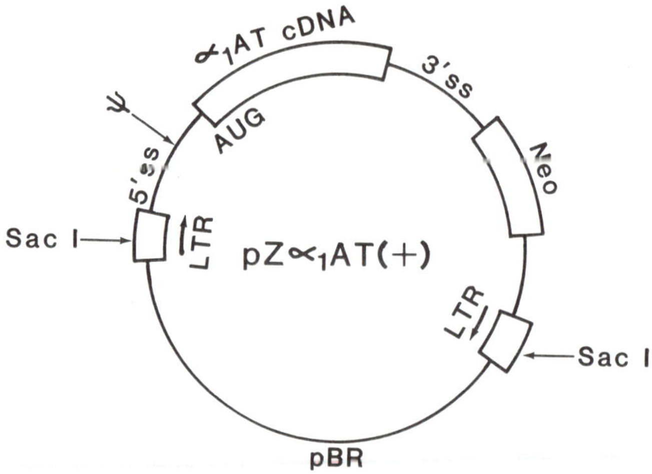

Figure 3 Construction of retroviral expression vector. The α_1-antitrypsin cDNA was inserted into the Bam site of (pZIPNEO-SVCx) provided by Dr R. Mulligan

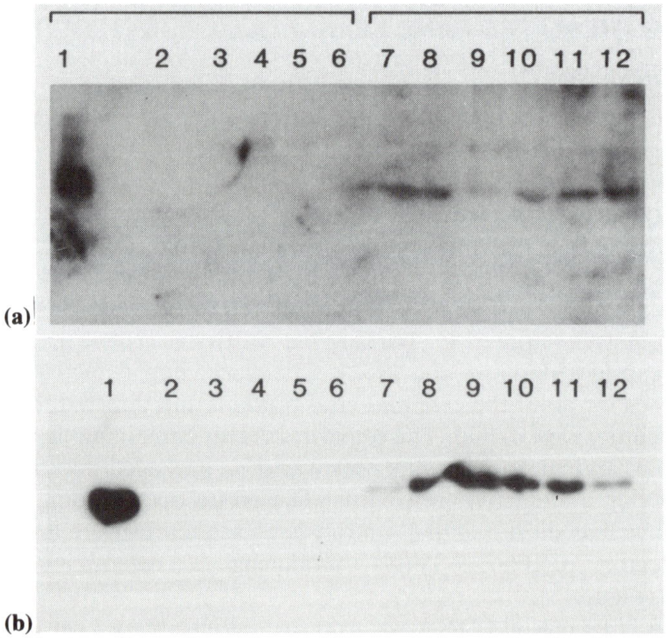

Figure 4 Synthesis and secretion of α_1-antitrypsin in infected cells. Western blot showing human α_1-antitrypsin **(a)** in cells and **(b)** secreted into the media of cells infected with the recombinant retrovirus (lanes 7–12), but not into control cells infected with pZIPNEO (lanes 1–6). α_1-Antitrypsin from the hep 362 cell line is shown in lane 1

for *neo* resistance were analysed for the ability to produce recombinant α_1-antitrypsin. DNA analysis demonstrated that each of the G418 resistant cells had an intact α_1-antitrypsin containing provirus. In addition RNA analysis indicated that the provirus was transcribed into a full length 6.0 kb proviral transcript which hybridized with an α_1-antitrypsin cDNA probe. More importantly, immunoblotting of infected cells and of media from infected cells indicated that α_1-antitrypsin was being synthesized (Figure 4a) and secreted (Figure 4b). These experiments provided conclusive evidence that recombinant retroviruses containing human α_1-antitrypsin have been generated which are capable of efficiently transmitting the capacity to synthesize and secrete the human protein into cultured mammalian cells.

CONCLUSION

Studies with cloned human α_1-antitrypsin have yielded considerable information about the structure of normal and mutant α_1-antitrypsin genes, have led to new methods of molecular genetic diagnosis of α_1-antitrypsin deficiency, and have demonstrated the feasibility of considering experiments in genetic replacement therapy of the deficiency state.

Continuing molecular genetic studies with α_1-antitrypsin should provide more information about the basic function and processing of the α_1-antitrypsin gene, and bring increasing benefits to physicians involved in the diagnosis and therapy of α_1-antitrypsin deficiency.

REFERENCES

Cepko, C. L., Roberts, B. E. and Mulligan, R. C. Construction and applications of a highly transmissible murine retrovirus vector. *Cell* 37 (1984) 1053–1062

Cox, D. N., Woo, S. L. C. and Mansfield, T. DNA restriction fragments associated with α_1-antitrypsin indicate a single origin for deficiency allele PiZ. *Nature* 316 (1985) 79–81

Fagerhol, M. K. and Laurell. The Pi system inherited variants of serum alpha-1 anti-trypsin. In Steinberg, A. B. and Bearn, A. (eds.) *Progress in Medical Genetics VIII*, 1970, 96–105

Kidd, W., Golbus, M. S., Wallace, R. B., Itakura, K. and Woo, S. L. C. Prenatal diagnosis of α_1-antitrypsin deficiency by oligonucleotide mapping of the gene. *N. Engl. Med. J.* 310 (1984) 639–642

Kidd, W., Wallace, R. B., Itakura, K. and Woo, S. L. C. α_1-Antitrypsin deficiency by direct analysis of the mutation site in the gene. *Nature* 304 (1983) 230–234

Kurachi, K., Chandra, T., Degen, S. J. F., White, T. T., Marchiorc, T., Woo, S. L. C. and Davie, E. W. Cloning and sequence of cDNA coding for α_1-antitrypsin. *Proc. Natl. Acad. Sci. USA* 78 (1981) 6826–6830

Ledley, F. D., Grenett, H. E., McGinnis, Shelnutt, M. and Woo, S. L. C. Retroviral mediated transfer of human phenylalanine hydroxylase into NIH3T3 and hepatoma cells. *Proc. Natl. Acad. Sci.* 83 (1986) 409–413

Long, G. L., Chandra, T., Woo, S. L. C., Kurachi, K. and Davie, E. W. Complete sequence of the cDNA for human α_1-antitrypsin and the gene for the S variant. *Biochemistry* 23 (1985) 4828–4837

Mann, R., Mulligan, R. C. and Baltimore, D. Construction of a retrovirus packaging mutant and its use to produce helper-free defective retrovirus. *Cell* 33 (1983) 153–159

Morse, J. O. α_1-Antitrypsin deficiency. *N. Engl. Med. J.* 299 (1978) 1045–1048

Owen, M. C. and Carrell, R. W. Sequence of the Z-variant typtic peptide. *FEBS Lett.* 79 (1977) 245–247

J. Inher. Metab. Dis. 9 Suppl. 1 (1986) 92–97

Direct Alteration of a Gene in the Human Genome

O. SMITHIES
Laboratory of Genetics, University of Wisconsin, Madison, WI, USA

Direct alteration of a gene in the human genome requires an understanding of the role of the gene in metabolism. A gene may need to be introduced into a specific tissue or alternatively it may be possible to use accessible tissue such as bone marrow. The level of gene expression required also needs to be known as does the position in the genome into which the gene is to be inserted. Insertion of DNA needs to be of high efficiency and accuracy. Various methods are available including virus, the use of inert adjuvant, microinjection and electroporation. The procedure with the most potential for accuracy is the use of specially designed plasmids. The example of the use of such a plasmid in achieving target modification of the β-globin gene is given. The method has high accuracy but low efficiency.

In the early sessions of this symposium the ways in which direct DNA analysis can be used to detect abnormal genes associated with inborn errors of metabolism were presented. A cautionary note was sounded on the need to become expert in Southern blot analysis and its interpretation before relying on one's own skill to identify carriers and embryos at risk for a given condition. While I endorse the need for caution, I nevertheless urge interested scientists to learn and use the technique themselves. Choose a condition that you are often called on to diagnose, and send DNA or the appropriate tissue sample to the experts – but if possible keep some for your own studies. Practise with this part of the sample after taking lessons from someone who does Southern blots frequently – and you will soon find that you can trust your own results and will rapidly be able to build up the necessary experience in interpreting the results (as judged by comparing them with those of the expert).

Time was also spent during the symposium on what can be done once a diagnosis (pre-natal or otherwise) has been obtained. Unfortunately, in many instances the possible actions are limited, and often they are less than satisfactory. It is not surprising therefore that the presentation by Professor Woo of his work with retroviruses that may eventually prove useful for the treatment by gene therapy of α_1-antitrypsin deficiency and phenylalanine hydroxylase deficiency was of great interest. Professor Woo was very careful to point out the various problems remaining to be solved before such therapy can be tried in humans – but he was also optimistic.

Journal of Inherited Metabolic Disease. ISSN 0141–8955.

In approaching the gene therapy of metabolic diseases it is essential to be specific. Some conditions are clearly more promising candidates for therapy than are others. Students of inborn errors of metabolism are better placed than I to evaluate which of the conditions encountered are potential candidates. For example, Professor Woo suggested that in the case of phenylhydroxylase deficiency it is probably necessary to introduce any corrective gene into hepatocytes, because in non-liver tissues the additional enzymes needed in the overall metabolic pathway of phenylalanine are not expressed. But it is also reasonable to expect that in some other conditions, it may not be necessary to introduce the corrective gene into the tissue nominally at risk. A more accessible tissue, such as bone marrow, may be adequate and it may not always be necessary to have a high level of expression of the introduced gene before useful results can be obtained. Yet there are conditions where both tissue specificity and a high level of expression are absolute prerequisites for usefulness. Haemoglobin for the treatment of a thalassaemic individual is only useful in a red cell, and a lot of it is needed! So in this case we need to introduce a globin gene into bone marrow stem cells in such a way that it is expressed at a high level in erythroid cells, but at an essentially zero level in non-erythroid cells.

Having chosen a gene, there is still a selection to be made of the method of introducing the DNA into the target cells, assuming that they are accessible. Probably the most efficient method of delivery currently available, as judged by the percentage of treated cells that will eventually incorporate the incoming DNA into their genomes, is to use viruses. RNA retroviruses of the sort discussed by Professor Woo are foremost in this regard. However, their apparent efficiency is not without a price – for at present the investigator cannot control the places in the genome where the resulting DNA proviruses will be inserted – they appear to be incorporated more or less randomly into the genomes of recipient cells. Furthermore, the incorporated sequences are often expressed at rather low levels. The overall result can be summarized in a somewhat oversimplified way by the statement that the system has *a high efficiency but a low accuracy*.

Why is accuracy (i.e. the site of incorporation of the exogenous DNA into the genome) desirable? At present, the answer to this question can only be stated as an assumption – that DNA sequences incorporated into the genome at their normal chromosomal locations are more likely to be normally controlled than are sequences incorporated randomly. This assumption is the guiding principle of my current work. Whether it is correct or not will only be determined by experiments which cannot be made until accurate insertion of appropriate sequences has been obtained.

Introduction of DNA into cells without the use of viruses is possible by several means. The most common until recently has been to co-precipitate the DNA with the genetically inert adjuvant calcium phosphate and to expose the recipient cells to the precipitate (Graham and van der Eb, 1973). This method is simple, and is capable of introducing DNA into many cells in a single experiment but only a small fraction of the treated cells (of the order of 1 in 10^5 – 10^6) subsequently incorporate the DNA into their genomes. Furthermore DNA sequences introduced by the calcium phosphate method are often incorporated into the genome at more than one site and usually there are several tandem copies of the inserted sequences at a given site.

Microinjection of DNA into single cells (Capecchi, 1980) has yielded many interesting results, particularly when the recipient cell is a fertilized egg (Palmiter *et al.*, 1982), but its use for gene therapy at the somatic level is likely to be quite limited.

Recently, electroporation (Neumann *et al.*, 1982) has proved promising. The method consists of exposing the recipient cells to a very short but high voltage electric pulse in the presence of DNA. The cells become porous for a brief time, and some of the DNA enters the cells, where it may then be incorporated into the genome of the recipient cells. Our experience with the method shows that under suitable conditions the method leads to the incorporation of single copies of the incoming DNA into the cellular genome at single sites. The efficiency of the method can be around 5×10^{-4}. This frequency of transformation is good, but it is still a long way from the efficiencies obtainable with retroviruses.

None of these procedures has intrinsic accuracy. So the question arises, is it possible to design into a method of introducing DNA into cells some features that will lead to the incorporation of the exogenous DNA into a specific place in the genome? Our work on this question forms the remainder of this paper.

About three and a half years ago we designed a plasmid with features aimed at facilitating its direct insertion into a specific gene in a preplanned way, while at the same time allowing us to assay the frequency of success. Figure 1, adapted from our recent article on the subject (Smithies *et al.*, 1985), illustrates the plasmid we used, pΔβ117, and helps in describing how it works.

The plasmid contains several important elements. The first is a 4.6 kb stretch of DNA taken from the human adult β-globin locus, which is the target gene. This DNA, shown by a heavy line in the figure, serves as a 'finder' sequence that enables the incoming DNA to find the equivalent sequence in the human chromosomal DNA. We expected that the finder sequence and the target sequence would recognize each other, and might then cross over to give rise to the desired gene modification. The expected recognition is by DNA-DNA interactions of the same type that enable accurate homologous crossing-over during meiosis. Homologous crossing-over involving exogenous DNA is increased in frequency in yeast cells (Orr-Weaver *et al.*, 1983) and in mammalian somatic cells (Kucherlapati *et al.*, 1984) by cutting the incoming DNA within the region of homology to generate ends that are recombinogenic. The incoming plasmid was therefore cut with the restriction enzyme *Bst*XI, as indicated.

A second feature in pΔβ117 is a single *Xba*I restriction enzyme to the *left* of the boxed letter S (explained below). (Notice that there is an *Xba*I site to the *right* of the normal chromosomal β-globin gene). If the plasmid crosses over homologously with its target sequence in the planned way it will be incorporated into the β-globin locus to give the modified chromosome shown in the lower part of the figure. When this occurs the left *Xba*I site from the plasmid will be next to the right *Xba*I site in the chromosome, and these two sites will be 7.7 kb apart. Consequently a novel 7.7 kb *Xba*I fragment will be potentially detectable in the genome of a correctly

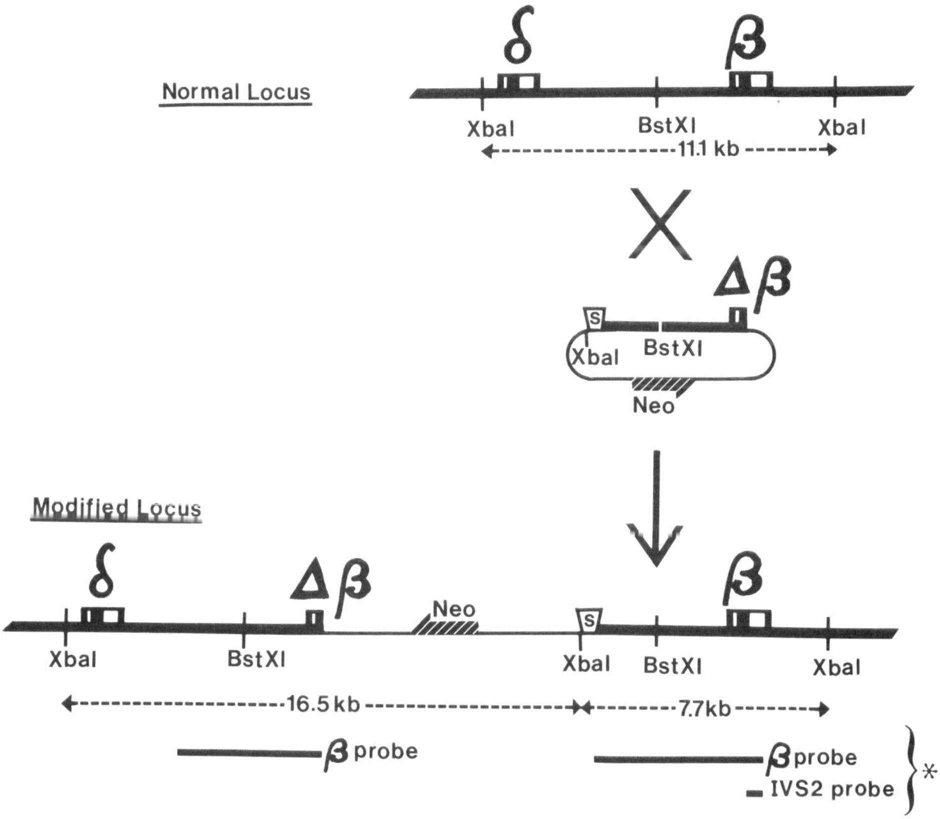

Figure 1 Test plasmid pΔβ117 (13.1 kb). ▬ Human DNA. —— Non-human DNA. [S] *supF* gene. * Diagnostic 7.7 kb *Xba*I fragment must hybridize to *both* probes Reproduced from Smithies *et al.* (1985), with permission.

modified cell. Rescuing this diagnostic *Xba*I fragment from the genomes of correctly modified cells forms the key to our assay for gene modification.

A third feature in the plasmid is indicated by the boxed letter S which signifies a suppressor gene, *supF*. Such suppressor genes will suppress (i.e. render unimportant) the amber mutations of certain mutant bacteriophages that are normally unable to grow on wild-type *E. coli*. So if bacteriophages that contain amber mutations are used to clone fragments of DNA from cells that have been treated with our plasmid, then only those bacteriophages that have rescued a fragment containing the *supF* gene should be able to grow. This procedure allows us to rescue DNA corresponding to the integrated copies of the pΔβ117 plasmid from many thousands of cells that have incorporated it into their genome. We can then ask whether any of the rescued integrants came from the correct site in the β-globin locus. If they did, they will be rescued in the form of 7.7 kb diagnostic *Xba*I fragment. If they are from elsewhere in the genome, they will be rescued as a fragment of some different size. The two classes of fragments can be distinguished in a more sophisticated way than by size alone, for only the diagnostic fragment will hybridize to a probe made from the IVS2 portion of the β-globin gene (see Figure 1).

In summary, recipient cells are treated with the test plasmid pre-cut with *Bst*XI, and allowed to grow. DNA is then prepared from them, cut with the restriction enzyme *Xba*I, packaged into the mutant bacteriophage and grown on *E. coli.*, and the resultant phages are blotted with the IVS2 probe. Only those that contain the 7.7 kb *Xba*I fragment will give a positive signal (showing that they are the result of accurate insertion of the incoming DNA into the β-globin locus). Thus we are rescuing the incorporated plasmids from the genomes of the treated cells and then asking how many of them came from the β-globin locus.

In this way we succeeded in demonstrating that targeted modification of the β-globin gene had occurred – as judged by the gene rescue assay – both in cells that were expressing the β-globin gene and in cells that were not expressing the gene. (Smithies *et al.*, 1985).

We then set out to isolate and clone one of the cells that had been modified in the correctly targeted way. To do this, we first used electroporation in the presence of the plasmid pΔβ117 to obtain pools of G418-resistant colonies (pΔβ117 contains a copy of the *neo* gene that confers G418-resistance on transformed cells and so G418 can be used to enrich treated cells for transformants). We tested each pool of cells by the assay, and only kept pools that scored positively for the diagnostic *Xba*I fragment. Re-pooling the positive cells into smaller and smaller pools, and keeping only positive pools, allowed us to identify a pool of only 20 colonies that still contained at least one colony having the correctly modified locus. At this stage we abandoned the assay, and directly tested the DNA of each of the individual colonies making up the 20-colony pool by the Southern blotting method. Two colonies were identified that had the modification, as judged by direct inspection of Southern blots of their genomic DNA after hybridizing *Xba*I digests of the DNA to the β IVS2 probe. (Correctly modified colonies will have the 7.7 kb diagnostic *Xba*I fragment (see Figure 1). Colonies modified at some other place in their genomes will have the 11 kb *Xba*I fragment characteristic of the unmodified normal β-globin locus. Our overall data showed that 1 in 300–1000 of the transformed (i.e. G418-resistant) colonies had a correctly modified β-globin gene. The other colonies had the plasmid incorporated elsewhere into their genomes.

These results show that DNA directly introduced into cells can be incorporated into the genome of a recipient cell in a planned manner at a planned site. The accuracy of the targeted modification appears to be perfect – but the efficiency (i.e. overall frequency) is still too low to be of practical value in gene therapy. Simply stated, we have achieved *high accuracy but low efficiency*.

The retrovirus method described above has high efficiency but low accuracy and what we all would like is to be able to devise a method that combines the better parts of these two procedures. When we have that – *high efficiency and high accuracy* – then gene therapy for the treatment of inborn errors of metabolism will begin to be really attractive.

ACKNOWLEDGEMENTS

This work was supported by National Institute of Health Grants AM20120 and GM20069. This is paper 2851 from the Laboratory of Genetics, University of WI, Madison, Wisconsin, USA.

REFERENCES

Capecchi, M. R. High efficiency transformation by direct microinjection of DNA into cultured mammalian cells. *Cell* 22 (1980) 479–488

Graham, F. L. and van der Eb, A. J. A new technique for the assay of infectivity of human adenovirus 5 DNA. *Virology* 52 (1973) 456–467

Kucherlapati, R. S., Eves, E. M., Song, K-Y., Morse, B. S. and Smithies, O. Homologous recombination between plasmids in mammalian cells can be enhanced by treatment of input DNA. *Proc. Natl. Acad. Sci. USA* 81 (1984) 3153–3157

Neumann, E., Schaefer-Ridder, M., Wang, Y. and Hofschneider, P. H. Gene transfer into mouse lyoma cells by electroporation in high electric fields. *EMBO J.* 7 (1982) 841–845

Orr-Weaver, T. L., Szostak, J. W. and Rothstein, R. J. Yeast transformation: a model system for the study of recombination. *Proc. Natl. Acad. Sci. USA* 78 (1981) 6354–6358

Palmiter, R. D., Brinster, R. L., Hammer, R. E., Trumbauer, M. E., Rosenfeld, M. G., Birnberg, N. C. and Evans, R. M. Dramatic growth of mice that develop from eggs microinjected with metallothionein-growth hormone fusion genes. *Nature* 300 (1982) 611–615

Smithies, O., Gregg, R. G., Boggs, S. S., Koralewski, M. A. and Kucherlapati, R. S. Insertion of DNA sequences into the human chromosomal β-globin locus by homologous recombination. *Nature* 317 (1985) 230–234

J. Inher. Metab. Dis. 9 Suppl. 1 (1986) 98–110

Diabetes Mellitus, Atherosclerosis, and the 5′ Flanking Polymorphism of the Human Insulin Gene

T. Mandrup-Poulsen[1], D. Owerbach[1,2], J. Nerup[1], K. Johansen[1] and A. Tybjærg Hansen[1]
[1]*Steno Memorial Hospital and Hagedorn Research Laboratory, Niels Steensensvej, DK-2820 Gentofte, Denmark*
[2]*University of Massachusetts, Medical Center, 55 Lake Avenue North, Mass. 01605, USA*

On the 5′ side of the human insulin gene is a highly polymorphic locus containing 2 major size classes of DNA restriction fragments which segregate in families as stable genetic elements. Fragments with an average size of about 600 base-pairs (bp) (the 'L-allele') seem to be a weak genetic marker for type 1 (insulin-dependent) diabetes mellitus, whereas fragments of an average size of about 2500 bp (the 'U-allele') have hitherto been associated with type 2 (non-insulin-dependent) diabetes mellitus and diabetic hypertriglyceridaemia. Recent evidence does not confirm the association between the U-allele and type 2 diabetes. Our own studies suggest that the U-allele is a fairly strong marker for the development of atherosclerosis with a relative risk for U-carriers of 3.36. The U-allele has not been associated with conventional cardiovascular risk factors such as body weight, blood pressure, or levels of blood glucose, triglycerides or lipoproteins. The putative functions of the polymorphic region in the aetiology of type 1 diabetes and atherosclerosis, and the relation of this region to other genetic markers for these disorders are not known.

In the last five years recombinant DNA technology as related to the insulin gene has been applied in the search for the genetic basis and possibly the aetiology of type 2 diabetes; as demonstrated in this review so far in vain. However, this work has revealed intriguing associations between a highly polymorphic DNA region flanking the human insulin gene and type 1 diabetes, but also a surprising relation between this region and atherosclerotic macrovascular disease in type 1 and type 2 diabetics as well as in non-diabetics.

THE HUMAN INSULIN GENE AND ITS FLANKING REGIONS

The amino acid sequence of human insulin has been known since 1959, but it was not until 1980 that the nucleotide sequence of the human insulin gene was deter-

Journal of Inherited Metabolic Disease. ISSN 0141–8955.

mined (Bell *et al.*, 1980a). The human insulin gene is located to the short arm of chromosome 11 in band p15 (Harper *et al.*, 1981; Owerbach *et al.*, 1981). The insulin gene proper consists of a coding sequence, interrupted by 2 intervening sequences of 179 and 786 nucleotides respectively (introns) (Figure 1), which codes for a 1430-nucleotide messenger RNA precursor. After excision of the 2 intervening sequences, the messenger RNA molecule for preproinsulin is formed.

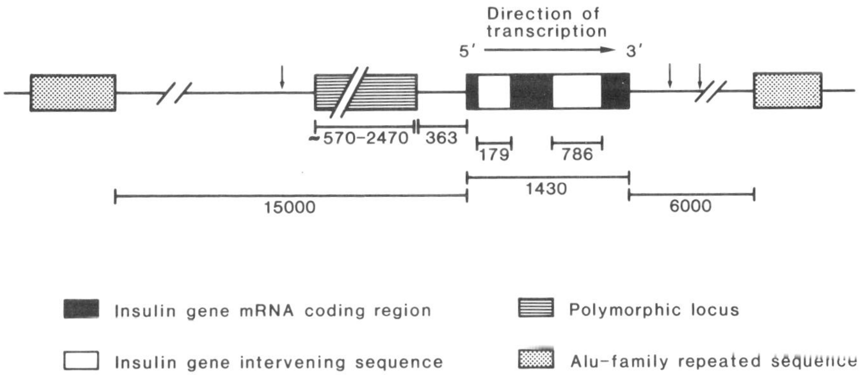

Figure 1 Organization of the insulin gene and flanking regions. Arrows indicate *Bgl*I restriction sites. Distances noted in base pairs. Modified after Bell *et al.* (1984)

The structure of the DNA-sequences flanking the insulin gene has also been determined recently (Figure 1). About 6000 base-pairs (bp) downstream (3′) and 15 000 bp upstream (5′) to the insulin gene are regions consisting of repetitive sequences, members of the so-called Alu-family (Bell *et al.*, 1980b; Harper *et al.*, 1981). The 3′ region is non-polymorphic, whereas the 5′ region is highly polymorphic, i.e. variable in length (Bell *et al.*, 1980b). The polymorphic 5′ region starts only 363 bp upstream to the insulin gene. Restriction fragments containing the 5′ region can be divided into 3 main size classes by their length.

The average sizes of the 3 major classes are 570 bp (class 1), 1320 bp (class 2), and 2470 bp (class 3) (Bell *et al.*, 1984). The length polymorphism is due to variation in the number of repetitions of a 14 bp oligonucleotide with the consensus sequence ACAGGGGTGTGGGG (Bell *et al.*, 1982; Ullrich *et al.*, 1982: Owerbach and Aagaard, 1984). This particular type of repetitive sequence is unique in the genome. On average class 1 fragments contain 40, class 2 95, and class 3 170 copies of this oligonucleotide.

Racial differences exist in the distribution of the size classes of the restriction fragments (Rotwein *et al.*, 1983; Bell *et al.*, 1984). Class 2 fragments occur in less than 1% of Caucasians in contrast to 22% of Negroes, and class 3 fragments are frequent in Caucasians but rare in Asians. Thus in Caucasians the 5′ region can be considered to be a locus with 2 'alleles', classes 1 and 3; or L-allele (for lower electrophoretic pattern) and U-allele (for upper electrophoretic pattern) respectively, in the terminology of Owerbach and Nerup (1982). The L- and U-alleles are stable genetic elements and they segregate in families according to mendelian laws (Figure 2) (Ullrich *et al.*, 1982; Owerbach and Nerup, 1982).

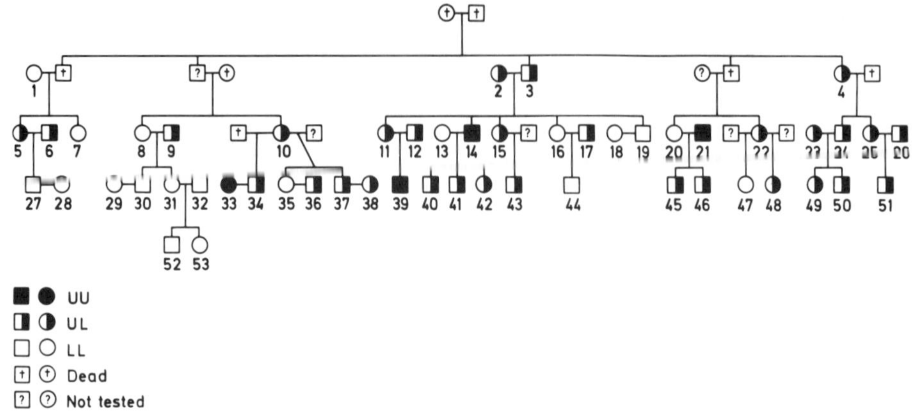

Figure 2 Distribution of U- and L-alleles in a large family. From Owerbach *et al.* (1982b)

Type 2 diabetes is probably a heterogeneous group of disorders, and since the polymorphic region starts close to the insulin gene coding sequence, it has been speculated that the two alleles influence the function of the insulin gene, e.g. by exerting different degrees of control on transcription. In both related and non-related non-diabetic members of a large family, the mean blood glucose concentrations as measured by glycosylated haemoglobin (haemoglobin A_{1c}, HbA_{1c}) were higher in U-allele carriers than in L-allele carriers (Owerbach *et al.*, 1982b). It is unknown whether this difference in the glucose regulation is due to a primary effect of the U-allele on the function of the insulin gene. However, the secretory capacity of the beta-cells was not found to be related to the U-allele in either type 2 diabetic or non-diabetic individuals (Permutt *et al.*, 1985).

We shall now review and discuss the development in the clinical associations of the restriction fragment length polymorphism flanking the insulin gene.

METHODS

The principles and procedures for the detection of DNA restriction length polymorphisms are described in detail elsewhere in this volume (Malcolm, 1986). In our studies, the restriction enzyme used was *Bgl*I, but other enzymes have been applied to the study of the insulin gene polymorphism, e.g. *Eco*RI, *Bgl*I, *Sac*I, etc. The recognition sites of *Bgl*I are indicated in Figure 1.

CLINICAL ASSOCIATIONS

Type 2 diabetes mellitus

Family and twin studies have indicated a strong heredity of type 2 diabetes but thus far it has not been possible to identify genetic markers for type 2 diabetes. Studies of the possible association between the polymorphic region 5′ to the insulin gene and type 2 diabetes were carried out almost simultaneously in San Francisco, USA

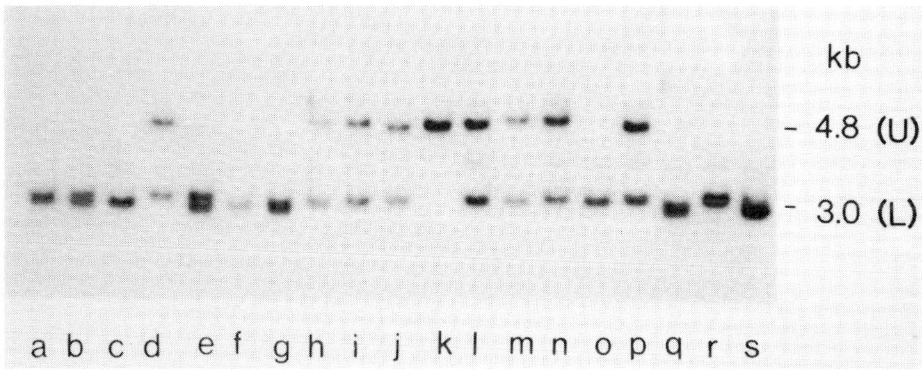

Figure 3 Autoradiogram of nitrocellulose filters with separated *BglI* restriction fragments hybridized with ^{32}P-labelled insulin gene probes. The two major size classes U and L are evident. The UU UL and LL genotypes are represented in lanes k, d and a, respectively

(Bell *et al.*, 1980b), St Louis, USA (Rotwein *et al.*, 1981), and Gentofte, Denmark (Owerbach and Nerup, 1982)

Bell and coworkers were unable to demonstrate differences in the distribution of U- and L-allele in a small series of type 2 and type 1 diabetics who were compared to non-diabetic controls (Bell *et al.*, 1980b). Two studies, published almost simultaneously, demonstrated an association between the U-allele and type 2 diabetes (Rotwein *et al.*, 1981, Owerbach and Nerup, 1982) (Table 1). This finding has recently been independently supported (Hitman *et al.*, 1984). However, in the combined series of Caucasian patients from San Francisco, St Louis, London and Gentofte, no significant association between the U-allele and type 2 diabetes can be demonstrated (Table 2). In addition, no association between the U-allele and type 2 diabetes was seen in 2 populations with high prevalences of type 2 diabetes; these were Nauruans (Serjeantson *et al.*, 1983) and Pima Indians (Knowler *et al.*, 1984).

Table 1 UU, UL and LL genotype frequencies in type 2 and type 1 diabetic patients and control groups

	UU	*UL*	*LL*
Type 2 diabetic patients ($n=47$)	8 (17%)	17 (36%)	22 (47%)
Type 1 diabetic patients ($n=37$)	1 (3%)	9 (24%)	27 (73%)
Normal glucose tolerance ($n=29$)	0 (0%)	16 (55%)	13 (45%)

UU+UL versus LL: Type 2 versus type 1 diabetic patients, $p=0.026$ (Fisher's exact test)
Type 2 diabetic patients versus normal glucose tolerance, $p=0.0333$
Type 1 diabetic patients versus normal glucose tolerance, $p=0.014$
Data from Owerbach and Nerup (1982), and Owerbach *et al.* (1982a)

Maturity-onset diabetes in the young

Maturity-onset diabetes in the young is a distinct disease entity characterized by a mild, non-insulin-dependent diabetes mellitus with few microvacular complications

Table 2 UU, UL and LL genotype frequencies in 4 series of Caucasian type 2 diabetic patients and non-diabetic control subjects

	Non-diabetics				*Type 2 diabetics*			
	UU	*UL*	*LL*	*Total*	*UU*	*UL*	*LL*	*Total*
San Francisco (Bell *et al.*, 1984)	8	38	37	83	4	24	48	76
St Louis (Rotwein *et al.*, 1983)	0	12	21	33	1	14	19	34
Copenhagen (Owerbach and Nerup, 1982; Owerbach *et al.*, 1982a)	0	16	13	29	8	17	22	47
London (Hitman *et al.*, 1984)	7	44	37	88	20	32	19	71
Total	15 (6.4%)	110 (47.2%)	108 (46.4%)	233 (100.0%)	33 (14.5%)	87 (38.2%)	108 (47.4%)	228 (100.0%)

UU+UL versus LL; Non-diabetic subjects versus type 2 diabetic patients: not significant
Allelic frequency of U: Non-diabetic subjects versus type 2 diabetic patients: not significant

and onset in youth. The disease is inherited as an autosomal dominant trait and thus it was obvious to look for an association between this disorder and the polymorphic insulin gene flanking region. Several studies have not been able to demonstrate an association between maturity-onset diabetes in the young and the U/L-alleles (Bell *et al.*, 1983; Owerbach *et al.*, 1983; Johnston *et al.*, 1984; Andreone *et al.*, 1985).

Type 1 diabetes mellitus

The genetic association between type 1 diabetes and the HLA-antigens D/DR3 and/or 4 is close to 100%. Thus it is unlikely that other disease susceptibility genes for type 1 diabetes should exist outside the HLA-region on the short arm of chromosome 6. Nevertheless, the LL-geneotype frequency in type 1 diabetic patients studied by Owerbach and Nerup (1982) was 73% as against 45% in non-diabetic controls tested for glucose intolerance ($p = 0.014$, Table 1) (Owerbach and Nerup, 1982; Owerbach *et al.*, 1982a). In a recent study of 113 type 1 diabetic patients a strong association between the L-allele and type 1 diabetes was demonstrated (Bell *et al.*, 1984) and by pooling of data on Caucasian type 1 diabetic patients from the 2 American and the Danish study populations, the statistical significance of this association was strengthened.

Hypertriglyceridaemia

A polymorphic region adjacent to the Apo-Al-lipoprotein gene on the long arm of chromosome 11 has been shown to be related to hypertriglyceridaemia and this particular polymorphism segregates with the disease in families. However, the Apo-Al-lipoprotein gene flanking DNA polymorphism is only part of the polygenic background of hypertriglyceridaemia. In the search for additional genetic markers for hypertriglyceridaemia, Jowett and coworkers (1984b) reported an association between hypertriglyceridaemia and the large size-class U-allele of the insulin gene flanking polymorphism. When these patients were subdivided on the basis of glucose tolerance, it was only hypertriglyceridaemic patients with impaired glucose tolerance who had an increased frequency of the U-allele (Jowett *et al.*, 1984b). Since analysis of the lipid and lipoprotein status of the type 2 diabetic patients included in the previously cited study populations had not been carried out in detail, Jowett and colleagues proposed that the association between the U-allele and type 2 diabetes was secondary to the association between the U-allele and diabetic hypertriglyceridaemia.

Atherosclerosis

Owerbach and Nerup (1982) noted a higher prevalence of atherosclerotic macrovascular disease (diabetic macroangiopathy) in type 2 diabetic patients carrying the UU- and UL-genotypes compared to type 2 diabetic patients with the LL-genotype. However, these investigators found a similar relation between macrovascular

Table 3 UU+UL and LL genotype frequencies in type 2 diabetic patients and non-diabetic control subjects in relation to macroangiopathy

	Type 2 diabetics		*Non-diabetic controls*	
	UU+UL	*LL*	*UU+UL*	*LL*
Total number of subjects	25	22	38	36
Number with macro-angiopathy	13 (52%)	6 (27%)	18 (47%)	4 (11%)
Number without macro-angiopathy	12 (48%)	16 (73%)	20 (53%)	32 (89%)

Frequency of genotypes UU+UL versus genotype LL in type 2 diabetic patients with macroangiopathy versus type 2 diabetics without macroangiopathy (13 : 6 versus 12 : 16) $p = 0.11$. UU versus LL in the same groups (6 : 6 versus 2 : 16): $p = 0.0483$
UU+UL versus LL in control subjects with macroangiopathy versus control subjects without macroangiopathy (18 : 4 versus 20 : 32): $p = 0.001$
UU+UL versus LL in type 2 diabetic patients without macroangiopathy versus control subjects without macroangiopathy (12 : 16 versus 20 : 32): not significant
Two-tailed Fisher's exact test. Data from Owerbach *et al.* (1982a)

disease and the U-allele in the non-diabetic control populations (Table 3) (Owerbach *et al.*, 1982a). These results indicated that the U-allele was associated with atherosclerosis and not only the diabetic subtype of macroangiopathy. This suggested that the type 2 diabetes/U-allele association was in fact due to the higher prevalence of atherosclerosis in type 2 diabetes and not, as previously thought, a primary association between type 2 diabetes and the U-allele. Since the prevalences of both atherosclerosis and type 2 diabetes increase with age, the selection of a study population of type 2 diabetic patients will necessarily select patients who have a high prevalence of atherosclerosis and *vice versa*.

The association between the U-allele and atherosclerosis was investigated in patients and controls, who were carefully characterized with regard to atherosclerosis and who had normal glucose metabolism. Of a group of 429 patients who had coronary angiography performed in the period 1977–1983 at the University Hospital of Copenhagen, Denmark, patients with verified coronary atherosclerosis i.e. intermediary or severe stenosis of two or three coronary vessels were randomly selected for this study.

Since previous studies had shown that a group of individuals selected as a random sample of the elderly background population would have a high prevalence of atherosclerosis (about 30% as assessed from questionnaires) and impaired glucose tolerance (about 30% as well, Owerbach *et al.*, 1982a), we chose as a control group all patients who had had coronary angiography performed in the period 1977–1983 at the University Hospital of Copenhagen and in whom the coronary vessels were found to be absolutely normal. The reasons for referring these patients for coronary angiography were heterogeneous, e.g. primarily valvular disease, non-characteristic chest pain or arrhythmias of unknown cause. The diagnosis of these patients at discharge from hospital were distributed in 9 different diagnostic categories (Table 4) (Mandrup-Poulsen *et al.*, 1984b). Thus selection of controls was not biased towards one type of non-atherosclerotic heart disease, which in itself might be associated positively or negatively with the genetic markers studied. The control subjects did not have symptoms or signs of macrovascular disease.

Table 4 Clinical diagnoses of non-atherosclerotic control subjects

Diagnoses	*N*
Variant angina	5
Stokes–Adams syndrome	1
Non-characteristic chest pain	5
Aortic insufficiency	4
Combined aortic–mitral insufficiency	1
Coarctation of the aorta	1
Abnormal exercise–ECG	1
Oesophageal spasm	2
Gallstone	1

Data from Mandrup-Poulsen *et al.* (1984b)

Subjects with elevated mean glucose concentrations as indicated by increased HbA_{1c} concentration or elevated fasting blood glucose concentrations were excluded from both atherosclerotic and non-atherosclerotic groups. The atherosclerotic patients were comparable to the control subjects with regard to age, body weight and blood pressure (Mandrup-Poulsen *et al.*, 1984a).

The U-allele frequency was 2.5 times higher in atherosclerotic patients than in controls (Table 5). Not surprisingly we found differences in sex distribution, smoking habits and lipoprotein fraction pattern (high VLDL and low HDL) between the 2 groups (Table 6). These data confirm that the 2 groups were representative of the atherosclerotic and non-atherosclerotic populations respectively. No association could be demonstrated between the U-allele and the known risk factors, e.g. body weight index, blood pressure, blood glucose, plasma triglyceride, plasma cholesterol or plasma lipoprotein fractions.

Table 5 Allelic frequency of U in atherosclerotic and non-atherosclerotic individuals

	Males	*Females*	*Total*
Atherosclerotic	0.29	0.42	0.30
($n = 41$)	(20/70)	(5/12)	(25/82)[a]
Non-atherosclerotic	0.15	0.09	0.12
($n = 21$)	(3/20)	(2/22)	(5/42)[a]
p-value (Fisher)	0.117	0.034	0.012

[a] The total number of alleles at the locus concerned is twice the number of subjects genotyped; the allelic frequency of U is the frequency of this allele expressed as a proportion of the total
Data from Mandrup-Poulsen *et al.* (1984a)

In Pima Indians it has recently been reported that there was no relation between ischaemic heart disease as assessed by resting electrocardiograms (ECG), and the UU+UL− genotypes, when small groups of type 2 diabetic and non-diabetic subjects were studied (Knowler *et al.*, 1984). If post myocardial infarction patients were compared to age-matched control subjects without clinical ischaemic heart disease, no differences in the distribution of UU+UL− genotypes were observed (Ferns *et al.*, 1985). Asymptomatic coronary artery disease in these controls was, however, not excuded by coronary arteriograms.

DISCUSSION

In summary, the U-allele has recently been associated with type 2 diabetes, diabetic hypertriglyceridaemia and atherosclerosis; and the L-allele with type 1 diabetes.

The L-allele and type 1 diabetes

Genetic markers for type 1 diabetes outside the HLA region have not been demonstrated previously and it seems unnecessary to assume that other major susceptibility genes exist outside the HLA region (Christy *et al.*, 1984). However, the possibility cannot be excluded that the L-allele is a weak genetic marker for type 1 diabetes in linkage disequilibrium with a hitherto unknown susceptibility locus on the short arm of chromosome 11. Family studies are needed to show a segregation of the L-allele with type 1 diabetes by formal linkage analysis.

The U-allele and type 2 diabetes, hypertriglyceridaemia and atherosclerosis

The apparently contradictory results regarding the clinical associations of the U-allele are probably primarily due to heterogeneity of the study populations with regard to racial composition, glucose tolerance and occurrence of atherosclerosis. If patients with atherosclerosis were excluded from the material of type 2 diabetics studied by Owerbach and colleagues (1982a), there were no longer statistically significant differences in the U-allele frequency when type 2 diabetic patients were

Table 6 Some cardiovascular risk factors in atherosclerotic and non-atherosclerotic subjects

	Study groups		
	Atherosclerotic	*Non-atherosclerotic*	*p*
Triglyceride before coronary angiography (mmol L^{-1})	2.4 (0.8–12.2) ($n = 41$)	1.4 (0.5–2.0) ($n = 17$)	<0.05
Triglyceride after coronary angiography (mmol L^{-1})	1.8 (0.6–5.4) ($n = 21$)	1.7 (0.9–2.9) ($n = 13$)	NS
Cholesterol before coronary angiography (mmol L^{-1})	7.0 (4.5–9.5) ($n = 41$)	6.6 (4.6–9.3) ($n = 20$)	NS
Cholesterol after coronary angiography (mmol L^{-1})	6.8 (4.4–11.0) ($n = 21$)	7.3 (5.3–9.8) ($n = 13$)	NS
HDL (mmol L^{-1})	1.3 (0.7–1.9) ($n = 21$)	1.6 (1.1–2.4) ($n = 13$)	<0.02
VLDL (mmol L^{-1})	1.7 (0–3.1) ($n = 21$)	0.9 (0.1–2.3) ($n = 13$)	<0.05
LDL (mmol L^{-1})	4.8 (2.5–7.5) ($n = 21$)	4.5 (2.3–7.2) ($n = 13$)	NS
$C3^F$ allelic frequency	0.17 (14/84) ($n = 42$)	0.26 (11/42) ($n = 21$)	NS
$HbA_{1}c$ (%)	5.69 (4.9–6.4) ($n = 42$)	5.65 (4.1–6.3) ($n = 21$)	NS
Fasting blood glucose (mmol L^{-1})	5.07 (3.8–6.3) ($n = 42$)	5.03 (4.1–6.6) ($n = 20$)	NS
Tobacco consumption (kg/lifetime)	231 (0–482) ($n = 38$)	148 (0–547) ($n = 21$)	<0.02
Sex ratio (M : F)	35 : 6	10 : 11	<0.002

Values are given as means (range)
NS: not significant
Data from Mandrup-Poulsen *et al.* (1984a)

Table 7 UU+UL genotype frequency in non-diabetic atherosclerotic patients and in non-atherosclerotic type 2 diabetic patients versus control subjects

	UU+UL genotype frequency (%)			
	Type 2 diabetic patients	*Control subjects*	*Relative risk*	*p (Fisher)*
Atherosclerosis study	49 ($n = 41$)	24 ($n = 21$)	3.36	0.037
Type 2 diabetes study[a]	43 ($n = 28$)	36 ($n = 33$)	1.31	NS

[a] Data from Owerbach *et al.* (1982a) and Mandrup-Poulsen *et al.* (1984a), corrected for presence of macroangiopathy (type 2 diabetic patients and control subjects), and impaired glucose tolerance (control subjects)
NS: not significant

compared with non-diabetic controls (Table 7). U-carriers have a relative risk of developing atherosclerosis which is 2–3 times higher than the relative risk for the same individuals of developing type 2 diabetes (Table 7). In the study of Mandrup-Poulsen and coworkers (1984a) the cardiovascular status of the patients and controls was evaluated by coronary angiography, whereas the prevalence of atherosclerosis in the type 2 diabetic patients (Owerbach *et al.*, 1982a) was assessed epidemiologically on the basis of questionnaires and hospital records. Thus it is likely that the relative risk of developing type 2 diabetes for U-carriers could in fact be lower than 1.31, if it were possible to exclude patients with abnormal coronary angiograms from the calculation.

Mandrup-Poulsen and coworkers did not find a correlation between the plasma triglyceride level and the U-allele. In the study of Jowett and colleagues (1984b) the patients were not characterized with regard to prevalence, extent or severity of atherosclerosis, and it is possible that the reported association between the U-allele and hypertriglyceridaemia in diabetics is secondary to a very high prevalence of macrovascular disease in these particular patients. That atherosclerosis and diabetes accompany each other seems to be established beyond doubt (Jarrett, 1984). There is no evidence, however, to support the concept of a causal relationship between chronic hyperglycaemia and atherosclerotic macrovascular disease. It is conceivable, however, that a common genetic background exists for these 2 diseases, predisposing to both atherosclerosis and type 2 diabetes (Jarrett, 1984).

Genes for a number of risk factors for the development of atherosclerosis have recently been mapped to 2 different chromosomes. The C3-complement type is associated with familial hypercholesterolaemia and the gene coding for the C3-complement phenotype has been localized to chromosome 19. Mandrup-Poulsen and colleagues (1984a) found no association between the U-allele and the $C3^F$-complement type. The gene for apolipoprotein E is situated on the same chromosome and this gene together with other factors causes familial type III hyperlipoproteinaemia. Both of these hyperlipoproteinaemias are well-known risk factors for the development of severe premature atherosclerosis. The Apo-A1-lipoprotein gene has been assigned to the long arm of chromosome 11. Apo-lipoprotein A1 is the major constituent of HDL, and low plasma HDL confers increased risk of developing atherosclerosis. The insulin gene flanking polymorphism and the Apo-A1-lipoprotein related polymorphism do not co-segregate (Jowett *et al.*, 1984a).

A gene product of the polymorphic insulin gene flanking region is not known. If this region is transcribed at all, the peptide formed would be of varying length, and every third amino acid would be glycine or proline depending on the direction of translation (Bell *et al.*, 1984). Interestingly, every third amino acid in the alpha-chain of collagen is in fact glycine (Prockop *et al.*, 1979) and an attractive hypothesis could be that differences in the structure of arterial vessel wall collagen may determine the susceptibility of an individual to atherogenic risk factors, assuming that the gene product of the polymorphic region is a collagen-like protein. However, the polymorphic region may be a genetic marker of atherosclerosis through linkage disequilibrium with an atherosclerosis-predisposing gene located close to the polymorphic region. The 45 000 bp restriction fragment containing the insulin gene and its flanking regions has not been shown to contain other genes.

LL-homozygous individuals seem to have a low risk for developing atherosclerosis. This group is particularly interesting, since a higher prevalence of macrovascular disease has previously been demonstrated in LL-homozygous males compared to LL-homozygous females (Owerbach *et al.*, 1982a). In addition, differences in the prevalence of atherosclerosis were observed in LL-homozygous individuals in the non-diabetic population, the group with impaired glucose tolerance, and the type 2 diabetic patients (8%, 15% and 27% respectively, Owerbach *et al.*, 1982a). In the study of the non-diabetic atherosclerotic patients (Mandrup-Poulsen *et al.*, 1984a) a significantly higher plasma triglyceride concentration and lower HDL concentration was found in LL-homozygous patients with atherosclerosis than in LL-homozygous non-atherosclerotic individuals. In other words, the 'pure' effects of the cardiovascular risk factors are easier to demonstrate in LL-homozygous 'low-risk' individuals. This implies that epidemiological studies of the influence of different risk factors on the development of atherosclerosis or intervention studies with impact on risk factors may give inconclusive results if the study populations are not genetically characterized.

CONCLUSIONS AND PERSPECTIVES

The studies reviewed here illustrate the epidemiological problems to be confronted when marker–disease associations are investigated in disorders of a mixed genetic–environmental etiology, present not only in a small group of patients, but also in a non-symptomatic form in the background population.

Genetic and clinical heterogeneity probably exists in atherosclerosis, and the application of DNA recombinant technology to the study of such inhomogeneous disorders demands a highly stringent selection and characterization of patients and controls. The previous studies of the insulin gene flanking polymorphism and atherosclerosis have been designed as case-control studies, but U/L-typing may help to identify high-risk individuals for the development of atherosclerosis in families or even in the general population in which intervention with impact on risk factors would be relevant.

ACKNOWLEDGEMENTS

The authors wish to thank A. Rafn for the preparation of this manuscript.

REFERENCES

Andreone, T., Fajans, S., Rotwein, P., Skolnick, M. and Permutt, M. A. Insulin gene analysis in a family with maturity-onset diabetes of the young. *Diabetes* 34 (1985) 108–114

Bell, G. I., Horita, S. and Karam, J. H. A polymorphic locus near the human insulin gene is associated with insulin-dependent diabetes mellitus. *Diabetes* 33 (1984) 176–183

Bell, G. I., Pictet, R. L., Rutter, W. J., Cordell, B., Tischer, E. and Goodman, H. M. Sequence of the human insulin gene. *Nature* 284 (1980a) 26–32

Bell, G. I., Pictet, R. and Rutter, W. J. Analysis of the regions flanking the human insulin gene and sequence of an Alu family member. *Nucleic Acids Res.* 8 (1980b) 4091–4109

Bell, G. I., Selby, M. J. and Rutter, W. J. The highly polymorphic region near the human insulin gene is composed of simply tandemly repeating sequences. *Nature* 295 (1982) 31–35

Bell, G. I., Wainscoat, J. S., Old, J. M., Chlouverakis, C., Keen, H., Turner, R. C. and Weatherall, D. J. Maturity onset diabetes of the young is not linked to the insulin gene. *Br. Med. J.* 286 (1983) 590–592

Christy, M., Mandrup-Poulsen, T. and Nerup, J. Genetic markers for insulin dependent diabetes mellitus. *Ann. Clin. Res.* 16 (1984) 53–63

Ferns, G. A. A., Stocks, J., Ritchie, C. and Galton, D. J. Genetic polymorphisms of apolipoprotein C-III and insulin in survivors of myocardial infarction. *Lancet* 2 (1985) 300–303

Harper, M. E., Ullrich, A. and Saunders, G. F. Localization of the human insulin gene to the distal end of the short arm of chromosome 11. *Proc. Natl. Acad. Sci.* 78 (1981) 4458–4460

Hitman, G. A., Jowett, N. I., Williams, L. G., Humphries, S., Winter, R. M. and Galton, D. J. Polymorphisms in the 5′-flanking region of the insulin gene and non-insulin-dependent diabetes. *Clin. Sci.* 66 (1984) 383–388

Jarrett, R. J. Type 2 (non-insulin-dependent) diabetes mellitus and coronary heart disease – chicken, egg or neither? *Diabetologia* 26 (1984) 99–102

Johnston, C., Owerbach, D., Leslie, R. D. G., Pyke, D. A. and Nerup, J. Mason-type diabetes and DNA insertion polymorphism. *Lancet* 1 (1984) 280

Jowett, N. I., Rees, A., Williams, L. G., Stocks, J., Vella, M. A., Hitman, G. A., Katz, J. and Galton, D. J. Insulin and apolipoprotein A-1/C-III gene polymorphisms relating to hypertriglyceridaemia and diabetes mellitus. *Diabetologia* 27 (1984a) 180–183

Jowett, N. I., Williams, L. G., Hitman, G. A. and Galton, D. J. Diabetic hypertriglyceridaemia and related 5′ flanking polymorphism of the human insulin gene. *Br. Med. J.* 288 (1984b) 96–99

Knowler, W. C., Pettitt, D. J., Vasquez, B., Rotwein, P. S., Andreone, T. L. and Permutt, M. A. Polymorphism in the 5′ flanking region of the human insulin gene. Relationships with non-insulin-dependent diabetes mellitus, glucose and insulin concentrations, and diabetes treatment in Pima Indians. *J. Clin. Invest.* 74 (1984) 2129–2135

Malcolm, S. Direct DNA analysis in family studies. *J. Inher. Metab. Dis.* 9 Suppl. 1 (1986) 32–37

Mandrup-Poulsen, T., Owerbach, D., Mortensen, S. A., Johansen, K., Meinertz, H., Sørensen, H. and Nerup, J. DNA sequences flanking the insulin gene on chromosome 11 confer risk of atherosclerosis. *Lancet* 1 (1984a) 250–252

Mandrup-Poulsen, T., Owerbach, D., Mortensen, S. A., Johansen, K., Meinertz, H., Sørensen, H. and Nerup, J. A genetic marker for atherosclerosis? *Lancet* 1 (1984b) 1131

Owerbach, D. and Aagaard, L. Analysis of a 1963-bp polymorphic region flanking the human insulin-gene. *Gene* 32 (1984) 475–479

Owerbach, D. and Nerup, J. Restriction fragment length polymorphism of the insulin gene in diabetes mellitus. *Diabetes* 21 (1982) 275–277

Owerbach, D., Bell, G. I., Rutter, W. J., Brown, J. A. and Shows, T. B. The insulin gene is located on the short arm of chromosome 11 in humans. *Diabetes* 30 (1981) 267–270

Owerbach, D., Johansen, K., Billesbølle, P., Poulsen, S., Schroll, M. and Nerup, J. Possible association between DNA sequences flanking the insulin gene and atherosclerosis. *Lancet* 2 (1982a) 1291–1293

Owerbach, D., Poulsen, S., Billesbølle, P. and Nerup, J. DNA insertion sequences near the insulin gene affect glucose regulation. *Lancet* 1 (1982b) 880–883

Owerbach, D., Thomsen, B., Johansen, K., Lamm, L. U. and Nerup, J. DNA insertion sequences near the insulin gene are not associated with maturity-onset diabetes of young people. *Diabetologia* 25 (1983) 18–20

Permutt, M. A., Rotwein, P., Andreone, T., Ward, W. K. and Porte, D. Islet beta-cell function and polymorphism in the 5′-flanking region of the human insulin gene. *Diabetes* 34 (1985) 311–314

Prockop, D. J., Kivirikko, K. L., Tuderman, L. and Guzman, N. A. The biosynthesis of collagen and its disorders. *N. Engl. J. Med.* 301 (1979) 13-23

Rotwein, P., Chyn, R., Chirgwin, J., Cordell, B., Goodman, H. M. and Permutt, M. A. Polymorphism in the 5′-flanking region of the human insulin gene and its possible relation to type 2 diabetes. *Science* 213 (1981) 1117–1120

Rotwein, P. S., Chirgwin, J., Province, M., Knowler, W. C., Pettitt, D. J., Cordell, B., Goodman, H. M. and Permutt, M. A. Polymorphism in the 5′ flanking region of the human insulin gene: a genetic marker for non-insulin-dependent diabetes. *N. Engl. J. Med.* 308 (1983) 65–71

Serjeantson, S. W., Owerbach, D., Zimmet, P., Nerup, J. and Thoma, K. Genetics of diabetes in Nauru: effects of foreign admixture, HLA antigens and the insulin-gene-linked polymorphism. *Diabetologia* 25 (1983) 13–17

Ullrich, A., Dull, T. J., Gray, A., Philips, J. A. and Peter, S. Variation in the sequence and modification state of the human insulin gene flanking regions. *Nucl. Acids Res.* 10 (1982) 2225–2230

J. Inher. Metab. Dis. 9 Suppl. 1 (1986) 111–114

WORKSHOP ON SCREENING FOR CONGENITAL ADRENAL HYPERPLASIA (STEROID 21-HYDROXYLASE DEFICIENCY)

Introduction

G. M. ADDISON
Royal Manchester Children's Hospital, Hospital Road, Pendlebury, Manchester M27 1HA, UK

Neonatal screening for several genetic and developmental diseases, in particular for phenylketonuria and congenital hypothyroidism, has become well established in many countries. Screening for other disorders occurs in a few countries. It has been assumed that since blood samples are already being collected for screening purposes the chief limitation to expanding the range of tests is technological i.e. it relies on the development of appropriate methodology. On this basis lists of diseases suitable for screening have been proposed (Bickel, 1980). This simplistic approach to screening needs critical evaluation to make neonatal screening practicable and beneficial.

Criteria have been well established with regard to the clinical, health care and laboratory aspects of screening. These criteria have been carefully reviewed by Sackett (1975) with particular reference to adult diseases. However, his observations and criticisms of screening programmes are equally pertinent to neonatal screening. In particular the advancement of the date of diagnosis is insufficient reason on its own to justify the introduction of a screening programme without real evidence of benefit to the patient or community.

Sackett and Holland (1975) classified screeners into 'evangelists' and 'snails'. The former, being convinced advocates of screening, use arguments which rely on pre-existing evidence, individual experience and 'common sense'. On the other hand, 'snails' believe that screening, like any other medical or scientific advance, should be subject to rigorous evaluation based on established criteria to ensure that the ultimate conclusion is correct. That arguments between these two opposite approaches occur is well illustrated by the paper of Dodge and Ryley (1982) on screening for cystic fibrosis and the subsequent correspondence in the *Archives of Disease in Childhood*.

The main problem in the evangelical approach is the absence of controlled trials which would compare the screening programme with the best current clinical and laboratory methods for achieving the diagnosis. In the case of neonatal hypothyroidism much of the clinical data on which the case for screening was established was obtained when it was technically very difficult to assess neonatal thyroid function biochemically, whereas modern methods require small quantities of blood and the tests are usually available rapidly and locally. It is generally

Journal of Inherited Metabolic Disease. ISSN 0141–8955.

accepted that this programme has justified itself even in the absence of controlled trials but the programmes themselves have raised important questions which cannot now be answered because of the ethical difficulties in going back and carrying out controlled studies.

One important area often overlooked when introducing neonatal screening for congenital disease is the psychological aspect for both parent and child. These will obviously differ if the child is affected from those in whom the screening test proves to be false positive or false negative. Equally, the absence of screening can produce psychological disturbances if the parent discovers that screening could have detected the disorder in his child at a time when it was more amenable to treatment (McNeil and Thelin, 1980).

Screening for the 21-hydroxylase variant of congenital adrenal hyperplasia (McKusick 20191) has been proposed and, following the report of Pang and co-workers (1977) of a pilot screening programme using the measurement of 17α-hydroxyprogesterone in dried blood spots, several groups in Europe, Japan and North America have carried out studies or developed screening programmes. These programmes have been applied to high risk groups such as the Alaskan Eskimo and the inhabitants of the island of La Réunion as well as in normal Caucasian populations. It seemed an appropriate time, therefore, to bring together representatives of interested laboratories, paediatric endocrinologists and geneticists to review the current status of screening for 21-hydroxylase deficiency. To this end a workshop was organized by The Society for the Study of Inborn Errors of Metabolism in conjunction with the 23rd annual meeting in Liverpool, September 1985.

Unlike PKU and congenital hypothyroidism, 21-hydroxylase deficiency does not cause mental retardation. However, the presentation of the disease is variable and, in the severe salt-losing forms, avoidable morbidity and mortality can occur if diagnosis is unduly delayed, particularly in males in the first two weeks of life. Missed diagnosis can also lead to assignment of incorrect gender or insidious and irreversible developmental changes with problems of growth and development. The arguments for screening in this disorder rely on the above observations. On the other hand many patients present clinically e.g. virilized females with ambiguous genitalia or, as with some salt-losing crises in the second week of life, too early to be detected in current screening programmes.

Retrospective analyses by various groups (Murtaza *et al.*, 1980; Werder *et al.*, 1980; Lebovitz *et al.*, 1984) have produced evidence that the diagnosis of males with 21-hydroxylase deficiency has often been missed or delayed. Preliminary evidence from two different approaches in Birmingham, presented at the workshop, has suggested on the other hand that this pattern of diagnosis may be changing and that there has been a substantial shift to much earlier diagnosis of 21-hydroxylase deficiency as the availability of assays for plasma 17α-hydroxyprogesterone has increased. This again emphasises the dangers of relying on retrospective analysis as used by Lebovitz and co-workers (1984) to justify a screening programme. Have these shifts in the age of diagnosis been enough to weaken the case for screening or will a significant number of children remain undiagnosed and at clinical risk? Another question which remains to be answered is: could at least some of the excess loss of males be pre- rather than postnatal and therefore already happened by the time of neonatal screening?

The variability of adrenal function in the neonate is an additional potential pitfall in screening if the programmme is based on the measurement of one particular steroid metabolite in a complex and rapidly changing pattern which is peculiar to the fetus and the newborn. As can be seen from the papers presented at the workshop there are problems of assay specificity and cross reaction between steroids. Alternative steroids to 17α-hydroxyprogesterone have been suggested, e.g. 21-deoxycortisol (Milevitz *et al.*, 1984).

The workshop heard two papers on the clinical (Dr Hughes) and biochemical (Dr Honor) backgrounds to screening followed by presentations on the results of screening programmes in Scotland, Italy and France. A discussion period followed in which the need for and current status of screening for 21-hydroxylase deficiency were debated. No overall conclusions could be reached (both 'evangelists' and 'snails' were well represented). Too few results are available to assess the performance of screening programmes and the different assays used. However, current evidence suggests that screening neonates for 21-hydroxylase deficiency could be useful and there is a strong case for the setting up of large controlled studies to see whether the actual performance of these programmes is of benefit. The need for these studies is urgent because it is difficult to conduct controlled studies once the procedure is regarded as routine.

In conclusion, following the initial reports of screening for 21-hydroxylase deficiency, a second phase of controlled studies of the cost effectiveness and clinical benefit of screening for 21-hydroxylase deficiency are needed in order to decide whether such procedures should be recommended for routine use.

ACKNOWLEDGMENTS

The financial sponsorship of Amersham International PLC, CIS (UK) Ltd, RIA (UK) Ltd and E. R. Squibb and Co Ltd towards the expenses of running the workshop on screening for congenital adrenal hyperplasia is gratefully acknowledged.

REFERENCES

Bickel, H. Rationale of neonatal screening for inborn errors of metabolism. In Bickel, H., Guthrie, R., Hammerson, G. (eds.) *Neonatal Screening for Inborn Errors of Metabolism*, Springer Verlag, Berlin, 1980, pp. 1–6

Dodge, J. A. and Ryley, H. C. Screening for cystic fibrosis. *Arch. Dis. Child.* 57 (1982) 774–779. See also Phelan, P. D. Commentary, *ibid* pp. 779–780 and correspondence in *Arch. Dis. Child.* 58 (1983) 317–318

Lebovitz, R. M., Pauli, R. M. and Laxova, R. Delayed diagnosis in congenital adrenal hyperplasia. Need for newborn screening. *Am. J. Dis. Child.* 138 (1984) 571–573

McNeil, T. F. and Thelin, T. Psychological considerations in screening for congenital diseases. In Böstrom, H. and Ljungstedt, N. (eds.) *Congenital Diseases in Childhood. Medical and Socio-Medical Aspects*, Almqvist and Wiksell International, Stockholm, 1980, pp. 196–219

Milevitz, A., Vecsei, P., Korth-Schütz, S., Haack, D., Kösler, A., Lichtwald, K., Lewicka, S. and Mittelstaedt, G. Development of plasma 21-deoxycortisol radioimmunoassay and application to the diagnosis of patients with 21-hydroxylase deficiency. *J. Steroid Biochem.* 21 (1984) 185–191

Murtaza, L., Sibert, J. R., Hughes, I. A. and Balfour, I. C. Congenital adrenal hyperplasia – a clinical and genetic survey. *Arch. Dis. Child.* 55 (1980) 622–625

Pang, S., Hotchkiss, J., Drash, A. L., Levine, L. S. and New, M. I. Microfilter paper method for 17-hydroxyprogesterone radioimmunoassay: its application for rapid screening for congenital adrenal hyperplasia. *J. Clin. Endocrinol. Metab.* 45 (1977) 1003–1008

Sackett, D. L. Laboratory screening: a critique. *Fed. Proc.* 34 (1975) 2157–2161

Sackett, D. L. and Holland, W. W. Controversy in the detection of disease. *Lancet* 2 (1975) 357–359

Werder, E. A., Siebenmann, R. E., Knorr Mürset, G. *et al.* The incidence of congenital adrenal hyperplasia in Switzerland: a survey of patients born in 1960–1974. *Helv. Paediat. Acta* 35 (1980) 5–11

J. Inher. Metab. Dis. 9 *Suppl.* 1 (1986) 115–123

Clinical Aspects of Congenital Adrenal Hyperplasia: Early Diagnosis and Prognosis

I. A. Hughes
Department of Child Health, University of Wales College of Medicine, Heath Park, Cardiff, CF4 4XN, UK

The neonatal presentation of congenital adrenal hyperplasia is either virilization of females or salt loss in both sexes. Early diagnosis is based on the rapid measurement of plasma 17α-hydroxyprogesterone. Milder forms of congenital adrenal hyperplasia can present later in life with abnormalities of somatic or sexual development. The majority of cases of congenital adrenal hyperplasia are clinically diagnosable in the first 2–3 weeks of life: the need for screening for the remaining missed cases and the late onset types remains to be established.

A Neopolitan anatomist, de Crecchio (1865), first described in detail the anatomical dissection of a 'man' who had died during an episode of vomiting and diarrhoea associated with salt-losing congenital adrenal hyperplasia (CAH). Although designated female at birth, a male gender was declared once and for all at four years of age, and he conducted his affairs, including sexual intercourse, as a man until his early demise. The autopsy showed a large phallus, hypospadias, empty labioscrotal folds, normal female internal genitalia and massively enlarged adrenal glands. Hence the alternative term, adrenogenital syndrome, for this condition.

The familial nature of the disorder was alluded to by Phillips (1887) who reported four children in one family who were described as hermaphrodite at birth and died during early infancy following a period of marked wasting. The last child, a female, was severely virilized. The author stated that it was fortunate for the community that these 'creatures do not survive, usually wasting and dying of inanition shortly after birth'. Perhaps this observation is one of the more persuasive reasons for the introduction of a newborn screening programme for CAH. The tragedy of inappropriate gender assignment is vividly illustrated in a transcript of a lecture delivered by H. W. Jones, Jr. (1979) on the history of the adrenogenital syndrome. He describes a child who was initially reared as a male. When a change to female gender was attempted it was refused by the parents and family priest. Subsequent disclosure to the patient of the true gender led to despair and eventual suicide. Fortunately such disasters of management are rarely encountered now that the wide spectrum of clinical abnormalities associated with CAH are increasingly recognised.

Journal of Inherited Metabolic Disease. ISSN 0141–8955.

CLINICAL PRESENTATION

The principal presenting features of CAH in the newborn and in later life are summarized in Table 1. The clinical hallmark of CAH is virilization. This is usually present at birth in affected females, but is delayed until the third or fourth year of life in boys. Excessive androgen production results from the accumulation of 17α-hydroxy-progesterone (17P) which is converted to androstenedione and subsequently to testosterone in the liver. More than 90% of cases are the result of a defect in 21-hydroxylation (Hughes, 1982); hence this is the subject of pilot CAH screening programmes at present. Fetal steroidogenesis is established by the end of the first trimester so that the anlagen for the development of the external genitalia (genital tubercle and folds) is exposed to increased serum androgen concentrations from early gestation. It is an unresolved question why the external genitalia of affected males are not virilized at birth.

Table 1 Clinical presentation of CAH

Newborn		*Later life*
Ambiguous genitalia:	complete	Pseudoprecocious puberty
	isolated clitoromegaly	Isolated pubarche
	isolated labial fusion	Isolated clitoromegaly
Cryptorchid, hypospadic 'male'		Rapid growth
Salt-wasting		Hirsutism
		Menstrual disorders
		Infertility
		Cryptic cases

The degree of virilization in affected females at birth can be quite variable ranging from isolated clitoromegaly or labial fusion to complete labial fusion ('scrotalization') and marked clitoromegaly with a phallic urethra. The apparent 'male' has bilateral 'cryptorchidism' with or without hypospadias. It is mandatory to question the sex of such an infant if the tragic consequences of inappropriate gender assignment are to be avoided. It is worth remembering that CAH is the commonest cause of ambiguous genitalia in the newborn and 21-hydroxylase deficiency is the most frequent enzymatic defect. The problem is a medical emergency and should be investigated urgently (Hughes and Davies, 1980).

More than half the infants with CAH also have an associated defect in aldosterone biosynthesis leading to salt-wasting. The onset of symptoms is usually delayed beyond the first week of life and after discharge from hospital. Delays in diagnosis have (and may still do) led to peripheral circulatory collapse and death. Newborn screening for CAH might detect affected male salt-losers who, contrary to affected females, do not display alerting signs of virilization.

Non-salt-losing male infants are not clinically detected at birth. Signs of virilization (penile growth, pubic hair, increased muscle bulk, rapid linear growth) appear later in infancy and childhood as a problem of pseudoprecocious puberty. The prepubertal size of the testes is a vital clinical sign of peripheral androgen production independent of central gonadotrophin stimulation. It is now recognized that CAH can masquerade as several different disorders presenting later in life (see Table 1). The term 'cryptic' refers to asymptomatic cases of CAH discovered from analysis of HLA haplotypes and plasma steroid responses to ACTH stimulation (New *et al.*, 1981).

EARLY DIAGNOSIS OF CAH

Immunoassays for plasma 17P are now readily available: it is widely accepted that measurement of this steroid soon after birth provides a rapid and reliable diagnostic test for 21-hydroxylase deficiency in the majority of affected cases. Figure 1 illustrates markedly elevated concentrations of plasma 17P within hours of birth

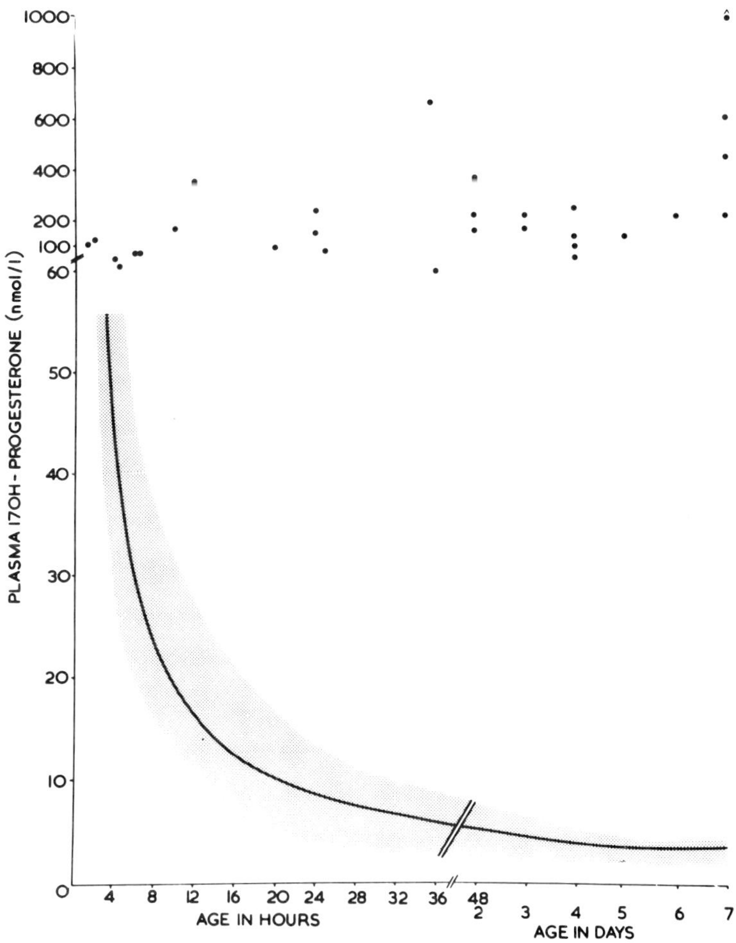

Figure 1 Plasma 17P concentrations in newborn infants. The line and shaded area represent the mean and range of values in normal term infants. Also shown are individual values obtained in infants with untreated CAH (Reproduced with permission of the editor of *Archives of Disease in Childhood*)

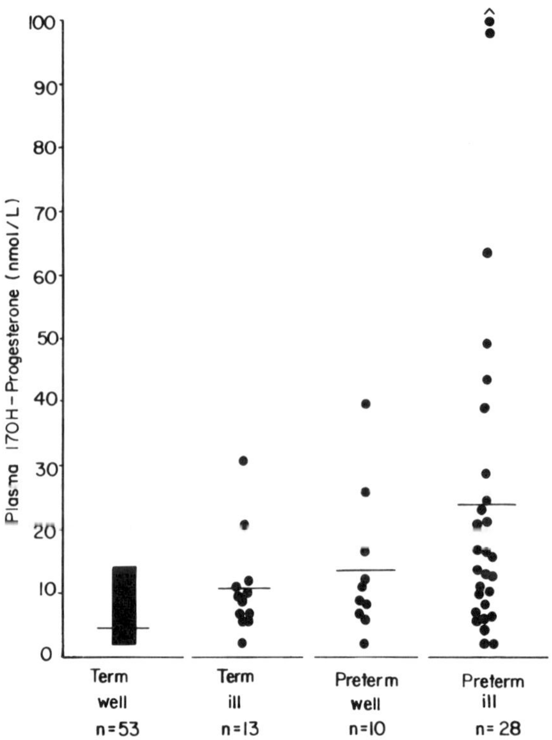

Figure 2 Mean and range for plasma 17P concentrations in term and preterm infants who were either healthy or ill (Reproduced with permission of the editor of *Archives of Disease in Childhood*)

in infants with CAH. There is a rapid decline in 17P levels in normal infants due to clearance of placental-derived 17P in the circulation. It is recommended that collection of diagnostic samples be delayed for 24 hours after birth to ensure adequate clearance of exogenous 17P (Youssefnejadian and David, 1975; Hughes *et al.*, 1979). Occasionally the rise in plasma 17P concentration is delayed (De Peretti and Forest, 1982) or the plasma 17P levels become extremely elevated (Figure 2) in infants who are ill from conditions other than CAH (Savage *et al.*, 1982; Murphy *et al.*, 1983). The latter category applies particularly to preterm infants who are often hyponatraemic as a result of a combination of inappropriate intravenous fluid replacement and transient renal tubular unresponsiveness to mineralocorticoids.

A previously affected sibling should ensure that the newborn infant is appropriately investigated, particularly if the sex is male. Prenatal diagnosis of CAH by measurement of amniotic fluid 17P concentration at 16–18 weeks gestation is also possible (Nagamani *et al.*, 1978; Hughes and Laurence, 1982). Consequently, the categories listed in Table 2 should readily identify most cases of CAH expected to present at birth.

Table 2 Cases of CAH readily identifiable in newborns

All affected females (theoretically)
Salt-losers
Cryptorchidism with hypospadias
Previous family history of CAH
Positive prenatal diagnosis

THE CASE FOR CAH SCREENING

Table 3 lists clinical situations which are potentially avoidable if screening is routinely practised. The symptoms of salt-wasting are invariably delayed beyond the immediate newborn period. A mistaken diagnosis of pyloric stenosis may be made in a male infant with vomiting and dehydration. The distinctive electrolyte patterns should distinguish the two disorders. A 19-year-old male salt-loser who attends the author's clinic permanently displays the distinctive pylorotomy scar of inappropriate surgery performed in infancy.

Table 3 Clinical problems potentially avoidable with CAH newborn screening

Salt-wasting crisis
Inappropriate diagnosis and treatment of 'pyloric stenosis'
Inappropriate gender assignment
Precocious puberty
Stunted growth
Sudden death

Late onset cases of CAH usually present with tall stature and advanced skeletal maturation. Ultimately adult height is often very short. Figure 3 depicts the linear growth chart of a female with non-salt-losing CAH whose diagnosis was delayed. Although initially tall for her age, she is now extremely short due to the combination of late diagnosis, excessive glucocorticoid medication, early puberty and subsequent premature epiphyseal fusion. It is possible that the unfavourable outcome in such cases could be improved if CAH screening identified the enzyme deficiency at birth.

The frequency of unexplained neonatal deaths in families of patients with CAH attests to missed diagnoses of the disorder, particularly in males. In a survey of CAH cases in Wales (Murtaza *et al.*, 1980), there was a significant deviation from the expected equal sex ratio and an excess number of female versus male salt-losers. In a more recent survey, Lebovitz and colleagues (1984) confirmed these findings and emphasized that the diagnosis of CAH was frequently delayed. Nevertheless it is the author's personal impression that there has been a reduction in both the number of missed cases and in delayed diagnoses with increasing awareness of the disorder by clinicians and the availability of rapid diagnostic tests.

PROBLEMS WITH CAH SCREENING

The technical problems associated with the development of an assay for 17P in blood spots is discussed in detail elsewhere in this issue. Ideally a direct assay (non-

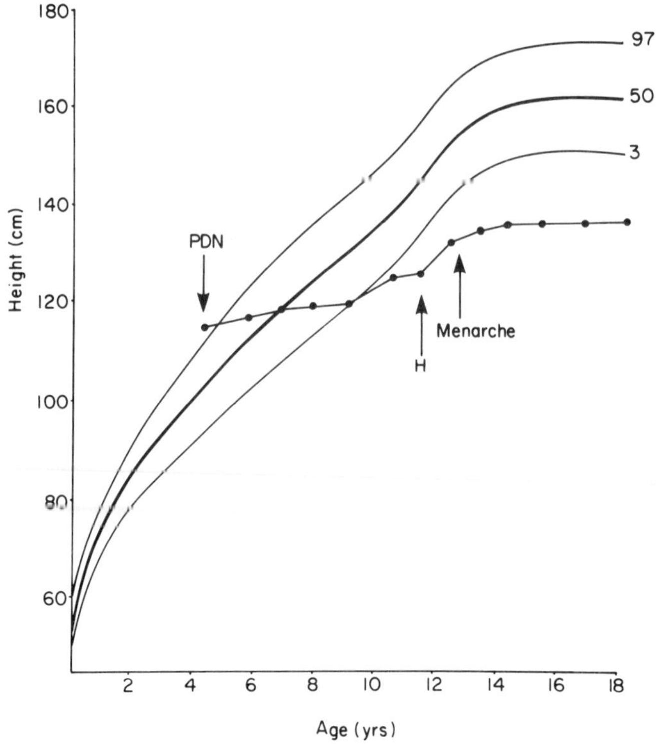

Figure 3 Linear growth in a girl with late onset CAH. Initial treatment with prednisone (PDN) was later changed to hydrocortisone (H) (Data from Hughes (1984) with permission of the editor, *Paediatric Endocrinology in Clinical Practice*)

extracted) capable of being automated should be developed which is simple, rapid and low in both false positive and recall rates. Previous studies using plasma samples have shown higher concentrations of 17P in preterm infants and in infants who are stressed due to a variety of non-adrenal disorders (Godo *et al.*, 1981; Murphy *et al.*, 1983). This is further confirmed from the results of several pilot screening programmes where the majority of false positive results have occurred in preterm infants and in infants with perinatal complications (Pang *et al.*, 1982; Cacciari *et al.*, 1983; Shimozawa *et al.*, 1984). The recall rate is considerably reduced when an additional microfilter assay for cortisol is performed and the result expressed as a ratio of the 17P value (Fujieda *et al.*, 1985).

Figure 4 shows data obtained on blood spot 17P values using a method adapted from an assay developed primarily to monitor treatment of CAH cases (Dyas *et al.*, 1984). The sensitivity of the method was 1.5 pg per 'spot' equivalent to 1 nmol/L 17P. The mean ±SD value for 17P in normal full-term infants was 7.5±2.7 nmol/L; there was no sex difference. Individual 17P values were higher in infants whose birth weights were less than 2500 g. Filter paper cards containing blood spots from five infants with CAH who had been screened for phenylketonuria and congenital hypothyrodism were retrieved from storage and blood spot 17P values measured retrospectively.

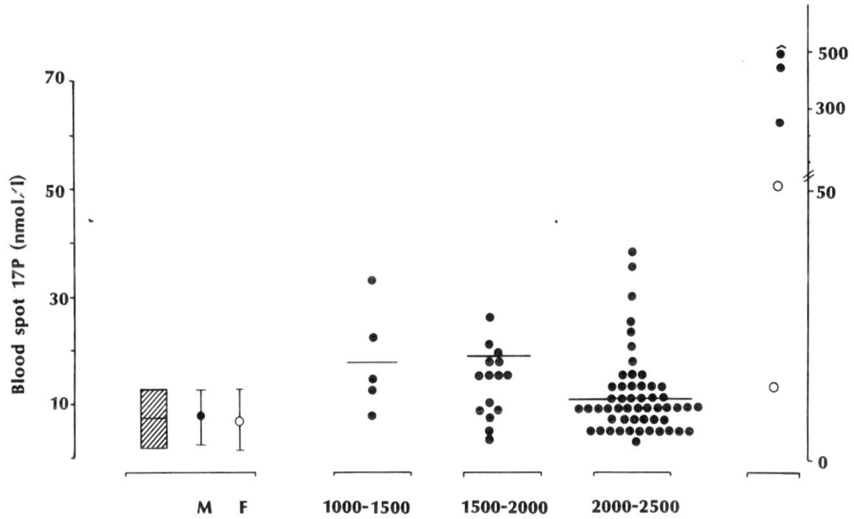

Figure 4 Blood spot 17P concentrations in newborn infants. The hatched bar indicates the mean ±SD in full term healthy infants. Birth weight categories are expressed in grams. There is a break in the right vertical axis to take account of the elevated 17P levels in CAH infants. ○ denotes 17P values in infants with 11β-hydroxylase deficiency. ● denotes a 17P concentration of 2400 nmol/L

In three infants with 21-hydroxylase deficiency, 17P levels were markedly elevated particularly in the two salt-losers. Two infants with 11β-hydroxylase deficiency showed only marginally elevated levels of 17P.

Clearly blood spot 17P assays currently available will accurately identify elevated 17P levels due to 21-hydroxylase deficiency. There is no information as yet on false negative rates. More data are required on blood spot 17P concentrations in relation to gestational age, birth weight, postnatal age and perinatal complications before CAH screening by this method is considered for routine use. The general criteria which should be considered for any newborn screening programme are shown in

Table 4 Criteria for screening a disorder at birth

Severe morbidity (possibly mortality) if undetected early	
Effective treatment readily available	
Improved prognosis with early treatment	
Clinical screening unreliable	
Incidence of the disorder relatively high (e.g. >1 in 15000)	
Screening test is	simple
	safe
	reliable
	rapid
Cost of screening programme is justifiable	

Table 4. While it can be argued that CAH is a disorder with significant morbidity and some mortality for which treatment is readily available, the incidence of cases that would not be detected clinically must be very low.

CONCLUSIONS

Blood spot 17P immunoassays currently available can readily identify both retrospectively and prospectively classical cases of CAH due to 21-hydroxylase deficiency. The false positive rate in infants who have perinatal complications, are preterm or both is presently high because data on the pattern of adrenal steroidogenesis in this age group are lacking. The number of infants with classical CAH whose diagnosis is missed on clinical criteria is small. However this minority has a significant morbidity and occasional mortality. Late onset and, in particular, cryptic cases are unlikely to be detected in a newborn screening programme. The question remains whether routine newborn screening is justified to detect a small minority of infants: clearly additional pilot screening programmes are required before a definite answer can be provided.

REFERENCES

Cacciari, E., Balsamo, A., Cassio, A., Piazzi, S., Bernardi, F., Salardi, S., Cicognani, A., Pirazzoli, P., Zappulla, A., Capelli, M. and Paolini, M. Neonatal screening for congenital adrenal hyperplasia. *Arch. Dis. Child.* 58 (1983) 803–806

de Crecchio, L. Sopra un case di apparenze virili in una donna. *Morgagni* 7 (1865) 151

Dyas, J., Read, G. F., Guha-Maulik, T., Hughes, I. A. and Fahmy, D. R. A rapid assay for 17OH-progesterone in plasma, saliva and amniotic fluid using a magnetisable solid-phase antiserum. *Ann. Clin. Biochem.* 21 (1984) 421–424

Fujieda, K., Matsuura, N., Fukushi, M. and Takasugi, N. Microfilter paper method for cortisol radioimmunoassay and its application to mass screening for congenital adrenal hyperplasia (CAH). *Ped. Res.* 19 (1985) 621

Godo, B., Visser, H. K. A and Degenhart, H. J. Plasma 17OH-progesterone in full term and preterm infants at birth and during the early neonatal period. *Horm. Res.* 15 (1981) 65–71

Hughes, I. A. Congenital and acquired disorders of the adrenal cortex. *Clin. Endocrinol. Metab.* 11 (1982) 89–125

Hughes, I. A. Medical and psychological management of congenital adrenal hyperplasia. In Aynsley-Green, A. (ed.) *Paediatric Endocrinology in Clinical Practice*, MTP Press, Lancaster, 1984, pp. 83–115

Hughes, I. A. and Davies, P. A. Neonatal endocrine and metabolic emergencies. *Clin. Endocrinol. Metab.* 9 (1980) 583–604

Hughes, I. A., Fahmy, D. R. and Griffiths, K. Plasma 17OH-progesterone concentrations in newborn infants. *Arch. Dis. Child.* 54 (1979) 347–349

Hughes, I. A. and Laurence, K. M. Prenatal diagnosis of congenital adrenal hyperplasia due to 21-hydroxylase deficiency by amniotic fluid steroid analysis. *Prenat. Diag.* 2 (1982) 97–102

Jones, H. W. Jr. A long look at the adrenogenital syndrome. *Johns. Hop. Med. J.* 145 (1979) 143–149

Lebovitz, R. M., Pauli, R. M. and Laxova, R. Delayed diagnosis in congenital adrenal hyperplasia. Need for newborn screening. *Am. J. Dis. Child.* 138 (1984) 571–573

In common with other inborn errors of metabolism the diagnosis of CAH due to 21-hydroxylase deficiency is generally established on the basis of elevated precursors in blood. A number of other biochemical tests for CAH are used though not all of these are appropriate for investigations in the neonatal period for reasons that will be demonstrated later. Even when using the technique of GC profile analysis without mass spectrometry the diagnosis is unreliable due to the delay in the appearance of an abnormal steroid pattern characteristic of the defect (Shackleton, 1976). Recent achievements in the analysis of steroids in urine are described in relation to the early diagnosis of the disorder. Interpretation of these data benefits from the experience of using this technology both in the diagnosis of salt-losing diseases of children and in a search for the role of the adrenal cortex in the fetus and neonate.

MATERIALS AND METHODS

The adrenal function of newborn infants with congenital adrenal hyperplasia has been characterized by using the analysis of steroids in single and sequential urine samples collected from day 1 to 3 months of age. Three infants (2 were 46XX and 1 46XY) had simple virilizing adrenal hyperplasia and 10 (8 were 46XX and 2 were 46XY) had the salt-losing form.

Steroids were extracted from urine by using Sep-Pak C_{18} cartridges (Waters Associates, Harrow, Middlesex) according to the method of Shackleton and Whitney (1980). In most cases steroids were further separated according to their conjugation (Figure 1) by using Sephadex LH-20 chromatography as described by Janne and colleagues (1969) using a 4 g column and a solvent system of methanol : chloroform (1 : 1 v : v, saturated with salt). Two fractions were collected: (1) a free and glucuronide fraction (eluted with 30 mL of the above solvent) and (2) a sulphate fraction eluted with 50 mL of ethanol. The first fraction was hydrolysed using the enzyme preparation of Helix pomatia. Free steroids were obtained by solvolysis of the sulphate fraction according to the method of Burstein and Liebermann (1958). The extracts were dissolved in 5 mL of ethyl acetate previously saturated with sulphuric acid. Solvolysis was allowed to proceed for 16 h at 37°C. The solvolysed fractions were washed with 0.5 mL of normal sodium hydroxide followed by 0.5 mL of water and dried over anhydrous sodium sulphate. When conjugates were not separated into groups the Helix pomatia enzyme preparation alone was used to liberate steroids from the total extract prior to re-extraction by using Sep-Pak cartridges.

Appropriate amounts of internal standards (5α-androstane-3α,17α-diol, stigmasterol and cholesteryl butyrate – labelled as A, S and C respectively in chromatographs) were added to the fractions. Methyloxime derivatives were prepared by heating the samples for 1 h at 60°C with 100 μL of 2% methoxyamine hydrochloride in pyridine. The samples were silylated by heating with trimethylsilylimidazole (TSIM) for 16 h. Pyridine was removed under nitrogen and the excess silylating reagents were removed by using the Lipidex procedure of Axelson and Sjovall (1974).

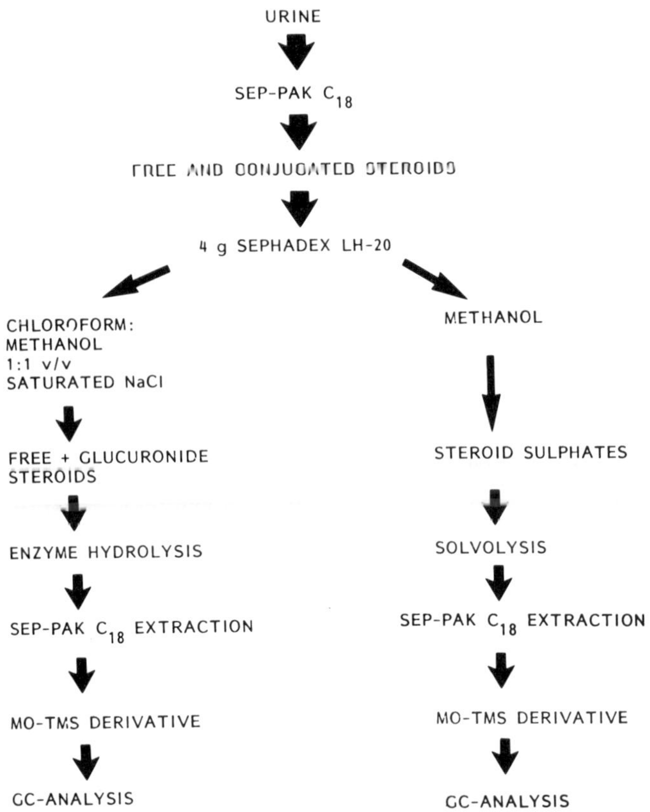

Figure 1 Analysis of steroids in neonatal urine to prepare two fractions of steroids containing (1) free and glucuronide conjugated steroids, and (2) steroid sulphates

Gas chromatography was carried out on a 25 m OV-1 fused silica column coupled with a solid injector and flame ionization detector. The sample was injected with the oven at 60°C. The temperature of the oven was then rapidly raised to 180°C and, following a 2 minute isothermal period, was programmed to rise at 2°C per min to 300°C. Steroids were quantified by measuring the peak height of individual compounds relative to a line joining the peaks of the internal standards. The identity of steroids was confirmed by combined gas chromatography–mass spectrometry with a VG Analytical MM-16 instrument with electron impact source (70 eV). The samples were introduced by on-column injection to a column similar to the one used for conventional gas chromatography. Mass spectra were acquired by repetitive scanning over the mass range 50–700 amu. Data were acquired and processed by PDP8 computer system.

RESULTS

In a normal adult the main steroids in urine can be assigned as androgen metabolites, progesterone metabolites and cortisol metabolites. CAH due to 21-hydroxylase deficiency can be recognized by the profile which displays high excretion of androgen metabolites, variable excretion of cortisol metabolites and extremely high excretion of 17α-hydroxypregnanolone and 5β-pregnane-3α,17α,20α-triol as two metabolites of 17α-hydroxyprogesterone. There is high excretion of 11-oxo-pregnanetriol, a metabolite of 21-deoxycortisol. This pattern can usually be straightforwardly regarded as the outcome of steroid production in the face of the enzyme deficiency. In order to avoid some doubt in interpretation of the profile it is important to pay attention to the derivatization procedure since unless the silylation reaction is left for at least 8 h the side chain of pregnanetriol and structurally related steroids will not completely derivatize. The partial derivatives have longer retention times than the fully silylated products and, for example, the presence of partially silylated forms of pregnanetriol gives rise to a peak with retention close to the fully silylated derivative of 11-oxo-pregnanetriol. This can be proved by mass spectrometry but if this detector is not being used, some doubt can be left in interpretation of a GC profile. It is also important to be sure of the identity of 17α-hydroxypregnanolone since this has the same retention time as 11β-hydroxyandrosterone. Certainly in some publications this distinction is not clear (Vierhapper *et al.*, 1985) but it is of immense importance since these metabolites derive from different hormones.

The steroid profile of a neonate is dominated by the steroids derived from the fetal adrenal zone. Thus in the GC profile of total steroids isolated from the urine of a newborn infant 16α-hydroxy-DHA is the first peak in the chromatograph. This is recognized as a double peak, the result of syn- and anti- forms of the oxime derivative. The retention times of these peaks and other 3β-hydroxy-5-ene steroids in urine at this time of life are summarized in Table 1. Even the pattern of cortisol metabolites is different from that seen in adults. Most of the metabolites are in the oxidized form of cortisol (cortisone) and are hydroxylated in the liver prior to their excretion in urine.

In the profile of steroids in urine of a newborn child suspected to have CAH due to 21-hydroxylase deficiency, two peaks are seen in the GC profile with retention times less than that of 16α-hydroxy-DHA (Figure 2) (the second steroid co-elutes with the first peak of 16α-hydroxy-DHA). Mass spectrometry has confirmed these to be 17α-hydroxypregnanolone and 3α,15β,17α-trihydroxy-5β-pregnan-20-one by comparison with spectra of reference compounds (Figure 3). The latter steroid has a very characteristic fragmentation pattern leading to a prominent peak at m/z 258. The high excretion of steroids derived by the fetal adrenal zones makes the interpretation of the remaining profile difficult, although when the profiles from several cases are compared with the pattern from a normal child a series of unusual peaks can be discerned. Particularly prominent is the peak due to 16α-hydroxypregnenolone.

The picture is considerably clarified by prior separation of steroids according to their conjugation. This effectively enables the steroid products of the fetal adrenal zone to be examined separately from steroids produced by the definitive zone. The production of cortisol metabolites at the expense of a high excretion of precursors by neonates with suspected congenital adrenal hyperplasia is confirmed from examination of the steroids in the fraction containing the free and glucuronide

Table 1 Steroids in urine of normal newborn infants, with their GC retention times relative to co-injected *n*-alkanes in temperature programmed analysis on OV-1 capillary column (25 m), and with the ranges of excretion in normal newborn infants

	GC retention times (methylene units)	*Normal excretion*(μg/day) mean±S.D. ($n=16$)
3β-hydroxy-5-ene steroids		
16α-hydroxy-DHA	27.38 27.42	300±290
16β-hydroxy-DHA	27.74	150±110
16-oxoandrostenediol	28.19	260±250
15β,16α-dihydroxy-DHA	28.20	
androstenetriol	28.46	200±140
16α,18-dihydroxy-DHA	28.65 28.81	420±340
16α-hydroxypregnenolone	29.38	420±380
21-hydroxypregnenolone	30.30 30.60	50± 20
5-androstene-3β,16α,17β,18-tetrol	29.72	50± 20
5-androstene-3β,15β,16α,17β-tetrol	29.64	80± 60
5-androstene-3β,15α,16α,17β-tetrol	30.25	40± 20
5-androstene-3β,15α,16β,17-tetrol	30.50	20± 10
5-pregnene-3β,20β,21-triol	30.72	20± 10
5-pregnene-3β,16α,20α,21-tetrol	31.00	20± 10
Cortisol metabolites		
tetrahydrocortisone	29.65	110± 80
α-cortolone	30.51	30± 25
6α-hydroxytetrahydrocortisone	30.80	90± 80
1β-hydroxytetrahydrocortisone	30.93	20± 10
β-cortolone	30.73	20± 10
6α-hydroxy-α-cortolone	31.60	10± 5
6α-hydroxy-β-cortolone	31.82	45± 40
1β-hydroxy-β-cortolone	32.60	25± 20

conjugates. Furthermore a pattern of 21-deoxysteroid metabolites has emerged from the data of these cases. Prominent steroids are 17α-hydroxypregnanolone and 3α,15β,17α-trihydroxy-5β-pregnane-20-one. The ion at *m/z* 258 in the spectrum of the latter steroid is seen also in other spectra associated with other 15β-hydroxylated metabolites of 17α-hydroxyprogesterone. Other 21-deoxysteroids were partially characterized by mass spectrometry. There are several steroids with the general structure of pregnenediolone (giving a mass spectrum with prominent ion at *m/z* 474) and of pregnanetriolone (*m/z* 564). Several of the steroids gave mass spectra which were not highly informative because of a prominent base peak at *m/z* 117 – a typical fragmentation of the side chain of 21-deoxysteroids. A shortage of reference compounds has restricted the precise identification of many such steroids. Nevertheless many of these serve as useful markers for the defect in the newborn period. The usual markers in the adult (pregnanetriol and 11-oxo-pregnanetriol) can be recognized in the profile but their contribution to the total metabolites of 17α-hydroxyprogesterone in the newborn period is very small (<10%).

The sulphate fraction largely resembles the same fraction of steroids in urine

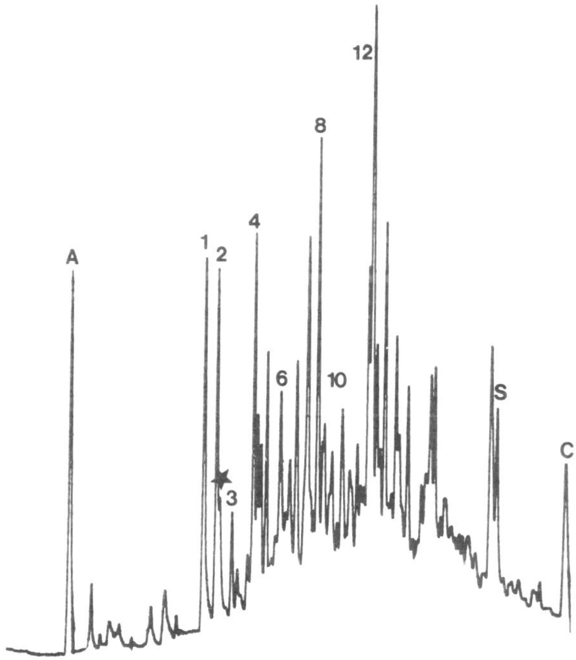

Figure 2 GC profile of steroids in free and glucuronide fraction of urine of a child with congenital adrenal hyperplasia due to 21-hydroxylase deficiency. A, S and C are internal standards (see text). Steroids are numbered according to the list in Table 2. * marks the second peak of 16α-hydroxy-DHA which is usually the first steroid seen in a neonatal profile

Table 2 Steroids in free and glucuronide fraction of urine of newborn infants with congenital adrenal hyperplasia due to 21-hydroxylase deficiency. For conditions of GC analysis see text

		GC retention time (methylene units)
1	17α-hydroxypregnanolone	27.00
2	3α,15β,17α-trihydroxy-5β-pregnan-20-one	27.35
3	androstanetriolone (see Steen *et al.*, 1982)	27.62
4	5β-hydroxy-3α,17α,20α-triol	28.00
5	3α,17α-dihydroxy-5β-pregnan-11,20-dione	28.30
6	3α,11β,17α-trihydroxy-5β-pregnan-20-one	28.25
7	3α,16α-dihydroxy-5β-pregnan-20-one	28.52
8	3α,17α,20α-trihydroxy-5β-pregnan-11-one	29.10
9	5-pregnene-3α,16α,20α-triol	29.20
10	3β,16α-dihydroxy-5-pregnen-20-one	29.38
11	3β,15β,17α-trihydroxy-5-pregnen-20-one	29.02
12	5-pregnene-3β,15β,17α,20α-tetrol	29.92

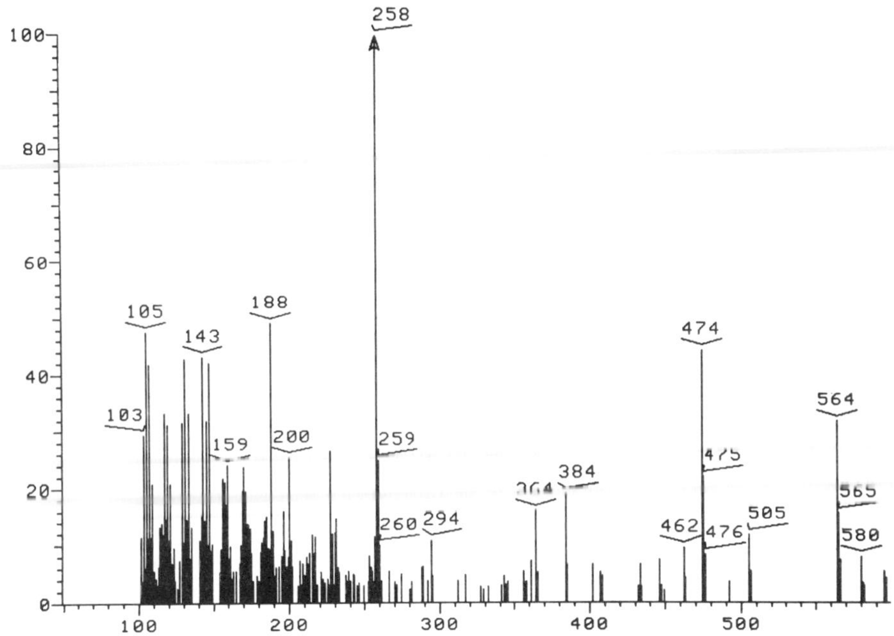

Figure 3 Mass spectrum of 3α,15β,17α-trihydroxy-5β-pregnan-20-one as methyloxime trimethylsilyl ether derivative

from a normal child, although the total daily excretion is greater in CAH and individual steroids may be elevated (e.g. 16α-hydroxypregnenolone). This presumably reflects the fetal adrenal zone response to the action of ACTH released from the pituitary in response to low cortisol production.

The above pattern of steroids seen in urine of children with CAH persists for several weeks. Even at 2 months pregnanetriol and 11-oxo-pregnanetriol (the classical markers for CAH) are not the most prominent steroids, but the excretion of other hydroxylated metabolites listed above is relatively less important than in the immediate newborn period.

DISCUSSION

In the present paper results are presented from the study of steroid excretion patterns in urine of infants in the neonatal period by using capillary column gas chromatography. A GC profile of steroids in urine aims to display in a single chromatogram the detector response with time as the steroids elute from the column. Internal standards are added to the extract before the analysis. These provide reference points for partial identification of the steroids in the extract and are quantitative markers for the measurement of the unknown steroids. Steroids can be partially identified by their retention times although in many instances, particularly with profiles from urine collected in the neonatal period, it is not always possible to rely on this data alone because of the complexity of the pattern.

Mass spectrometry is thus essential for the structural identity though clearly this is only available in a few centres.

The steroid profile of a neonate is dominated by the steroids derived from the fetal adrenal zone. It is worth recalling that the adrenal gland of a newborn human is as large as that of an adult. Histologically the bulk of the fetal adrenal gland is taken up by a zone of cells unique to this time of life. In the fetus this zone increases in size to a maximum at term and following delivery this zone regresses during the first 6 to 9 months of life. The fetal adrenal zone largely produces steroids with 3β-hydroxy-5-ene configuration-like dehydroepiandrosterone, which are metabolized by the placenta to oestrogens. In the normal neonate the steroids of the fetal adrenal zone tend to be excreted in urine as sulphate conjugates. Their production declines with age over the first year in parallel with the morphological changes of the adrenal. The definitive adrenal zones produce accepted adrenal glucocorticoid and mineralocorticoid steroids. The steroids derived from the adult adrenal zones tend to be excreted in urine as free-steroid or as glucuronide conjugates.

The data presented here not only reveal the complexity of steroid production at this time but demonstrate the suitability of unique marker steroids for the neonatal diagnosis of congenital adrenal hyperplasia which differ from the accepted metabolite markers. In an adult, CAH due to 21-hydroxylase deficiency can be recognized by the profile which displays high excretion of 17α-hydroxypregnanolone and 5β-pregnane-3α,17α,20α-triol as two metabolites of 17α-hydroxyprogesterone. There is also high excretion of 11-oxo-pregnanetriol, a metabolite of 21 deoxycortisol. Using these criteria, Shackleton (1976) examined the steroid excretion pattern of newborn infants with suspected congenital adrenal hyperplasia. Shackleton used the selectivity of a GC MS to reveal the presence of pregnanetriol and 11-oxo-pregnanetriol. These steroids could be detected on the third day of life. When using GC analysis alone the diagnosis, based on identification of these markers, was not certain until the second or third week. At that time Shackleton used a weak silylation reaction which did not fully protect pregnanetriol and similar steroids.

In the present study a chromatographic separation has been introduced into the analytical procedure routinely used for neonatal samples. This effectively enables the steroid products of each adrenal zone to be examined separately. In this way the low excretion of cortisol metabolites by neonates with suspected congenital adrenal hyperplasia can be confirmed. Furthermore a pattern of 21-deoxysteroid metabolites has emerged from the data of several cases. The identification of three such steroids was aided by a publication by Joannou (1981) who used a microbiological approach to synthesize a number of steroids hydroxylated at the C-15 position. A characteristic MS fragmentation of such steroids was noted and this has enabled a number of related steroids to be identified in the steroid profile for the first time. In some publications 3α,15β,17α-trihydroxy-5β-pregnan-20-one has been called 3α,11β,17α-trihydroxy-5β-pregnan-20-one despite the presentation of a mass spectrum and a GC retention time different from those given by the latter reference compound (Steen *et al.*, 1980; van der Ploegg *et al.*, 1982). These 15β-hydroxylated products of 17α-hydroxyprogesterone are important markers for CAH due to 21-hydroxylase deficiency in the neonatal period. They are among a number of steroids which should be tested for interference in any radioimmunoassay for 17α-hydroxyprogesterone applied to a screening programme. The polar nature of these metabolites may mean, however, that assays which include a solvent extraction step can be made to be more specific than assays where the steroids are extracted into buffer before RIA. These 15β-hydroxylated steroids may also serve in the prenatal diagnosis of CAH by analysis of amniotic fluid or maternal urine. To date these steroids have not been detected in these biological fluids (Homoki *et al.*, 1983).

Over the last 20 years a number of steroids have been proposed as indicators for

Table 3 Urinary steroids recommended as indicators for steroid 21-hydroxylase deficiency in newborn children

Steroid(s)	*Author(s)*
16α-hydroxypregnenolone/16α-hydroxy-DHA	Reynolds (1965)
21α-hydroxypregnenolone/16α-hydroxypregnenolonc	Mitchell and Shackleton (1969)
	Joannou (1981)
16α-hydroxypregnenolone	Shackleton and Mitchell (1967)
	Homoki and Teller (1981)
5-ene-steroids	Gustafsson *et al.*, (1982)
pregnanetriol and 11-oxo-pregnanetriol	Shackleton (1976)
	Viinikka *et al.*, (1973)
pregnanetriol and 17-oxosteroids	Viinikka *et al.*, (1973)
17α-hydroxypregnanolone	Holsboer and Knorr (1977)
3α,15β,17α-trihydroxy-5β-pregnan-20-one	Joannou (1981)

steroid 21-hydroxylase deficiency in children (Table 3). From the results of the present investigations we are able to confirm that all of these steroids can be found in the urine of affected infants but individually one steroid may predominate over others at different ages so that caution must be taken in relying upon the use of a single steroid. In the knowledge of the present findings the measurement of pregnanetriol alone or of 17-oxosteroids is not recommended in the neonatal period. These findings are endorsed by the results of Peretti and Forest (1982) from longitudinal studies of plasma hormone concentrations in newborns with CAH. In 1980 Steen and co-workers suggested that 17α-hydroxypregnanolone was a good indicator of 21-hydroxylase deficiency in the neonatal period. This observation is confirmed in the present study. One advantage of this steroid as a marker is its short GC retention time – preceding that of the usual steroids in urine of a neonate. This obviates the need for the conjugate separation proposed in the present work. However by including this separation the presence of other 21-deoxysteroids can be revealed to add confidence to the diagnosis.

In the diagnosis of CAH due to 21-hydroxylase deficiency the majority of the biochemical investigations which are used today are directed to the radioimmunoassay determination of 17α-hydroxyprogesterone in blood as a means of revealing substrate accummulation prior to the enzyme blockage (Murphy *et al.*, 1983).

Any method for neonatal screening needs to be evaluated in the context of the endogenous steroid milieu of the newborn infant. This disorder represents the commonest of the inborn areas of steroid metabolism, with incidences in different populations ranging between 1 in 5000 and 1 in 15 000. CAH should be suspected clinically in most females with the disorder at birth. Males with the salt-losing form should be detected at a very young age. Thus a screening programme will, in principle, be most effective for the detection of males with simple virilizing CAH. The incidence of heterozygosity for congenital adrenal hyperplasia due to 21-hydroxylase deficiency may be as high as 1 in 50 of the population. The recent literature pertaining to the late onset of congenital adrenal hyperplasia should not be ignored. These may present as problems in the menstrual cycle and of unwanted hair growth during reproductive years. Should a screening programme aim to achieve an early prediction for these forms in addition to the classical form of CAH? Other causes of congenital adrenal hyperplasia are rare and in no way can screening be profitable since this would require the simultaneous measurement of a number of other precursors with limited success. Furthermore this would be impractical because in using the blood spot approach there is insufficient sample available for further investigations. Pang and co-workers (1985) have recently demonstrated a relatively high incidence of 3β-hydroxysteroid dehydrogenase deficiency in similar patients: the defect being recognized by the ratio of 3β-hydroxy-5-ene steroids relative to the 3-keto-4-ene steroids following adrenal stimulation with ACTH is thus impractical in a screening programme.

Since CAH is a disease which may require life-long therapy it is important that a diagnosis based on a blood spot analysis for 17α-hydroxyprogesterone is confirmed by a proper follow-up. This is probably best achieved by the use of a GC profile of steroids in urine since this is applicable to the diagnosis of congenital adrenal hyperplasia regardless of the enzyme defect (see Honour *et al.*, 1983) and in a single analysis will exclude other causes for the raised 17α-hydroxyprogesterone concentration in the blood spot.

ACKNOWLEDGEMENTS

I am grateful for the collaboration of my former colleagues, C. H. L. Shackleton and N. F. Taylor, and to the following for their co-operation and permission to publish data relating to their patients: J. Anderson, Wolverhampton; P. Betts, Southampton; A. W. Blair, Kirkcaldy; C. G. D. Brook, Middlesex Hospital, London; B. Clayton, Southampton; I. Hughes, Cardiff; I. G. Jefferson, Northampton; B. M. Laurence, Queen Elizabeth Hospital, London; M. O. Savage, St Bartholomews Hospital, London; D. W. Stevens, Gloucester; D. Thistlethwaite, Burnley and J. G. Winwick, Cambridge. The technical support of W. Tsang and M. Madigan is also much appreciated.

REFERENCES

Axelson, M. and Sjovall, J. Separation and computerised gas chromatography – mass spectrometry of unconjugated neutral steroid in plasma. *J. Steroid Biochem.* 5 (1974) 733–738

Burstein, S. and Liebermann, S. Hydrolysis of keto steroid hydrogen sulphates by solvolysis procedures. *J. Biol. Chem.* 233 (1958) 331–335

Gustafsson, J.-A., Gustafsson, S. and Olin, P. Steroid excretion patterns in urine from two boys in the neonatal period with congenital adrenal hyperplasia due to 21-hydroxylase deficiency. *Acta Endocrinol. (Kbh)* 71 (1972) 353–364

Holsboer, F. and Knorr, D. Determination of urinary 17α-hydroxypregnanolone by gas chromatography – mass spectrometry in patients with congenital adrenal hyperplasia. *J. Steroid Biochem.* 8 (1977) 1197–1199

Homoki, J., Roitman, E. and Shackleton, C. H. L. Characterization of the major steroids present in amniotic fluid obtained between 15 and 17 weeks of gestation. *J. Steroid Biochem.* 19 (1983) 1061–1068

Homoki, J. and Teller, W. M. Increased urinary excretion of total 16α-hydroxypregnenolone in newborn infants with congenital adrenal hyperplasia due to 21-hydroxylase deficiency. *Klin. Wochenschr.* 60 (1982) 409–410

Honour, J. W., Anderson, J. M. and Shackleton, C. H. L. Difficulties in the diagnosis of congenital adrenal hyperplasia in early infancy: the 11β-hydroxylase defect. *Acta Endocrinol. (Kbh)* 103 (1983) 101–109

Janne, O., Vihko, R., Sjovall, J. and Sjovall, K. Determination of steroid mono-and disulphates in human plasma. *Clin. Chim. Acta* 23 (1969) 405–412

Janoski, A. H., Roginsky, M. S., Christy, N. P. and Kelly, W. G. On the metabolism of 16α-hydroxy-C_{21}-steroids. III. Evidence for high rates of production of 16α-hydroxypregnenolone in the salt-losing form of congenital adrenal hyperplasia. *J. Clin. Endocrinol.* 29 (1969) 1301–1309

Joannou, G. E. Identification of 15β-hydroxylated C_{21} steroids in the neonatal period: the role of 3α,15β,17α-trihydroxy-5β-pregnan-20-one in the perinatal diagnosis of congenital adrenal hyperplasia due to 21-hydroxylase deficiency. *J. Steroid Biochem.* 14 (1981) 901–912

Mitchell, F. L. and Shackleton, C. H. L. The investigation of steroid metabolism in early infancy. *Adv. Clin. Chem.* 12 (1969) 141–215

Murphy, J. P., Joyce, B. S., Dyas, J. and Hughes, I. Plasma 17α-hydroxyprogesterone concentrations in ill newborn infants. *Arch. Dis. Child.* 58 (1983) 532–534

Pang, S., Lerner, A. J., Stoner, E., Levine, L. S., Oberfield, S. E., Engel, I. and New, M. I. Late onset adrenal 3β-hydroxysteroid dehydrogenase deficiency. I. A cause of hirsutism in pubertal and post-pubertal women. *J. Clin. Endocrinol. Metab.* 60 (1985) 428–439

de Peretti, E. and Forest, M. G. Pitfalls in the etiological diagnosis of congenital adrenal hyperplasia in the early neonatal period. *Hormone Res.* 16 (1982) 10–22

van der Ploegg, K., Wolthers, B. G., Nagel, G. T., Volmer, M. and Drayer, N. G. The diagnosis of 21-hydroxylase deficiency in a prematurely born infant on the basis of the urinary steroid excretion pattern. *Clin. Chim. Acta* 120 (1982) 341–353

Reynolds, J. W. The excretion of two 3β-hydroxy-5-ene, 16α-hydroxysteroids by patients with congenital adrenal hyperplasia. *Pediatrics* 36 (1965) 583–591

Shackleton, C. H. L. Congenital adrenal hyperplasia caused by defect in steroid 21-hydroxylase: establishment of definitive urinary steroid excretion pattern during the first weeks of life. *Clin. Chim. Acta* 67 (1976) 287–298

Shackleton, C. H. L. and Mitchell, F. L. The measurement of 3β-hydroxy-5-ene steroids in human fetal blood, amniotic fluid, infant urine and adult urine. *Steroid* 10 (1967) 359–385

Shackleton, C. H. L. and Whitney, J. O. Use of Sep-pak cartridges for urinary steroid extraction: evaluation of the method for use prior to gas chromatographic analysis. *Clin. Chim. Acta* 107 (1980) 231–243

Steen, G., Tas, A. C., de Brauw, M. C., ten Noever, Drayer, N. M. and Wolthers, B. C. The early recognition of the 21-hydroxylase deficiency variety of congenital adrenal hyperplasia. *Clin. Chim. Acta* 105 (1980) 213–224

Vierhapper, H., Nowotny, P., Waldhauser, W. and Frisch, H. Capillary gas chromatography as a tool for characterization of urinary steroid excretion in patients with congenital adrenal hyperplasia. *J. Steroid Biochem.* 22 (1985) 363–369

Viinikka, L., Janne, O., Perheentupa, J. and Vihko, R. Congenital adrenal hyperplasia. Plasma and urinary steroid conjugates in seven children with steroid 21-hydroxylase deficiency. *Clin. Chim. Acta* 48 (1973) 359–365

J. Inher. Metab. Dis. 9 Suppl. 1 (1986) 135–141

Large Scale Pilot Studies

The following three papers describe the assays for 17α-hydroxyprogesterone used in and the results of neonatal screening programmes for steroid 21-hydroxylase deficiency in Scotland, Italy and France. Specific assays are achieved by prior extraction of 17α-hydroxyprogesterone from the blood spots by organic solvents. This method is complex and unsuitable for large assays. Non-extraction or direct assays using ^{125}I steroid label in the assay are less specific but are simple to perform and capable of being automated. Results with the relatively small numbers so far detected would suggest that the lack of specificity does not confer a serious disadvantage although a higher reference range is needed. The quantity of 17α-hydroxyprogesterone in the blood spots depends on gestational age and birthweight, and cut-off limit must be adjusted accordingly. The majority of false positive tests occur in premature infants.

Very small numbers of patients are reported in the preliminary accounts of mass screening programmes (5 in Scotland; 7 in Italy; 2 in France excluding La Réunion). Of these, six had the diagnosis established by the screening programmes, and six were diagnosed clinically before the results of screening were available. The remaining two were reported to have the late onset or cryptic form of 21-hydroxylase deficiency (raised 17α-hydroxyprogesterone and no clinical signs or symptom). Whether early detection of this type is clinically useful remains to be evaluated.

Review of CAH Screening Programmes and the Scottish Experience

A. M. Wallace
Department of Clinical Biochemistry, Glasgow Royal Infirmary, Glasgow, UK

Recent advances in immunoassay techniques have heralded a new era in neonatal screening and it is now possible to detect endocrine disorders by blood spot hormone analysis. For instance, congenital hypothyroidism is now diagnosed by measuring TSH or thyroxine in blood spots, permitting early treatment of this potentially debilitating condition, and this procedure is now accepted as a worthwhile part of most neonatal screening programmes (Delange *et al.*, 1980; Sutherland *et al.*, 1981). Stimulated partly by this success neonatal screening has been advocated for congenital adrenal hyperplasia (CAH) and assays for 17α-hydroxyprogesterone (17-OHP) in blood spots have been developed to detect 21-hydroxylase deficiency (Pang *et al.*, 1977; Solyom 1981; Riordan *et al.*, 1984; Shimozawa *et al.*, 1984; Hofman *et al.*, 1985). The first screening programme was conducted in Alaska where an exceptionally high incidence of the condition occurs amongst Yupik

Journal of Inherited Metabolic Disease. ISSN 0141–8955. Queen Square, Lancaster, UK. Printed in Great Britain by Titus Wilson & Son Ltd., Kendal.

Eskimos (Pang *et al.*, 1982). Subsequent pilot programmes have been started in areas of lower incidence and information has been published from Italy (Cacciari *et al.*, 1983; Natoli *et al.*, 1983), Japan (Shimozawa *et al.*, 1984), the State of Washington, USA (Hofman *et al.*, 1985) and Scotland (Wallace *et al.*, 1986). Thus worldwide interest has occurred despite the fact that no one, to date, has produced conclusive evidence either that such screening is cost-effective or that it provides valuable clinical information. The timing of this workshop is opportune in that I believe that this vital information is only now becoming available.

METHODOLOGICAL CONSIDERATIONS

Are suitable methods available for large scale measurement of 17-OH-progesterone (17-OHP) in neonatal blood spot samples? Due to the large sample throughput the method should be simple, easy to operate and inexpensive. Solvent extraction which is extremely labour-intensive, time-consuming and expensive should be avoided. Tritium, the traditional label for steroid immunoassay, has the disadvantage of requiring expensive scintillation fluid and long counting times. The screening method must be precise and extremely robust. Sufficient sample may not be available for repeat determination and obtaining a further sample can be difficult and time-consuming to organise, is unpleasant for the baby and may upset the mother. For practical reasons it is essential that any screening system clearly differentiates positive cases from normals. Other considerations such as assay sensitivity and specificity will be discussed later. A number of screening methods have been published, some with solvent extraction of the steroid prior to radioimmunoassay (Pang *et al.*, 1977; Cacciari *et al.*, 1983) and some without (Hofman *et al.*, 1985; Shimozawa *et al.*, 1985; Wallace *et al.*, 1985). In addition a variety of steroid

Table 1

Labels	*Separation procedures*
tritium	dextran coated charcoal
iodine-125	second Ab
luminescence	polyethyleneglycol
fluorescence	solid phase first Ab
enzyme	solid phase second Ab
	microencapsulated Ab

labels and separation procedures have been used (Table 1). To some extent method selection is dependent on available equipment and expertise.

SCOTTISH SCREENING PROGRAMME

The aim of our study was to determine whether neonatal screening for CAH is possible and if so whether it contributes to health care. A high emphasis was placed on the development of a cheap and simple blood spot assay for 17-OHP. At the outset there were three essential requirements: the method must not involve solvent extraction; the separation of antibody bound from free fraction must be robust and efficient; and for fast and cost effective detection a gamma emitting label would be required. A direct screening procedure was developed tailored to these needs.

Iodinated 17-OHP label (17-OHP-3-CMO-iodohistamine) and rabbit antibody (raised against 17OHP-3CMO-BSA) were both produced in the Department of Clinical Biochemistry, Glasgow Royal Infirmary. The antibody was sheathed within semipermeable nylon microcapsules before use. Within such capsules the antibody is protected from interference by compounds of large molecular weight, and the capsules serve as a vehicle in which the antibody can be sedimented and washed prior to the counting of the antibody bound fraction (Wallace and Wood, 1984).

Initially it was important to establish the limits of normality for blood spot 17-OHP. Account was taken of the reports that 17-OHP concentrations are higher in premature infants (Pang *et al.*, 1982; Cacciari *et al.*, 1983; Murphy *et al.*, 1983), and results were analysed for mature and premature babies (from and before 37 weeks gestation respectively). In the direct assay, samples from 3567 mature and 376 premature babies were analysed. Median levels of 17-OHP were 17.5 (range: undetectable–90) and 31 (range: undetectable–120)nmol/L respectively. In the extraction assay, samples from 480 mature and 118 premature samples were examined. Results were considerably lower. Median levels of 17-OHP obtained were 5.0 (range: undetectable–55) and 13.5 (range: undetectable–75)nmol/L respectively. These results illustrate that as well as 17-OHP, some water soluble compound – probably 17-OH-pregnenolone sulphate or related conjugated steroid – is detected in the direct assay. As illustrated by Honour (1986) the fetal zone of the adrenal immediately post partum is exceptionally active in producing delta 5 steroids such as 17α-OH-pregnenolone, pregnenolone, dehydroepiandrosterone and their sulphates. We have also studied urinary steroid patterns in the neonate and obtained indirect evidence that in the preterm the fetal zone is exceptionally active. Therefore the high blood spot levels in the direct compared to the extraction assay, plus even higher levels in preterms compared to terms, can both be explained by lack of antibody specificity. All direct screening methods are likely to suffer from this lack of specificity since all 17-OHP antibodies reported to date show small but significant 17α-OH-pregnenolone cross reaction. It could be argued that this lack of specificity negates the use of the direct procedure for screening. In practice our experience is that this is not the case and the fact that we are measuring other related steroids may actually be to our advantage.

The upper cut-off for the direct assay was arbitrarily set at 100 nmol/L. This classed 0.3% of samples from mature cases and 2.5% of samples from premature babies as abnormal. Samples showing these high concentrations were re-examined using the extraction assay. This served both to confirm the elevated level and to improve specificity. The upper cut-off for the extraction assay was set at 50 nmol/L, and 0.2% of mature and 1.5% of premature cases exceeded this limit. From these findings an initial safe action limit was defined, and a follow-up sample and clinical history requested if a result of over 100 nmol/L in the direct assay was confirmed as being over 50 nmol/L after solvent extraction. These action limits were later reset to 140 nmol/L and 70 nmol/L respectively in the light of experience gained from screening 50 000 babies. Confirmation of 21-hydroxylase deficiency was obtained by urinary steroid scans performed as described by Shackelton and Honour (1976).

A flow diagram of our overall screening procedure is shown in Figure 1.

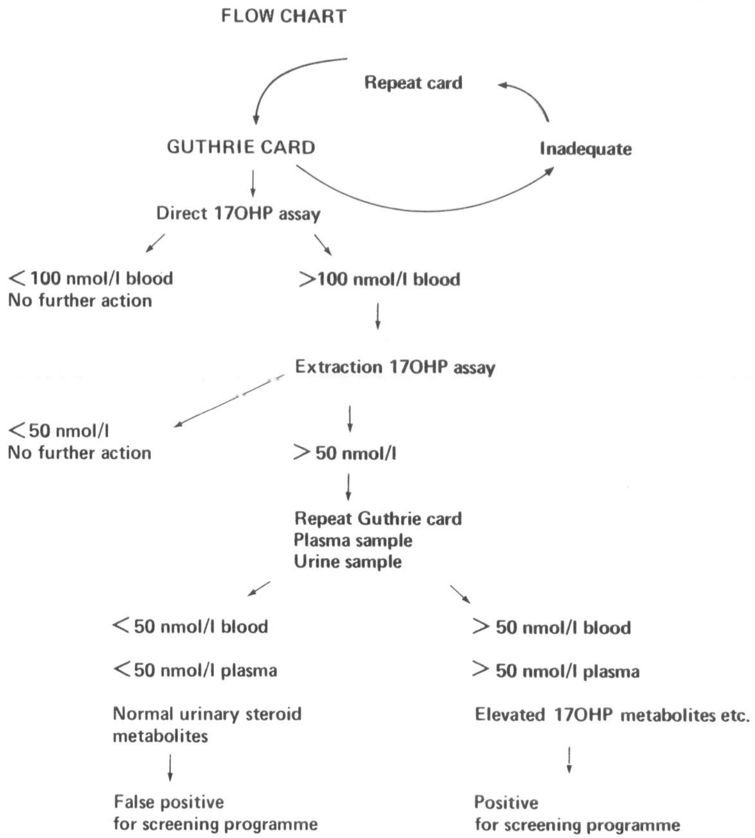

Figure 1 Neonatal screening for congenital adrenal hyperplasia: flow chart

There are continuing reports of delays in diagnosis of CAH. Hughes (1986) has reviewed the clinical advantages of early diagnosis. Theoretically neonatal screening for CAH should eradicate delayed diagnosis. As part of our screening study we have attempted to find out whether this is, in fact, the case in practice.

The Endocrine Laboratory at Glasgow Royal Infirmary offers a national service for the measurement of 17-OHP in plasma samples for infants with suspected CAH. Details of most Scottish cases are therefore available within the laboratory. A retrospective study of 15 cases diagnosed between 1978 and 1984 was conducted. In at least half the cases the condition was not suspected within three weeks of birth and in one instance the diagnosis was not made until the age of six. The original Guthrie card blood samples, which were stored at the neonatal screening laboratory, Stobhill Hospital, were located and retrospective analysis revealed elevated blood spot 17-OHP levels in all cases. Thus it can be anticipated that a national screening programme would provide useful diagnostic information in over half the CAH cases. The prevalence of CAH as calculated from this retrospective study is 1 in 20097 with a range of 1 in 12675 to 1 in 32604 (n = 301455). Retrospective studies, however, are subject to a number of limitations. In particular, we cannot know the prevalence of undiagnosed cases of CAH from the period 1978–1984. It is possible, for instance, that one or more babies may have died from a severe but undiagnosed instance of CAH. The prospective trial began in December 1983 and over 100000 neonates have now been screened for 21-hydroxylase deficiency. The current false positive rate is 0.04% and as far as we are aware there are no false negative cases (Table 2). Most of the false positives were preterm infants. In most cases a diagnosis of CAH was eliminated simply by the detection of normal 17-OHP levels in a repeat blood spot sample. In total, five CAH cases were detected. In each case a grossly elevated level of blood spot 17-OHP was detected

Table 2 Screening efficacy

	Initial action limit	*Current action limit*
blood spot 17-OHP (direct)	>100 nmol/L	>140 nmol/L
blood spot 17-OHP (extraction)	>50 nmol/L	>70 nmol/L
false positives	0.099%	0.042%
false negatives	0	0
sensitivity	100%	100%
specificity	99.9%	99.96%
predictive value of a positive result	3.9%	14.3%

and the paediatrician in charge was immediately informed (Table 3). All cases had evidence of salt loss and by examining the pattern of urinary steroid metabolites obtained by capillary column gas chromatography a definitive diagnosis of adrenal 21-hydroxylase deficiency was made. In cases 1 and 4 CAH was clinically suspected soon after birth but in three infants (cases 2, 3, and 5) there was no suspicion of any abnormality and these babies had been allowed home. Unfortunately in case 2 the initial blood sample was insufficient and the screening result was not available until day 21 at which time the infant was admitted as an emergency. This male infant had a history of persistant and progressive vomiting since birth and was extremely ill upon admission. In cases 3 and 5 the results were available by days 12 and 9 respectively. Both these cases lived some distance from a major hospital and were fortunately quickly admitted on our recommendation. Upon admission both infants had electrolyte abnormalities of a serious nature. Case 3 suffered a short collapse soon after admission and the child's life was probably saved by the immediate availability of a paediatric intensive care unit. Steroid replacement stabilized the condition in all cases: the time taken to stabilize was directly related to the extent of salt loss at time of diagnosis. The prevalence of CAH as calculated from the information gained in the prospective trial was 1 in 18401 with a range of 1 in 7422 to 1 in 50006. The efficacy of our screening programme is outlined in Table 2.

Table 3 Details of CAH positive cases

Case No.	*Abbreviated clinical history*	*Na* (mmol/L)	*K* (mmol/L)	*Direct blood spot 17-OHP* (nmol/L)	*Extract blood spot 17-OHP* (nmol/L)	*Plasma 17-OHP* (nmol/L)
1	Well but jaundiced Asian infant. Genitalia male in appearance. Female karyotype. FH of CAH uncovered	128	6	>300	750	1205
2	Critically ill male. First blood spot card insufficient. 2nd card processed by day 21	103	9	>300	600	4185
3	Male term infant. Transferred to hospital on day 12 in response to raised blood spot 17-OHP. Penis and scrotum pigmented. Na fell to 123 mmol/L during subsequent adrenal crisis	127	7.4	480	400	1210
4	Male term infant (sibling with CAH). Dehydrated, jaundiced, lethargic	134	7.9	392	187	310
5	Male term infant. Transferred to hospital on day 9 in response to high blood spot 17-OHP. Replacement therapy took some time to stabilize the condition	129	8.8	483	508	600
	(upper limit of normal			140	70	50)

Our findings are in agreement with others and indicate that neonatal screening for CAH is possible. Our major expense is the employment of one operator and running costs are in the region of £10 000 per year (15p per birth). Initially we were unsure as to the clinical value of screening, but as the project progressed we became more and more certain that we were making a positive contribution to health care. The procedure is so inexpensive if added to an already operating neonatal screening programme that the question is: can we now afford not to screen?

ACKNOWLEDGEMENTS

The author is extremely grateful to all who contributed to this study. In particular thanks are due to many paediatricians throughout Scotland. The Greater Glasgow Health Board and Serono Diagnostics provided financial support that was greatly appreciated.

REFERENCES

Cacciari, E., Balsamo, A., Cassio, A., Piazzi, S., Bernardi, F., Saladi, S., Cicognani, A., Pirazzoli, P., Zappulla, F., Capelli, M. and Paolini, M. Neonatal screening for congenital adrenal hyperplasia. *Arch. Dis. Child.*, 58 (1983) 803–806

Delange, F., Beckers, C., Hofer, R., Konig, M. P., Monaco, F. and Varome, S. Progress report on neonatal screening for congenital hypothyroidism in Europe. In Burrow, G. N. and Dussault, J. H. (eds.), *Neonatal Thyroid Screening*, Raven Press, New York, 1980, p. 107

Hofman, L. F., Klanieki, J. E. and Smith, E. K. Direct solid-phase radioimmunoassay for screening 17α-hydroxyprogesterone in whole-blood samples from newborns. *Clin. Chem.* 31 (1985) 1127–1130

Honour, J. Biochemical aspects of congenital adrenal hyperplasia. *J. Inher. Metab. Dis.* 9 Suppl. 1 (1986) 124–134

Hughes, I. A. Clinical aspects of congenital adrenal hyperplasia: early diagnosis and treatment. *J. Inher. Metab. Dis.* 9 Suppl. 1 (1986) 115–123

Murphy, J. F., Joyce, B. G., Dyas, J. and Hughes, I. A. Plasma 17α-hydroxyprogesterone concentration in ill newborn infants. *Arch. Dis. Child.* 58 (1983) 532–534

Natoli, G., Moschini, L., Asconia, P., Albino, G., Costa, P. and Pansa, G. Neonatal screening by microassay of 17α-hydroxyprogesterone in congenital adrenal hyperplasia. In Chiumello, G. and Sperling, M. (eds.) *Recent Progress in Pediatric Endocrinology*, Raven Press, New York, 1983, pp. 285–290

Pang, S., Hotchkiss, J., Drash, A. L., Levine, L. S. and New, M. I. Microfilter paper method for 17-hydroxyprogesterone radioimmunoassay: its application for rapid screening for congenital adrenal hyperplasia. *J. Clin. Endocrinol. Metab.* 45 (1977) 1003–1008

Pang, S., Murphey, W., Levine, L. S., Spence, D. A., Leon, A., LaFranchi., Surve, A. S. and New, M. I. A pilot newborn screening for congenital adrenal hyperplasia in Alaska. *J. Clin. Endocrinol. Metab.* 55 (1982) 413–420

Riordan, F. A. I., Wood, P. J., Wakelin, K., Betts, P. and Clayton, B. E. Bloodspot 17α-hydroxyprogesterone radioimmunoassay for diagnosis of congenital adrenal hyperplasia and home monitoring of corticosteroid replacement therapy. *Lancet* 2 (1984) 708–710

Shackleton, C. H. L. and Honour, J. W. Simultaneous estimation of urinary steroids by semi-automated gas chromatography. Investigation of neonatal infants and children with abnormal steroid synthesis. *Clin. Chim. Acta* 69 (1976) 267-278

Shimozawa, K., Saisho, S., Saito, N., Yata, J., Igarashi, Y., Hikita, Y., Irie, M. and Okada, K. A neonatal mass-screening for congenital adrenal hyperplasia in Japan. *Acta Endocrinol.* 107 (1984) 513–518

Solyom, J. Blood-spot 17-hydroxyprogesterone radioimmunoassay in the follow-up of congenital adrenal hyperplasia. *Clin. Endocrinol. (Oxford)* 14 (1981) 547–553

Sutherland, R. M., Ratcliffe, J. G., Kennedy, R., Stevenson, J. S., Patrick, M. J. and Ferguson-Smith, M. A. Neonatal screening for hypothyroidism in Scotland. *Scot. Med. J.* 26 (1981) 229–234

Wallace, A. M. and Wood, D. A. Development of a simple procedure for the preparation of semipermeable antibody-containing microcapsules and their analytical performance in a radioimmunoassay for 17-hydroxyprogesterone. *Clin. Chim. Acta* 140 (1984) 203–212

Wallace, A. M., Beastall, G. H., Cook, B., Ross, A. M., Kennedy, R. and Girdwood, R. W. A. Neonatal screening for congenital adrenal hyperplasia: a programme based on a novel direct radioimmunoassay for 17-hydroxyprogesterone in blood spots. *J. Endocrinol.* 108 (1986) 299–308

J. Inher. Metab. Dis. 9 Suppl. 1 (1986) 142–146

Neonatal Screening Programme for Congenital Adrenal Hyperplasia in a Homogenous Caucasian Population

E. Cacciari[1], A. Balsamo[1], A. Cassio[1], S. Piazzi[2], F. Bernardi[1], S. Salardi[1], A. Cicognani[1], P. Pirazzoli[1], F. Zappulla[1], M. Capelli[2], M. Paolini[2] and C. I. Cordaro[1]

[1]2nd Pediatric Clinic and [2]Central Laboratory, University of Bologna, S. Orsola Hospital, via Massarenti 11, Bologna, 40138, Italy

The considerable variation in the reported incidence of congenital adrenal hyperplasia (CAH 1, McKusick 20191) (Childs *et al.*, 1956; Prader, 1958; Hubble, 1966; Rosenbloom and Smith, 1966; Hirschfield and Fleshman, 1969; Qazi and Thompson, 1972; Pang *et al.*, 1981) may be explained partially by the lack of a valid screening method. To evaluate the true prevalence of CAH, we examined all the newborns in the Emilia Romagna region of Italy during a period of approximately three years. Emilia Romagna is situated in northern Italy and our sample there was of a homogenous Caucasian population. For the screening programme we took advantage of the specimens collected on filter paper for neonatal screening of hypothyroidism and phenylketonuria. For the 17-OH-progesterone assay, the microfilter paper method modified from that of Pang and colleagues (Pang *et al.*, 1977; Cacciari *et al.*, 1982; Piazzi *et al.*, 1981; Cacciari *et al.*, 1983) was used.

After statistical analysis of the results and the clinical examination of subjects during the first period of the screening procedure, we established 20 pg/disc as the recall value. Where values were higher than this, they were confirmed by a second microfilter paper assay and then the serum 17-OH-progesterone concentration was determined. 73 000 newborn babies were examined. 132 (0.18%) had a value above the threshold of 20 pg/disc and were retested. Among those recalled, 7 demonstrated a pathological value, with a CAH prevalence of 1 case in 10 428.

Table 1 represents the frequency of the various forms of 21-hydroxylase deficiency and the 95% confidence limits as well as the heterozygote and gene frequencies (Diem and Leutner, 1972; Fristrom and Spieth, 1980). Recently Natoli and colleagues (1984) found a similar incidence of 21-hydroxylase deficiency in a population of 94 121 newborns from central and southern Italy using the same method of screening for CAH (estimated incidence of homozygous affected population 1 in 9412; heterozygous carrier population 1 in 49; gene frequency 0.0003).

Day of sampling, gestational age, and birthweight were all considered in the analysis of results. With regard to gestational age, infants were divided into two groups, namely term (delivered between 37 and 42 weeks of gestation) or preterm (delivered before 37 weeks gestation). 17-OH-progesterone values in relation to

Journal of Inherited Metabolic Disease. ISSN 0141–8955.

Table 1 Frequencies of the various forms of 21-hydroxylase deficiency

Prevalence of CAH	1:10428
salt-losing forms	1:18250
simple virilizing forms	1:73000
non-classical forms	1:36500
95% Confidence limits	
lower	1:21978
upper	1:5062
Heterozygote frequency	1:51
Gene frequency	0.010

Table 2 Relation between 17-OHP values and day of sampling

Day	*Number of cases*	*Value* (pg/disc) (*mean±SD*)
2	219 (0.3%)	5.62±1.01
3	1460 (2.0%)	6.03±2.10
4	11534 (15.8%)	6.42±2.43
5	34456 (47.2%)	6.31±2.58
6	14819 (20.3%)	6.98±3.02
7	2555 (3.5%)	8.84±8.39
7	7957 (10.9%)	7.83±7.74

the day of sampling are reported in Table 2. No statistically significant differences were found between the various days. What might be surprising is the low mean value of 17-OH-progesterone given by infants examined on their second day of life. This finding might be ascribed to the fact that sampling was usually done before the baby left the obstetric ward, and it is possible that the infants examined and considered fit to be moved on days 2 and 3 of life were the most mature, and therefore showed lower 17-OH-progesterone values.

Table 3 Number and percentage of retests according to gestational age

	Patients tested		*Patients retested*	
	number	*percentage*	*number*	*percentage*
Term infants	66503	91.1	53	0.08*
Preterm infants	6497	8.9	79	1.22*

* $\phi^2 = 418$ ($p<0.0000001$)

Table 3 represents the number and percentage of the neonates recalled, according to gestational age. The percentage recalled among preterm infants was significantly higher than that of term infants. This justifies the setting of a higher recall threshold for the preterm infants. Furthermore, it must be pointed out that in spite of the fact that the number recalled turned out to be high in the premature infants, the

17-OH-progesterone values rapidly became normal even in these subjects, as could be seen in the first follow-up which was usually made within the third week of life.

The 17-OH-progesterone values according to gestational age (term and preterm)

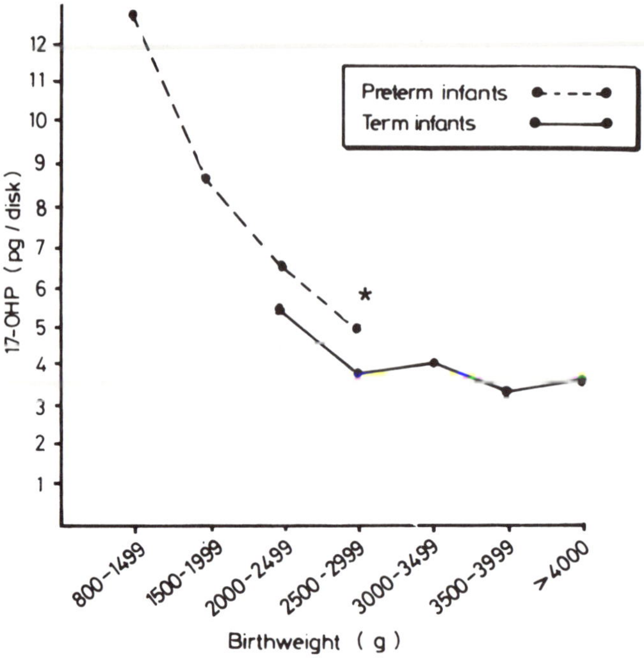

* $P<0{\cdot}05$ between term and preterm children in the group with birthweight 2500–3000 g.

Figure 1 17-OH-progesterone values (pg/disc) according to gestational age (term and preterm) and birthweight

and birthweight, show significant differences (Figure 1). Among the term infants, a significant difference was found between the groups with birthweights of less than 2500 g and the groups with birthweights of more than 3500 g. Another significant difference was evident between the term and preterm infants in the weight range 2500–3000 g, while no such difference was present between the groups with birthweights of 2000–2500 g. From these data it would seem that the gestational age has greater influence on adrenal enzymatic maturity in infants having a birthweight greater than 2500 g, whereas birthweight seems to be more important in infants of less than 2500 g.

The seven infants affected by 21-hydroxylase deficiency (four females and three males) included four with salt wasting (Table 4, cases 1, 4, 5 and 7), one simple virilizing form (Table 4, case 2), and two patients (Table 4, cases 3 and 6) with late onset or cryptic form of CAH, based on a high 17-OH-progesterone value with no clinical signs (Levine *et al.*, 1978; Zachmann and Prader, 1978; New *et al.*, 1979; Blankstein *et al.*, 1980). Six of them were born at term and one preterm.

In cases 1 and 4 the screening enabled us to make a diagnosis and begin therapy immediately. In the other infants, with the exception of the two having the non-

Table 4 Clinical and hormonal features of the 7 infants with CAH

Case	*Age* (days)	*Gestation*	*Birthweight* (g)	*17-OH-progesterone*		*External genitalia*
				1st spot (pg/disc)	*serum* (ng/dL)	
1 (M)	4	term	4000	250		mild macrogenito-
	24				5000	somia
2 (F)	5	term	3300	28*		ambiguous
	150				5000	
3 (F)	5	term	3870	47		normal
	30				1400	
4 (F)	4	term	3000	250		ambiguous
	14				5000	
5 (F)	3	term	3200	250		ambiguous
	7				5000	
6 (M)	2	preterm	1350	150		normal
	2				560	
7 (M)	3	term	3250	250		mild macrogenito-
	16				5000	somia

* This patient's blood, collected on filter paper, was stored in unfit conditions, which may explain her relatively low 17-OH-progesterone value

typical form, the results of the screening did nothing but confirm the diagnostic suspicion of the physician.

In the last six months, because of technical reasons, CAH screening has been restricted to 'at risk' subjects only, after an intense educational campaign especially in the obstetric and newborn environment. Using this method, two more cases of CAH have been diagnosed, and this is practically just what we expected. Naturally, the non-typical forms may have missed by this approach to screening.

In conclusion we can say that (1) neonatal screening for CAH by means of 17-OH-progesterone assay on filter paper discs is a reliable method for diagnosing 21-hydroxylase deficiency, and it is convenient to carry it out in the same laboratory that screens for phenylketonuria and hypothyroidism, (2) the maturity of the neonates and the particular day of sampling affect the values of 17-OH-progesterone but not the validity of the screening, and (3) although these data alone do not justify wide scale or even national scale screening for CAH, further experience is needed before definite conclusions may be drawn.

REFERENCES

Blankstein, J., Faiman, C., Reyes, F. I., Shroeder, M. L. and Winter, J. S. D. Adult onset familial adrenal 21-hydroxylase deficiency. *Am. J. Med.* 68 (1980) 441–448

Cacciari, E., Balsamo, A., Cassio, A., Piazzi, S., Bernardi, F., Salardi, S., Cicognani, A., Pirazzoli, P., Zappulla, F., Capelli, M. and Paolini, M. Neonatal screening for congenital adrenal hyperplasia using a microfilter paper method for 17α-hydroxyprogesterone radioimmunoassay. Experience gained from the study of 22 233 cases. *Horm. Res.* 16 (1982) 4–9

Cacciari, E., Balsamo, A., Cassio, A., Piazzi, S., Bernardi, F., Salardi, S., Cicognani, A., Pirazzoli, P., Zappulla, F., Capelli, M. and Paolini, M. Neonatal screening for congenital adrenal hyperplasia. *Arch. Dis. Child.* 58 (1983) 803–806

Childs, B., Grumbach, M. M. and Van Wyk, J. J. Virilizing adrenal hyperplasia. A genetical and hormonal study. *J. Clin. Invest.* 35 (1956) 213–221

Diem, K. and Lentner, C. *Scientific Tables*, 7th edn. Ciba Geigy, Switzerland, 1982, p. 188

Fristrom, J. W. and Spieth, P. T. *Principles of Genetics*, Chiron Press, New York, 1980, p. 533

Hirschfield, A. J. and Fleshman, J. K. An unusually high incidence of salt-losing congenital adrenal hyperplasia in the Alaskan Eskimo. *J. Pediatr.* 75 (1969) 492–494

Hubble, D. Congenital adrenal hyperplasia. In Holts, K. S. and Raine, D. N. (eds.) Basic Concepts of Inborn Errors and Defects of Steroid Biosynthesis, *Proceedings of the 3rd Symposium Society for the Study of Inborn Errors of Metabolism*, Livingstone, Edinburgh, 1966, pp. 68–75

Levine, L. S., Zachmann, M. and New, M. I. Genetic mapping of the 21-hydroxylase-deficiency gene within the HLA linkage group. *N. Engl. J. Med.* 299 (1978) 911–915

Natoli, G., Angeloni, P., Costa, F., Pausa, G., Moschini, L., Stara, B., Maggioni, G. Neonatal screening for 21-hydroxylase deficiency congenital adrenal hyperplasia: our experience on 94 121 newborns. Satellite Symposium, 7th International Congress of Endocrinology, 1984, New York (In press)

New, M. I., Lorenzen, F., Pang, S., Gunczler, P., Dupont, D., and Levine, L. S. 'Acquired' adrenal hyperplasia with 21-hydroxylase deficiency is not the same genetic disorder as congenital adrenal hyperplasia. *J. Clin. Endocrinol. Metab.* 48 (1979) 356–369

Pang, S., Hotchkiss, J., Drash, A. L., Levine, L. S. and New, M. I. Microfilter paper method for 17α-hydroxyprogesterone radioimmunoassay: its application for rapid screening for congenital adrenal hyperplasia. *J. Clin. Endocrinol. Metab.* 45 (1977) 1003–1008

Pang, S., Murphy, W. and Levine, L. S. A pilot newborn screening for congenital adrenal hyperplasia (CAH) due to 21-hydroxylase deficiency at New York Hospital and Alaska. 1st Joint Meeting LWPES–ESPE, Geneva, 1981

Piazzi, S., Capelli, M., Paolini, M., Perugini, D., Grossi, G., Balsamo, A., Salomoni, P., Cassio, A., Bugiardini, G. and Cacciari, E. Neonatal screening for 21-hydroxylase deficiency: a microfilter paper method for 17α-hydroxyprogesterone assay. *J. Endocrinol. Invest.* 5 (1982) 87–90

Prader, A. Die Hauefigkeit des kongenital adrenogenital Syndroms. *Helv. Paediatr. Acta* 13 (1958) 426–431

Qazi, Q. H. and Thompson, W. M. Incidence of salt-losing form for congenital virilizing hyperplasia. *Arch. Dis. Child.* 47 (1972) 302–307

Rosenbloom, A. L. and Smith, D. W. Congenital adrenal hyperplasia (letter). *Lancet* 1 (1966) 660

Zachmann, M. and Prader, A. Unusual heterozygotes of congenital adrenal hyperplasia due to 21-hydroxylase deficiency. *Acta Endocrinol.* 87 (1980) 557–565

J. Inher. Metab. Dis. 9 Suppl. 1 (1986) 147–151

Neonatal Screening for Congenital Adrenal Hyperplasia: a Pilot Study in France

J. L. DHONDT[1], C. DORCHE[2], J. P. FARRIAUX[1] and C. COURTE[3]
[1]*Regional Centre for Neonatal Screening, Faculté de Médecine, 59045 Lille, France;*
[2]*Hopital Debrousse, 69322 Lyon, France;*
[3]*BioMerieux, 69260 Charbonnieres-les-Bains, France*

Congenital adrenal hyperplasia (CAH) due to a deficiency of 21-hydroxylase is the most common inborn error of the adrenal steroid biosynthetic pathway. The considerable increase of 17α-hydroxyprogesterone (17-OHP) in the serum of CAH patients has been shown to be already evident at the neonatal period (Chaussain *et al.*, 1974). Consequently, radioimmunoassays have been developed to measure 17-OHP in dried blood samples and have made neonatal screening programmes possible.

Two French regional centres for neonatal screening, Lille and Lyon, set up a pilot programme in 1981 to study the different problems raised by CAH mass screening. The present report summarizes the results of CAH screening in different populations and some technical improvements of the RIA determination of 17-OHP in dried blood samples.

METHOD

Capillary blood samples were collected on the filter paper routinely used for the neonatal screening of phenylketonuria and congenital hypothyroidism, usually on the fifth day of life. 17-OHP was measured by two RIA methods developed in collaboration with Biomerieux (Marcy l'Etoile, France):

Tritium method: 17-OHP was eluted from 6 mm diameter discs with 1 mL of phosphate buffer for 30 min and then extracted with 5 mL of ethyl ether using a Sepex apparatus (Biomerieux). Organic phase separation was obtained by freezing the watery phase. The organic phase was evaporated under nitrogen. The extract was dissolved in 100 μL of buffer, then 100 μL of ^{3}H-tracer and 100 μL of antiserum were added. After a 30 min incubation, at room temperature, separation of bound and free was achieved with dextran-charcoal.

Iodine-125 method: 17-OHP was eluted from 3 mm diameter discs with 100 μL of phosphate buffer, 100 μL of ^{125}I-labelled 17-OHP and 100 μL of antiserum. After 1 hour at 37°C, the bound phase was separated using a further 30 min incubation with a polyethyleneglycol second antibody mixture.

Journal of Inherited Metabolic Disease. ISSN 0141–8955.

Standard solutions or standard discs prepared with spiked blood samples were used for the calibration curve (0–800 pg/tube).

RESULTS

CAH screening with the tritium RIA method (Table 1)

Three different pilot programmes have been conducted:

(1) In the Lyon region during 1981–1982, 27 857 tests were performed on male newborns only, since clinical diagnosis was initially thought to be easier for girls. With a recall value of 24 nmol/L (80 pg/disc), 30 infants (0.11%) were recalled. 27 were born prematurely. One patient was found to have a mild form of CAH.

(2) A systematic sample was made of 17 466 infants born in the Lille area during 1981–1982 and 1984. With a recall value of 40 pg/disc, the recall rate was 0.4%. Approximately two thirds of the recalled infants were premature or low birthweight babies. One female infant was found to have a mild form of CAH.

(3) 10 617 samples were collected from infants born in the island of La Réunion, a French overseas department with a high incidence of CAH, four patients were proven to have CAH.

Table 1 17-OHP values obtained in 16 patients

Patient	*Sex*	*Area of origin*	*Circumstance of testing*	*Tracer*	*17-OH-P* (pg/disc)	*Day of sampling*	*Remark*
1	F	La Réunion	systematic screening	^{3}H	1024	5	—
2	F	Lille	virilization	^{3}H	409	1	—
3	F	Lille	systematic screening	^{3}H	173	5	mild CAH
4	M	La Réunion	salt-losing	^{3}H	1406	20	—
5	F	La Réunion	virilization	^{3}H	912	2	—
6	M	La Réunion	systematic screening	^{3}H	1035	5	died on day 41
7	M	La Réunion	systematic screening	^{3}H	1051	5	died on day 30
8	M	La Réunion	systematic screening	^{3}H	1143/1127	5/21	—
9	M	La Réunion	salt-losing	^{3}H	95	5	mild CAH
10	M	Lyon	systematic screening	^{3}H	297	6	—
11	F	Lyon	salt-losing	^{3}H	450	5	—
12	F	Lyon	salt-losing	^{3}H	800	23	—
13	F	Lyon	salt-losing	^{3}H	800	25	—
14	M	Outside Lyon	salt-losing	^{3}H	300	5	—
15	F	Lyon	systematic screening	^{125}I	160	5	mild CAH
16	M	Lille	systematic screening	^{125}I	300	5	—

In addition to the systematic screening, eight clinically suspected neonates from other areas were submitted to this test.

CAH screening with the iodine RIA method (Table 1)

Evaluation of the assay: The sensitivity was usually 10 pg/tube and 50% of displacement obtained for 50 pg/tube. No significant difference was observed when the standard curve was established with either liquid standard solution or spiked blood spots. Intra-assay and inter-assay coefficients of variation were below 10%. The cross-reaction with other steroids was calculated at 50% displacement of ^{125}I-labelled 17-OHP and was 2.1% for 17-OH-pregnenolone, 1.3% for 11-deoxycortisol, 0.02% for progesterone and less than 0.003% for cortisol, pregnenolone, testosterone, estriol and Δ4-androstenedione. However, cross-reactivity with water soluble 17-OH-pregnenolone-3-sulphate has not been yet measured.

In order to check the method accuracy, 52 dried blood samples obtained from treated CAH patients were analysed with the direct ^{125}I method, and sera collected at the same time were assayed by a conventional ^{3}H method after ether extraction. Results were expressed in nmol/L of serum: the linear regression equation was $y(^{125}\mathrm{I}) = 1.13\ (^{3}\mathrm{H}) + 3.66$, $r = 0.966$. In addition, dried blood samples from 78 neonates were analysed with the two methods; the linear regression equation was $y(^{125}\mathrm{I}) = 2.80\ (^{3}\mathrm{H}) + 42.7$, $r = 0.859$.

APPLICATION TO MASS SCREENING

A pilot programme was initiated on 1st January 1985. According to the distribution of 17-OHP values in the first 6788 neonates examined, the threshold value was fixed at 65 pg/disc (99th centile).

During the initial period, 5687 tests were performed and 81 submitted to a retest procedure including ^{3}H and ^{125}I assay from the original filter paper: 28 (35%) were above 40 pg/6 mm disc with the ^{3}H method and 39 (48%) above 65 pg/3 mm disc with the direct ^{125}I method. Following the demonstration that the two methods were highly correlated, and in order to keep the time between sampling and final result as short as possible, it was decided that for samples with initial values above 65 pg/disc a repeat determination would be performed only with the direct ^{125}I method, but on duplicates to minimize intra-assay error.

A total of 38 541 newborn infants had been tested by 30th May 1985 ; 483 (1.3%) had values above 65 pg/disc and were checked by a second assay in duplicate on the same card, and 212 (44%) were confirmed as above 65 pg/disc: 77% were from premature babies. These subjects were either recalled to obtain a second specimen or immediately recommended for medical evaluation for suspected CAH, depending on the 17-OHP level and clinical information (prematurity, intercurrent disease etc.). Usually infants in whom 17-OHP remained high presented with severe illness (i.e. cardiac or diaphragmatic malformation). One male infant with a non-salt-losing form of CAH and a girl with a virilizing and salt-losing form have been recognized: at the time of screening 17-OHP values were respectively 160 and 300 pg/disc.

DISCUSSION

CAH associated with a deficiency of the 21-hydroxylase enzyme (EC 1.1.1.151) is the most common inborn error of the adrenal steroid biosynthetic pathway, accounting for 91.5% of such defects in France (Bois *et al.*, 1985). The feasibility of a reliable newborn screening programme for CAH utilizing the microfilter paper test for 17-OHP determination has been demonstrated by several groups (Cacciari *et al.*, 1982; Pang *et al.*, 1982; Riordan *et al.*, 1984; Shimozawa *et al.*, 1984; Solyom, 1981; Tsuji *et al.*, 1983). The incidence of CAH in France has recently been estimated as 1 in 23 000 (Bois *et al.*, 1985), a figure in agreement with that which we obtained in the metropolitan population (1 in 20 966). The higher frequency in the island of La Réunion (1 in 2650) can be explained by a higher incidence of consanguinity.

The tritium method can be considered as a reference method, but organic extraction and liquid scintillation counting are difficult to handle when a large number of samples have to be tested each day. For these reasons we have developed a direct assay using a ^{125}I-tracer. The method fits the usual requirements for a screening test, directness, speed (~3 h) and cheapness (~0.35US$), by eliminating the costly and time consuming steps due to extraction and liquid scintillation counting. Three to four batches of 200 blood spots could be routinely analysed per day. A high significant correlation was observed between disc 17-OHP and plasma concentrations. In neonates however, the former were significantly higher than the latter, a figure already described when direct methods are used and presumably secondary to interference of 17-OH-pregnenolone and its sulphate derivative (Shimozawa *et al.*, 1984; Tsuji *et al.*, 1983).

In the present study samples have been taken mostly on day 5 of life (90% being collected between days 4 and 9). Consequently results are not influenced by the dramatic changes of steroids concentration during the perinatal period (Forest and Cathiard, 1978; Tapanainen *et al.*, 1984). However, as expected from previous studies (Godo *et al.*, 1981), there were many premature infants among the false positive cases. The choice of a threshold value which would reduce the incidence of false positive remains difficult. 17-OHP values are appreciably higher in ill term and healthy preterm babies. In some cases, values approaching those seen in untreated CAH infants have been reported (Hughes *et al.*, 1979; Murphy *et al.*, 1983). On the other hand, some patients have been reported with either 'borderline' or normal values (Deperetti and Forest, 1982; Shimozawa *et al.*, 1984). A larger trial would give additional information on difficulties of interpretation and on the risks of raising the cut-off value. At present it appears crucial to maintain a low alarm threshold and to take account of gestational age and presence of stress-related illness for the recall decision.

ACKNOWLEDGEMENTS

We are grateful to Dr M. Forest for the tritium determination of 17-OH-progesterone for tests found positive with the iodine method. This work was supported by the Association Regionale pour le Depistage et la Prevention des Maladies Metaboliques et des Handicaps de l'Enfant (Lille) and by the Association Regionale pour le Depistage et l'Etude des Maladies Metaboliques de l'Enfant (Lyon).

REFERENCES

Bois, E., Mornet, E., Chompret, A., Feingold, J., Hochez, J. and Goulet, V. L'hyperplasie congenitale des surrenales (21-OH) en France. *Arch. Fr. Ped.* 42 (1985) 175–179

Cacciari, E., Balsamo, A., Cassio, A., Piazzi, S., Bernardi, F., Salardi, S., Cicognani, A., Pirazzoli, P., Zappulla, F., Capelli, M. and Paolini, M. Neonatal screening for congenital adrenal hyperplasia using a microfilter paper method for 17α-hydroxyprogesterone radioimmunoassay. *Horm. Res.* 16 (1982) 4–9

Chaussain, J. L., Estrada, Y., Roger, M., Tea, N. T., Scholler, R., Canlorbe, P. and Job, J. C. La 17-OH-progesterone plasmatique. Mesure chez l'enfant normal et dans les hyperplasies surrenales congenitales par bloc de la 21-hydroxylation. *Nouv. Presse Med.* 3 (1974) 2621–2624

Forest, M. G. and Cathiard, A. M. Ontogenic study of plasma 17α-hydroxyprogesterone in the human. I. Postnatal period: evidence for a transient ovarian activity in infancy. *Pediatr. Res.* 12 (1978) 6–11

Godo, B., Visser, H. K. A and Degenhart, H. J. Plasma 17-OH-progesterone in fullterm and preterm infants at birth and during early neonatal period. *Horm. Res.* 15 (1981) 65–71

Hughes, I. A., Riad-Fahmy, D. and Griffiths, K. Plasma 17-OH-progesterone concentrations in newborn infants. *Arch. Dis. Child.* 58 (1981) 65–71

Murphy, J. F., Joyce, B. G., Dyqs, J. and Hughes, I. A. Plasma 17-hydroxyprogesterone concentrations in ill newborn infants. *Arch. Dis. Child.* 58 (1983) 532–534

New, M. I., Dupont, B., Pang, S., Pollack, M. and Levine, L. S. An update of congenital adrenal hyperplasia. *Recent Prog. Horm. Res.* 37 (1981) 105–182

Pang, S., Murphy, W., Levine, L. S., Spence, D. A., Leon, A., La Franchi, S., Surve, A. S. and New, M. I. A pilot newborn screening for congenital adrenal hyperplasia in Alaska. *J. Clin. Endocrinol. Metab.* 55 (1982) 413–420

De Peretti, E. and Forest, M. G. Pitfalls in the etiological diagnosis of congenital adrenal hyperplasia in the early neonatal period. *Horm. Res.* 16 (1982) 10–22

Riordan, F. A. I., Wood, P. J., Wakelin, K., Betts, P. and Clayton, B. E. Bloodspot 17α-hydroxyprogesterone radioimmunoassay for diagnosis of congenital adrenal hyperplasia and home monitoring of corticoidsteroid replacement therapy. *Lancet* 1 (1984) 708–710

Shimozawa, K., Saisho, S., Saito, N., Yata, J., Igarashi, Y., Hikita, Y., Irie, M. and Okada, K. A neonatal mass-screening for congenital adrenal hyperplasia in Japan. *Acta Endocrinol.* 107 (1984) 513–518

Solyom, J. Blood-spot 17α-hydroxyprogesterone radioimmunoassay in the follow-up of congenital adrenal hyperplasia. *Clin. Endocrinol.* 14 (1981) 547–553

Tapanainen, J., Huhtaniemi, I., Koivisto, M., Kujansuu, E., Tuimala, R. and Vihko, R. Hormonal changes during the perinatal period: FSH, prolactin and some steroid hormones in the cord blood and peripheral serum of preterm and fullterm female infants. *J. Steroid Biochem.* 20 (1984) 1153–1156

Tsuji, A., Maeda, M., Arakawa, H., Naruse, H., Suzuki, E. and Kambegawa, A. Fluorescence enzyme immunoassay of 17α-hydroxyprogesterone and its application to mass screening for congenital adrenal hyperplasia. In Naruse, H. and Irie M. (eds.) *Neonatal Screening. Excerpta Medica*, 1983, pp. 324

J. Inher. Metab. Dis. 9 Suppl. 1 (1986) 152–155

Existing Clinical Diagnoses

The following two short communications summarize the changes in ages of patients diagnosed to have congenital adrenal hyperplasia and show a distinct improvement in detection at an early age (<1 month) since 1970. Incidence figures also suggest that few patients are being missed.

Congenital Adrenal Hyperplasia in Birmingham: a Retrospective Analysis (1958–1985)

N. K. Virdi and A. Green
Department of Clinical Chemistry, The Children's Hospital, Birmingham B16 8ET, UK

Recent estimates of the prevalence of congenital adrenal hyperplasia (CAH) are 1 in 8000–9000 by neonatal screening (Cacciari *et al.*, 1983) and 1 in 12 000–13 000 by case report (Murtaza *et al.*, 1980; Werder *et al.*, 1980). Up to two thirds of the cases suffer from the more severe salt-losing form of the disease (Murtaza *et al.*, 1980; Werder *et al.*, 1980; Lebovitz *et al.*, 1984).

The purpose of our study was to review retrospectively the presentation and age at diagnosis of all known patients with CAH under the care of paediatricians at the Birmingham Children's Hospital between 1958 and 1985. There is no neonatal screening programme for CAH at Birmingham, and all cases had been diagnosed because of clinical presentation. The following information was collected: patient's sex, date of birth, age at diagnosis, presenting clinical features, diagnosis (salt-losing or non-salt-losing) and relevant family history.

RESULTS

117 cases were reviewed. In some cases not all the information was available.

Sex distribution: There were 44 males and 71 females (male : female ratio 2 : 3).

Prevalence of salt loss: 27 of 44 males (61.4%) and 38 of 67 females (56.7%) were salt losers.

Age at diagnosis and presenting features: The age at diagnosis of males and females is shown in Figure 1. 31 female patients presented within 24 h of birth with ambiguous external genitalia. Of these, 22 (71%) were salt-losers. The remaining female patients were diagnosed at ages ranging from 5 d to 13.5 y. The age range for diagnosis of male patients was 3 d to 7 y. All salt-losers were diagnosed within 6 months of life, with 90% of the diagnoses being made by 1 month of age.

Journal of Inherited Metabolic Disease. ISSN 0141–8955. Printed in Great Britain by Titus Wilson & Son Ltd., Kendal.

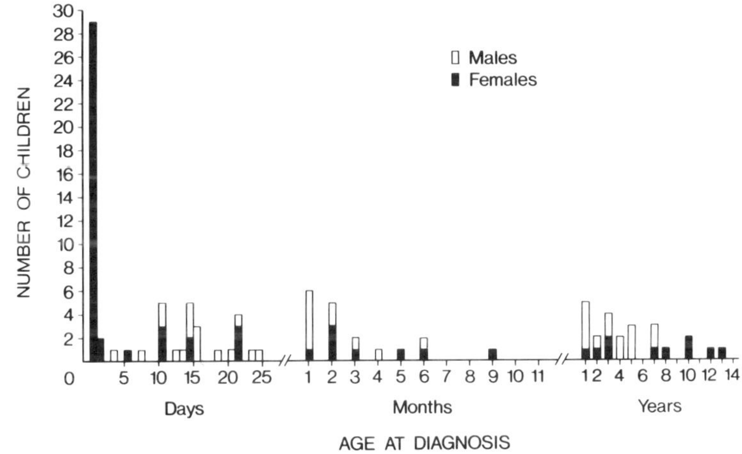

Figure 1 Patients with CAH: age at diagnosis

Table 1 Presenting clinical features of CAH in females

Diagnosis	*Total number*	*Presentation*	
Salt-losers	38	ambiguous genitalia	38
		adrenal crisis hyponatraemia	7 (2 designated male at birth)
		vomiting, dehydration failure to thrive	6
Non-salt-losers	29	ambiguous genitalia	29 (2 designated male at birth)
		vomiting, dehydration failure to thrive	2
		precocious puberty	6

Tables 1 and 2 summarize the clinical presentation of female and male patients respectively. Ambiguous genitalia were noted in all female patients on presentation. Four of these had been incorrectly assigned the male sex at birth.

Figure 2 shows age at diagnosis related to year of birth. The mean age at diagnosis is lower for children born after 1970 (7.6 months) than for those born before 1970 (21.5 months). For children born between 1970 and 1980, 74.3% of all diagnoses were made before the patient was 1 month of age, whereas for children born before 1970, the corresponding figure was 53.3%. The improvement was predominantly in the diagnosis of males. Children born after 1980 could not be compared as they were not old enough to include all potential late presenting cases.

CONCLUSION

Our figures show that there has been an improvement in the clinical pick-up rate of CAH in the 1970s compared to previous years. Additional data in the

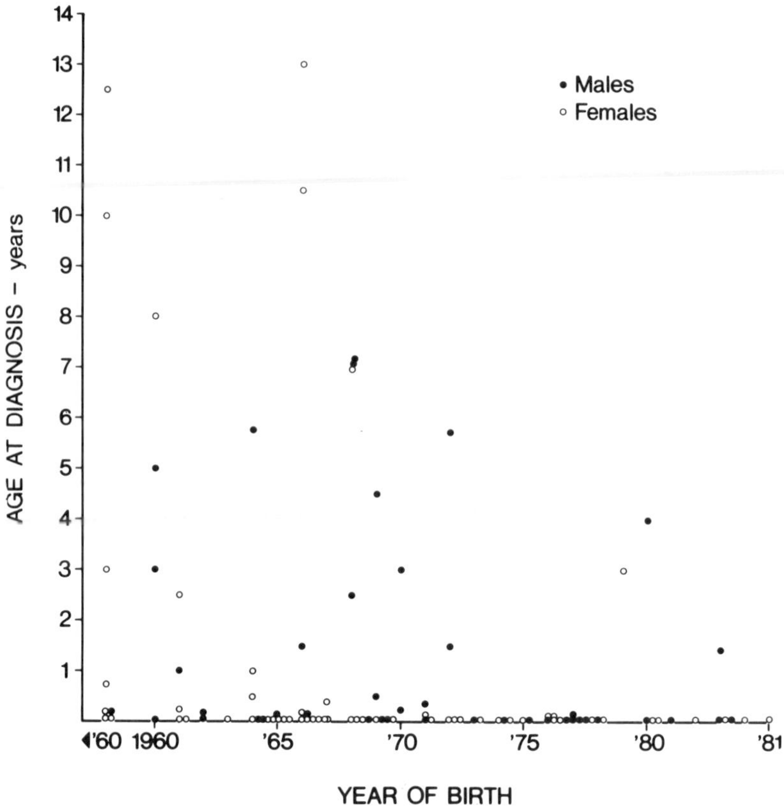

Figure 2 Patients with CAH: age at diagnosis

Table 2 Presenting clinical features of CAH in males

Diagnosis	*Total number*	*Presentation*	
Salt-losers	27*	adrenal crisis hyponatraemia	3
		vomiting, dehydration failure to thrive	21
Non-salt-losers	17*	precocious puberty	15
		comatose	1

* Adequate information was not available in 3 salt-losers and 1 non-salt-loser

accompanying report from Birmingham (B. T. Rudd) shows that the number of cases picked up in the absence of neonatal screening in Birmingham in 1984 was consistent with the number expected from knowledge of the incidence of the disease. The reasons for improvement in diagnosis are probably a combination of improved clinical awareness and better diagnostic tests. We are therefore not convinced of the need for a neonatal screening programme for CAH in Birmingham.

EDITORIAL NOTE

The data in Figure 1 would suggest that the male : female ratio has approached unity in the last decade.

REFERENCES

Cacciari, E., Balsamo, A., Cassio, A., Piazzi, S., Bernardi, F., Salardi, S., Cocognani, A., Pirazzoli, P., Zappulla, F., Capelli, M. and Paolini, M. Neonatal screening for congenital adrenal hyperplasia. *Arch. Dis. Child.* 58 (1983) 803–806

Lebovitz, R. M., Pauli, R. M. and Laxova, R. Delayed diagnosis in congenital adrenal hyperplasia. *Am. J. Dis. Child.* 138 (1984) 571–573

Murtaza, L., Sibert, J. R., Hughes, I. and Balfour, I. C. Congenital adrenal hyperplasia: a clinical and genetic survey. *Arch. Dis. Child.* 55 (1980) 622–625

Werder, E. A., Siebenmann, R. E., Knorr-Mürset, G., Zimmermann A., Sizonenko, P. C., Theintz, P., Girard, J., Zachmann, M. and Prader, A. The incidence of congenital adrenal hyperplasia in Switzerland: a survey of patients born in 1960 to 1974. *Helv. Paediatr. Acta.* 35 (1980) 5–11

J. Inher. Metab. Dis. 9 *Suppl.* 1 (1986) 155–156

Prevalence of Adrenal 21-Hydroxylase Deficiency in Neonates Born in the West Midlands: a Retrospective Study

B. T. Rudd

Department of Clinical Endocrinology, Birmingham and Midland Hospital for Women, Showell Green Lane, Birmingham B11 4HL, UK

In 1980 a simple procedure for the measurement of serum 17α-hydroxy progesterone (17-OHP) was introduced that was suitable for monitoring 17-OHP concentrations in infants and children (Davila *et al.*, 1980). Experience with this method to 1984 has demonstrated that it is useful for identifying infants at risk due to congenital adrenal hyperplasia (CAH), providing due care is taken in interpreting the results. In particular, prematurity and the rapid decrease in 17-OHP after birth must be considered (Rudd *et al.*, 1984). This study presents our experience in 1984 with the assay when applied to sera received from infants suspected of CAH. The data relates to samples sent by eight major maternity units in the West Midlands to whom the service is offered. The protocol adopted was a non-screening procedure and relied on obstetric and paediatric clinical assessment of the neonates and a knowledge of the electrolyte status of the infants.

Figure 1 illustrates the criteria that were used before any 17-OHP value was considered abnormal and consistent with the clinical diagnosis of CAH. The birth total for all eight maternity units was 24 750.

Using the criteria illustrated in Figure 1, four infants (three females, one male) were identified as patients with CAH (Figure 2). The prevalence for the population

Journal of Inherited Metabolic Disease. ISSN 0141–8955.

CAH PREVALENCE (1984)

WMRHA - MATERNITY UNITS

NON-SCREEN METHOD

17OHP CRITERIA FOR INCLUSION

ALL VALUES EXCEEDING 30NMOL/L ON ONE OR MORE OCCASIONS FROM DAY 3 TO FIRST MONTH OF LIFE.
ALL BORN BETWEEN 31ST DEC 1983 - JAN 1ST 1985

MATERNITY HOSPITALS N=8
TOTAL LIVE BIRTHS 24,750

Figure 1

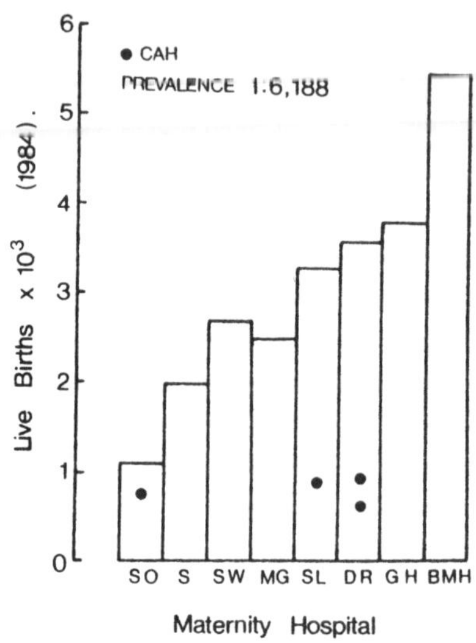

Figure 2 Originating maternity units for the four cases of CAH

studied was 1 in 6188. There was no relationship between birth rates in a given maternity unit and the detection of infants with CAH. The prevalence of CAH reported in the literature from screening studies varies according to methods used and populations studied. The data presented from this study does, however, suggest the pick-up rate by a non-screening procedure is consistent with the expected incidence in the UK. The problem of male patients with CAH that may be missed in retrospective studies still remains.

REFERENCES

Davila, N., Rudd, B. T., Morris, R., Kandeel, F., Bodden, J. and London, D. R. A simple procedure for the radioimmunoassay of 17α-hydroxyprogesterone in serum: comparison with an immunological purification technique. *Ann. Clin. Biochem*, 17 (1980) 31–37

Rudd, B. T., Holder, G. and Wharton, B. Serum 17α-hydroxyprogesterone (17-OHP) as an index of 21-hydroxylase deficiency in the neonate. *ACB National Meeting, Abstract 37.* Buxton, May 1984

J. Inher. Metab. Dis. 9 Suppl. 2 (1986) 157–158

Introduction and Explanation

J. T. Ireland

To mark the occasion of my retirement from official SSIEM duties, Scientific Hospital Supplies Ltd., through Mr Brian Gill, kindly offered to sponsor an event of my own and the Society's choosing. The main symposium of the meeting was scientifically biased and to complement this a half-day 'clinical' symposium was selected. The subject of the symposium, phenylketonuria, was of interest to paediatricians and scientists alike, to dieticians and nutritionists who were invited to attend and to Scientific Hospital Supplies who have a longstanding interest in this aspect of inborn errors of metabolism.

Phenylketonuria has now been treated for some thirty years: results overall have been excellent. There remain, however, a number of problems in diagnosis and management of PKU. These include the treatment of maternal PKU as the earliest treated patients reach reproductive maturity and the growing belief in the continuous maintenance of diet in older patients with PKU. Four groups of professionals have their own special problems; the laboratories, special food manufacturers, paediatricians and most of all the dieticians and nutritionists directly in touch with the patients.

In the time available only four could be discussed at the symposium: (1) problems of diagnosis in relationship to treatment, (2) regression in older children off treatment, (3) maternal phenylketonuria and (4) dietary management. Additional problems are listed in Table 1.

Over the years whilst arranging SSIEM symposia I have been in receipt of much hospitality and friendship both at home and abroad. It was intended that the invitation to contribute to this symposium should be regarded as a part return for all the kindness shown to me. The number of speakers was obviously limited and I hope that the four speakers taking part will be looked upon as the representatives of a much wider group of friends whom I would also have liked to invite. The four papers which follow are contributed by experts in this particular field to whom I am deeply grateful for their acceptance of my invitation and the excellence of their contribution. Problems of the kind discussed here also exist in many of the treatments of other inborn errors of metabolism besides PKU and I would like to suggest that there is a need later for a wider symposium along these lines.

Journal of Inherited Metabolic Disease. ISSN 0141–8955.

Table 1 Problems with management of phenylketonuria

(1)	*Laboratory*
	Measurement of plasma phenylalanine and metabolites in blood and urine
	Identification of PKU variants
	Assessment of nutritional status
(2)	*Special food manufacturer*
	Source, e.g. purified amino acids, hydrolysis of proteins
	Removal of phenylalanine, D forms
	Additional nutritional requirements, e.g. calories, carbohydrate, fat, vitamins, trace elements and additional tryptophan and tyrosine
	Acceptability to patient, taste, osmolality
	Variability of nutritional requirement with age
	Cost
(3)	*Paediatrician*
	Correct identification of PKU variant
	Genetic counselling
	Monitoring of treatment
	Dietary discontinuation
	Psychological problems, parental guilt, adolescence
	Transfer to adult physicians, maternal PKU
(4)	*Nutritionist*
	Choice of product, type, palatability
	Dietary instruction of patient and parent
	Provision of balanced diet
	Effects of elemental diet on absorption

J. Inher. Metab. Dis. 9 Suppl. 2 (1986) 159–168

Maternal Phenylketonuria

R. Koch, E. Gross Friedman, E. Wenz, K. Jew, C. Crowley and G. Donnell
Medical Genetics Division of The Childrens Hospital of Los Angeles, 4650 Sunset Boulevard, Los Angeles, California, 90027, USA; and Department of Pediatrics of the University of Southern California, School of Medicine, Los Angeles, California, USA

Pregnant women with untreated phenylketonuria (PKU) with blood phenylalanine levels greater than 1200 μmol/L usually give birth to offspring with congenital birth defects, including microcephaly, cardiac defects and mental retardation. According to Mabry and Levy, hyperphenylalaninaemic (HPA) women with blood phenylalanine levels between 600 and 1200 μmol/L also have an increased risk to their offspring. To study this problem further, the National Institute of Child Health and Human Development has established a collaborative study for 7 years to elucidate a proper treatment programme for these women.

Pregnancy in women with metabolic disorders such as diabetes has been well studied, but relatively little is known about the reproductive ability of women with inborn errors of metabolism. This is due to the fact that identification and treatment for these diseases have only been accomplished within the last 2 decades. The best known and well studied of the inborn errors is phenylketonuria (PKU) (McKusick 26160). Most women with PKU who have normal intelligence are still too young for marriage and child bearing. Thus the natural history of the maternal PKU syndrome, as we know it today, deals primarily with pregnancy outcome in a group of mentally retarded PKU women who conceived while on an unrestricted phenylalanine intake (Woolf *et al.*, 1961; Mabry *et al.*, 1963; Fisch *et al.*, 1966; Forbes *et al.*, 1966; Frankenburg *et al.*, 1968; Zaleski *et al.*, 1979). The excellent reviews by Mabry (1978) and Lenke and Levy (1980) have detailed the natural history of poor reproductive outcome in these women. The clinical challenge today is to develop an approach which could assure an improved child bearing experience for women with PKU.

Our experience suggests that maternal phenylalanine levels of 240–480 μmol/L are not detrimental to fetal outcome (Koch and Blaskovics, 1982). Three mothers in this range gave birth to 9 children with intelligence within the normal range. On the other hand, the one woman with phenylalanine concentrations above this range (600–900 μmol/L) had 4 retarded children.

During pregnancy there is a positive gradient of phenylalanine from mother to fetus. This has been documented with simultaneous maternal and cord blood specimens for amino acid analysis. Since the PKU woman does not provide sufficient tyrosine to the fetus, tyrosine supplementation has been recommended in addition to restricting phenylalanine intake to achieve successful pregnancy outcome (Komrower *et al.*, 1979).

DIETARY THERAPY

There remain many unsolved problems (Buist *et al.*, 1979; Levy and Waisbren 1983) and there is legitimate divergence of opinion concerning dietary therapy for maternal HPA. The reports by Allen (1968), Komrower and colleagues (1979), Smith and colleagues (1979), Nielson and colleagues (1979) and Tenbrink and Stroud (1982) showed improved fetal outcome when treatment with the phenylalanine restricted diet was instituted shortly before or after conception. The recent summary of the outcome of 34 such pregnancies by Lenke and Levy (1982) is not conclusive about the efficacy of dietary therapy.

Lenke and Levy (1980) reported results of their international survey of 524 pregnancies in 155 women with PKU and HPA. Restriction of phenylalanine intake prior to conception occurred in 3 pregnancies and 31 received therapy after pregnancy was established. Among the 121 untreated women the frequency of mental retardation associated with microcephaly in their offspring was increased over those born to women treated during pregnancy. 95% of mothers with blood phenylalanine levels greater than 1200 μmol/L had at least one mentally retarded child. However, the information on the treated pregnancies was fragmentary, often incomplete and largely retrospective. Thus is was not possible to conclude that dietary therapy post-conception was therapeutic (Lenke and Levy, 1982).

Based on the reported evidence, the prudent course is to institute the phenylalanine restricted diet prior to conception as suggested by Nielson and colleagues (1979).

GENERAL ASPECTS OF THERAPY

Providing care for a pregnant PKU woman includes medical and dietary treatment, health education and emotional support. Close supervision of the diet, frequent monitoring of serum phenylalanine and serial obstetrical evaluations are essential to document the progress of a woman's pregnancy. Health education should emphasize the effects of maternal PKU on the unborn infant, as well as the physiological changes during pregnancy. The mother's level of intelligence and her emotional maturity should be taken into account when counselling. Providing the mother with support and encouragement during the pregnancy establishes positive rapport helpful in maintaining appropriate dietary treatment and compliance with clinical care. Cooperation between the obstetrician and the nearest medical centre offering clinical PKU services is preferred for the provision of comprehensive care. Members of the clinical team managing a pregnant woman with PKU can establish positive rapport through ongoing education and support, to encourage successful dietary therapy and pregnancy outcome.

A protocol for the nutrition support of maternal PKU was recently developed for the Maternal PKU Collaborative Study between the United States and Canada, sponsored by the National Institute of Child Health and Human Development. General nutritional guidelines had been developed and published earlier (Acosta *et al*., 1982).

The role of trace elements in the diet of PKU women treated with the phenylalanine restricted diet is unclear because the requirements for normal pregnancy are not well established (Metcoff *et al*., 1981). Recommended dietary allowances for man have been determined for 3 (iodine, iron and zinc), and ranges of 'estimated safe and adequate daily dietary intakes' for 6 others (chromium, copper, fluoride, manganese, molybdemun and selenium) (Dairy Council Digest, 1982). Some of these data are based on animal data and thus their application to pregnancy outcome is difficult to assess. Recently data on zinc requirements in pregnancy suggested that this element may play a critical role (Mertz, 1981; Sever, 1982). Zinc levels during pregnancy are lower than those in non-pregnant women. The 25% decrease in zinc levels in the last trimester of pregnancy is probably physiological because of increased blood volume, decline in serum albumin in levels and raised levels of endogenous oestrogens (Hambidge and Mauer, 1978).

In addition to these decreases in zinc levels, the pregnant woman with PKU is restricted in meat intake and other dietary sources of available zinc: supplementation of zinc to the recommended intake during pregnancy is therefore indicated. Further research and prospectively collected data are required to determine the significance of trace elements in the treatment of maternal PKU.

EXPERIENCE AT THE CHILDRENS HOSPITAL OF LOS ANGELES

Publications prior to 1970 delineated the course of women with hyperphenylalaninaemia cared for at this institution (Forbes *et al*., 1966; Frankenburg *et al*., 1968). The outcome despite our best efforts at treatment were poor. Since those publications appeared, 5 additional pregnancies in PKU women have been treated. It is gratifying to report that the most recent therapeutic efforts have been more rewarding. The better results seen in our last 5 pregnancies are no doubt related to earlier institution of the phenylalanine restricted diet, but may also be due to more careful attention to nutritional care, trace element and tyrosine supplementation.

Case Report 1

The mother is a 19-year-old in whom PKU was diagnosed and treated at 5 days of age. She continued diet restriction until aged 8 years and her intelligence quotient on the Wechsler Intelligence Scale for Children (WISC) at age 15 was 90. After dietary discontinuation, her blood phenylalanine levels usually ranged above 1200 μmol/L. She attended public school classes for the educationally handicapped and graduated from high school at the age of 18 years.

At the time of the suspected pregnancy, a blood phenylalanine level of 1308 μmol/L was noted. The pregnancy was not confirmed until 7 weeks later because of failure to keep clinic appointments. This woman therefore did not begin the phenylalanine restricted diet until about 12 weeks gestation.

Initially Phenyl-Free* was offered: this product made her nauseous and subsequently Lofenalac* was prescribed. Thereafter, she was able to tolerate the phenylalanine restricted diet for the remainder of her pregnancy.

Blood phenylalanine levels were usually between 600–780 μmol/L and were consistently above the recommended range. Every effort made to lower these high levels was unsuccessful. She was not competent in keeping dietary records: thus it was unclear what her protein intake was during the pregnancy. Supplementation of the mother's diet with tyrosine (50 mg kg^{-1} day^{-1}) was started at the beginning of the 14th week of pregnancy. Serum tyrosine levels rose to 200 μmol/L and she exhibited a maculopapular rash. The dose was reduced and the rash disappeared. Subsequently she tolerated 50 mg kg^{-1} day^{-1} until delivery. The maternal phenylalanine level on the day of delivery was 344 μmol/L. In contrast, the infant's cord blood level was 786 μmol/L, but dropped sharply within 19 hours to 78 μmol/L. Simultaneous amniotic fluid phenylalanine level was 276 μmol/L on the day of delivery. Arterial cord blood was 93 μmol/L. Simultaneous plasma tyrosine level at delivery was 47 μmol/L, and the amniotic fluid level was 33 μmol/L. Physical examination of the newborn infant revealed a slightly lethargic male who appeared normal. The head circumference measured 31.5 cm, length 50 cm and weight 2863 g. The anterior fontanelle was small, measuring only 1.5 cm in width.

An ultrasound evaluation suspected a small fetal head circumference at the end of the 2nd trimester. A small head circumference (−2 SD) persisted to 4 years of age. Developmental assessment at the time reported an IQ of 89 and immature speech development. This child is now nearly 5½ years of age. There are no other abnormal physical findings.

Case Report 2

She was an only child born to young, unstable parents. Her mother was mildly retarded with an IQ of 71 on the Wechsler Adult Intelligence Scale (WAIS). At 5½ months of age, a routine diaper screening test for phenylpyruvic acid was reported as positive and subsequently a blood phenylalanine level of 1860 μmol/L was recorded. Due to problems with dietary treatment, she was placed in foster care. At age 13 years she removed herself from the phenylalanine restricted diet. She attended regular public school, but did not graduate from high school.

At age 18 years, she returned to our clinic when she discovered that she was pregnant. This pregnancy ended in a spontaneous abortion at 10–12 weeks gestation. Although she was aware of the need for the phenylalanine restricted diet and was sexually active, she was reluctant to start dietary treatment prior to conception.

She subsequently became pregnant at age 20. She notified our staff when she was about 12 weeks pregnant and resumed dietary restriction at that time. The

* Phenyl–Free and Lofenalac are the 2 low-phenylalanine formulae produced by Mead–Johnson and Co., Evansville, Indiana

initial blood phenylalanine level was 1080 μmol/L. During this pregnancy, the phenylalanine concentrations averaged 492 μmol/L (range 264–708). Ultrasonography on several occasions revealed a normal sized fetus. Tyrosine supplementation of 4 g/day was started at 20 weeks gestation. This was arbitrarily increased to 6 g/day by 26 weeks and to 8 g/day at 35 weeks gestation. In addition to the tyrosine, a mineral supplement was commenced at 20 weeks gestation. Serum zinc, iron and copper were monitored monthly. Labour was induced during the 38th week of pregnancy. The baby was delivered in good condition, weighing 3062 g and measuring 51 cm in length with a normal head circumference of 34 cm.

This infant appeared normal at birth and continued to grow normally in both height and weight. There were no physical findings of microcephaly or cardiac disorders. The last developmental assessment at 30 months of age reported a DQ of 84 on the Gesell Developmental Test. This child is currently 3 years old.

Case Report 3

This pregnancy occurred in the same woman as reported in case 2. This time however, the mother initiated the phenylalanine restricted diet when she realized she was pregnant, at 6 weeks gestation. Her blood phenylalanine levels averaged 588 μmol/L (range 126–1062 μmol/L). She went into spontaneous labour at 35 weeks gestation and delivered a 2551 g male infant at home. His head circumference was 32 cm and his length was 44 cm. These birth measurements were consistent with the gestational age. The infant appeared normal at birth and no abnormal physical findings have been identified to date.

The child is now 22 months old. Growth measurements for length, height and head circumference have consistently been less than the 5th percentile, but are proportional for size. His small size is probably related to the mother's small stature.

Case Report 4

This woman was born to an unstable marriage. When it became clear that she was mentally retarded, she was evaluated in a child development clinic at age 2½ years, when the diagnosis of PKU was made and a phenylalanine restricted diet initiated. At age 4 years her estimated IQ on the Stanford–Binet Intelligence Scale was 40. Because of her unstable family environment since early infancy, she was subsequently placed in a foster home where she continued on phenylalanine restriction and attended special classes in school. She continued to improve intellectually and by age 14 years her IQ on a WISC was 98. She discontinued dietary therapy at age 13 years. She attended special education classes and completed the 12th grade.

She conceived twice off dietary therapy at age 19 years and elected to have therapeutic abortions. Her blood phenylalanine levels off treatment ranged between 1014–1710 μmol/L. Shortly thereafter, she had a spontaneous abortion while starting on a phenylalanine restricted diet. She remained on dietary treatment and conceived 3 months later. Her blood phenylalanine levels during the pregnancy averaged 528 μmol/L (range 324–1208). Ultrasound at 26 weeks revealed twins, one of whom had a possible congenital cardiac defect. The twins were delivered by caesarian section at 35 weeks gestation due to premature onset of labour.

At birth, twin A appeared developmentally normal for physical growth, with a weight of 1729 g, length 43 cm, and head circumference 29.5 cm. No cardiac disorders or microcephaly were identified in this child. He required a tracheostomy at 2 months of age due to tracheal stenosis following severe bronchitis and pneumonia. Additionally, he had an endotracheal tube placed for less than 24 hours, a short time after birth. Gesell testing at 13 months of age reported a DQ of 98. He is currently 27 months old.

At birth, twin B exhibited a loud systolic murmur, but the infant appeared normal otherwise. The weight was 1843 g, length 43 cm and head circumference 29.5 cm. Further diagnostic cardiac studies confirmed the presence of an endocardial cushion defect with marked mitral valve deformity. Surgical correction was attempted when his cardiac condition could not be managed. Post-operatively, his condition deteriorated. He had a severe lesion involving the outflow tract of the left ventricle. This infant died at 5 months of age.

Case Report 5

The mother in this case was the mother of the twins reported above. She had a therapeutic abortion within 3 months of the birth of the twins. During the subsequent year, she became pregnant with case 5. She restarted the phenylalanine restricted diet at 3 weeks gestation and maintained fairly good control, averaging 552 μmol/L (range 222–960). At 39 weeks gestation, she delivered a healthy-seeming boy weighing 3298 g, measuring 50 cm in length and 33 cm in head circumference.

A fetal echocardiagram revealed an atrial septal defect at 22 weeks gestation. However, it was thought not to be as severe as in the previous twin. On physical examination at birth, no audible murmur was detected. An echocardiagram completed during the 1st week of life did confirm a small atrial septal defect: however, by 1 month of age the defect resolved without medical or surgical intervention. This child is currently 7 months old. He has been referred for a neurological evaluation due to persistent poor head control. Developmental assessment has not been completed. The child is alert, socially responsive and is growing well.

SUMMARY OF CLINICAL FINDINGS

The 3 PKU women reported here gave birth to 6 liveborn males. The PKU mother who started dietary treatment post-conceptionally had one child with severe cardiac defect and one with mild cardiac defect which resolved without intervention. However, this infant may have delayed neurological development and needs further evaluation. The PKU mother with blood phenylalanine above 600 μmol/L during her pregnancy had a son with persistent small head circumference at −2 SD. The children of the remaining PKU mother appear to be developing normally.

The 4 children who completed developmental testing are functioning in the borderline to average range of intelligence. However, the offspring will require long-term follow-up for accurate developmental assessment. School performance and learning disorders are difficult to determine from the early developmental assessments. Environmental factors such as parenting skills and socio–economic status will also have an impact on the outcome of these offspring.

DISCUSSION

It is clear that maternal PKU poses a serious risk to fetal development in the absence of dietary restriction of phenylalanine. The degree of fetal risk with therapy is as yet unclear, but most believe that phenylalanine restriction is beneficial. To assess the degree of risk, the National Institute of Child Health and Human Development has initiated a study involving the United States and Canada. The Medical Genetics Division at Childrens Hospital of Los Angeles was selected as the coordinating centre for the project, with 4 regional contributing centres encompassing 50 States and the District of Columbia (Figure 1).

The research design is prospective, longitudinal and observational in nature, and will attempt to include 200 hyperphenylalaninaemic (HPA) pregnancies and their offspring. Women with blood phenylalanine levels persistently greater than 240 μmol/L, on an unrestricted diet, would be eligible.

The treatment plan will consist of:

(1) provision of adequate nutrition during pregnancy
(2) offering the phenylalanine restricted diet to HPA women with blood phenylalanine concentrations consistently greater than or equal to 600 μmol/L
(3) aiming to maintain blood phenylalanine concentrations between 120–600 μmol/L
(4) supplementation with tyrosine and trace elements as medically indicated.

The research questions that the study is designed to answer are the following:

(1) does the phenylalanine restricted diet reduce the frequency of mental retardation, spontaneous abortion, low birth weight, congenital malformations, neurological and behavioural impairment reported in pregnancies of HPA mothers who were on unrestricted phenylalanine intake during pregnancy?
(2) is pregnancy outcome in HPA women who restrict phenylalanine intake during pregnancy comparable to that of non-HPA women?
(3) is pregnancy outcome in HPA women related to maternal phenylalanine levels during pregnancy?
(4) is gestational age, at the onset of intervention, predictive of fetal outcome?
(5) are there beneficial effects of starting diet prior to conception?
(6) what are the levels of tyrosine and trace elements during pregnancy and what are the effects on pregnancy outcome of supplementation if levels are found to be reduced?

In order to have demographically and genetically similar groups of non-HPA women to whom subjects may be compared, the study will follow prospectively

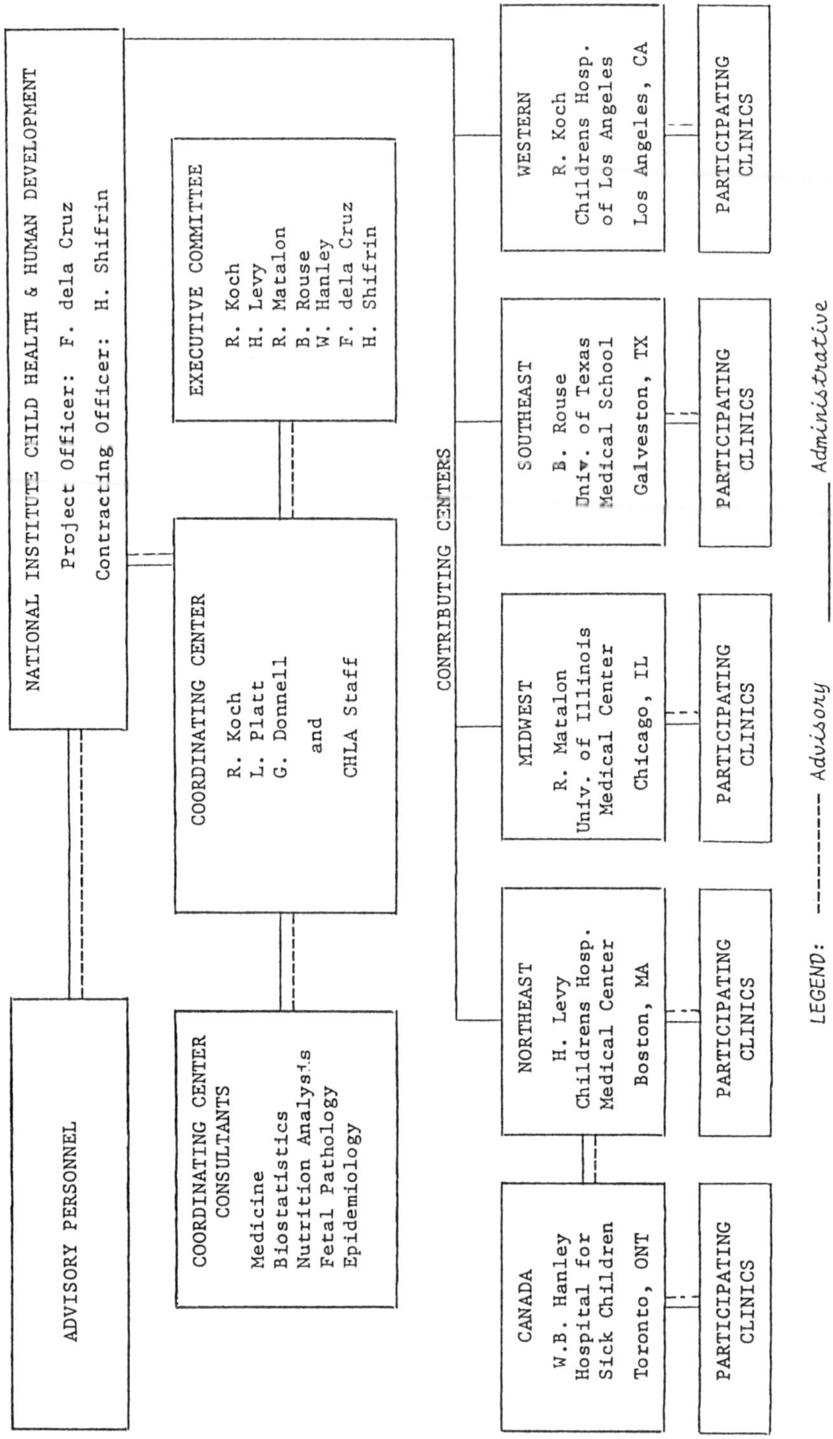

Figure 1 Maternal PKU collaborative study organization and administrative structure

(1) normal controls matched for race, age, gestation and parity, and (2) familial controls obtained from the sibship of the HPA woman or her mate, or first cousins of the HPA woman or her mate.

Additional comparison groups will include (1) prospective evaluation of the pregnancies of the mates of HPA males, (2) prospective evaluation of offspring from previous pregnancies of HPA subjects, and (3) historical data on untreated HPA pregnancies from the 1980 Lenke–Levy survey.

In an observational study such as the present one, many extraneous factors could contribute to observed differences between subjects and comparison groups. Some are accounted for in matching criteria for controls. Others will need to be routinely assessed and controlled for at the time of data analysis. Among this latter group are parental intelligence and head circumference, socio–economic status of the family, nutritional status apart from phenylalanine level prior to and during pregnancy, and maternal exposure to teratogens, such as drugs, tobacco and alcohol.

The very nature of long-term collaborative studies calls for dedication and self-sacrifice for the research effort, by the families and many individuals contributing to the data collection and analysis. The present study began on 1st May 1984, and has completed its organizational phase. Subject enrollment commenced on 1st November 1984. To date, 15 pregnancies have been followed and 25 more PKU women enrolled who are planning pregnancies.

It is hoped that the study will allow us to determine what phenylalanine level during pregnancy will maintain normal fetal development, whether preconceptual phenylalanine restriction is necessary, and whether supplementation with tyrosine and various trace elements such as zinc are necessary for normal pregnancy outcome.

In this early phase of the study most of the enrolled women are mildly retarded or borderline in intelligence. This problem hopefully will resolve as the study progresses and more women are enrolled with normal intellectual ability.

ACKNOWLEDGEMENT

This study is supported by NICHD Contract N01–HD–4–3807.

REFERENCES

Acosta, P. B., Blaskovics, M., Cloud, H., Lis, E., Stroud, H. and Wenz, E. Nutrition in pregnancy of women with hyperphenylalaninemia. *J. Am. Diet. Assoc.* 80 (1982) 443–450

Allen, J. D. Maternal phenylketonuria. In Holt, K. S. and Coffey, V. P. (eds.) *Some Recent Advances in Inborn Errors of Metabolism.* E and S Livingston Ltd., Edinburgh and London, 1968, pp. 14–38

Bickel, H. *Maternal Phenylketonuria.* Frankfurt: Maizena. Diat Gesellschaft MBH, 1980

Buist, N. R. M., Lis, E. W., Tuerck, J. M. and Murphy, W. H. Maternal phenylketonuria. *Lancet* 2 (1979) 589

Fisch, R. O., Walker, W. A. and Anderson, J. A. Prenatal and postnatal developmental consequences of maternal phenylketonuria. *Pediatrics* 37 (1966) 979–986

Forbes, N. P., Shaw, K. N. F., Koch, R., Coffelt, R. W. and Strauss, R. Maternal phenylketonuria. *Nurs. Outlook* 14 (1966) 40–42

Frankenburg, W. K., Duncan, B. R., Coffelt, R. W., Koch, R., Coldwell, J. G. and Son, C. D. Maternal phenylketonuria implications for growth and development. *J. Pediatr.* 73 (1968) 560–570

Hambidge, K. M. and Mauer, A. M. In *Indices of Nutritional Status in Pregnancy* NRC Nat. Acad. of Science, Washington DC 1978, pp. 157–193

Koch, R. and Blaskovics, M. Four cases of hyperphenylalaninemia: studies during pregnancy and of the offspring produced. *J. Inher. Metab. Dis.* 5 (1982) 11–15

Komrower, G. M., Sardharwalla, I. B., Couts, J. M. and Ingham, D. Management of maternal phenylketonuria: an emerging clinical problem. *Br. Med. J.* 1 (1979) 1383–1387

Lenke, R. and Levy, H. L. Maternal phenylketonuria and hyperphenylalaninemia. *N. Eng. J. Med.* 303 (1980) 1202–1208

Lenke, R. and Levy, H. L. Maternal phenylketonuria: results of dietary therapy. *Am. J. Ob. Gyn.* 142 (1982) 548–552

Levy, H. L., Lenke, R. R. and Crocker, A. C. Maternal PKU. DHHS Publication no (HSA) 81–5299. US Department of Health and Human Services, Rockville, Maryland 20857

Levy, H. L. and Waisbren, S. E. Effects of untreated maternal phenylketonuria and hyperphenylalaninemia on the fetus. *N. Eng. J. Med.* 309 (1983) 1269–1274

Mabry, C. Presentation on maternal phenylketonuria. Fourteenth General Medical Conference, Collaborative Study for the Treatment of Children with Phenylketonuria. Stateline, Nevada, March 16, 1978

Mabry, C., Denniston, J. C., Nelson, T. L. and Son, C. D. Maternal phenylketonuria. *N. Eng. J. Med.* 269 (1963)1505

Mertz, W. The essential trace elements. *Science* 213 (1981) 1332–1338

Metcoff, J., Costiloe, J. P., Crosby, W., Beltle, I., Seshachalam, D., Sandstead, H. H., Bodwell, C. E., Weaver, F. and McClain, P. Maternal nutrition and fetal outcome. *Am. J. Clin. Nutr.* 34 (1981) 708–721

Nielsen, K. B., Wamberg, E. and Weber, J. Successful outcome of pregnancy in a phenylketonuric woman after low phenylalanine diet introduced before conception. *Lancet* 1 (1979) 1245

Sever, I. E. Zinc deficiency and birth defects. *Int. J. Environ. Studies* 18 (1982) 273–274

Smith, I., McCartney, F. J., Erodohazi, M., Pincott, J. R., Woolf, O. H., Brenton, D. P., Biddle, S. A., Fairweather, D. V. I. and Dobbing, J. Fetal damage despite low-phenylalanine diet after conception in a phenylketonuric woman. *Lancet* 1 (1979) 17–19

Tenbrinck, M. S. and Stroud, H. W. Normal infant born to a mother with phenylketonuria. *JAMA* 247 (1982) 2139–2140

Trace elements in human nutrition. *Dairy Council Digest* 53 (1982) 1–3

Woolf, L. I., Ounsted, D. L., Lee, M., Humphrey, N., Cheshire, and Steed, G. R. Atypical PKU in sisters with normal offspring. *Lancet* 2 (1961) 464

Zaleski, L. A., Casey, R. E. and Zaleski, W. Maternal phenyl-dietary treatment during pregnancy. *Can. Med. Assoc. J.* 121 (1979) 1591

J. Inher. Metab. Dis. 9 Suppl. 2 (1986) 169–177

Dietary Problems of Phenylketonuria: Effect on CNS Transmitters and their Possible Role in Behaviour and Neuropsychological Function

F. GÜTTLER and H. LOU
The John F. Kennedy Institute, DK–2600 Glostrup, Denmark

Thirty years ago it was observed that the synthesis of serotonin, dopamine and norepinephrine was impaired in untreated phenylketonuria (PKU) as judged either by a decreased concentration in the blood or decreased excretion in the urine of these neurotransmitters, or of their metabolites, 5-hydroxyindoleacetic acid (5-HIAA) and homovanillic acid (HVA). Fifteen years later, when early treatment of PKU with a phenylalanine restricted diet was routinely introduced, an inverse relationship was found between phenylalanine levels and the urinary excretion of dopamine and serotonin. An inverse relationship between blood phenylalanine levels and cerebrospinal fluid (CSF) concentrations of HVA and 5-HIAA has repeatedly been reported during the past 10 years. Recently, the effect of the discontinuation of diet in PKU on the synthesis of dopamine, norepinephrine and serotonin has been examined, and the possible relationship between low levels of these neurotransmitters and impaired performance on neuropsychological tests has been evaluated. In some PKU patients the performance on neuropsychological tests of higher integrative function is impaired after discontinuation of diet, especially when blood phenylalanine values exceed 1200 μmol/L, and the patients often complain of lack of concentration and emotional instability. When these patients return to a 'relaxed' phenyalanine restricted, tyrosine enriched diet, the impaired neuropsychological and behavioural functions appear to be reversible. One mechanism may involve an impaired synthesis of dopamine and serotonin, as the improvement is accompanied by an increase in dopamine and serotonin excretion and a significant increase in CSF concentrations of HVA and 5-HIAA. Quite recently it has been observed that supplementation of a free diet with tyrosine (approximately 150 mg/kg) seemed to improve personality, behaviour, reaction time or reaction time variability in patients off diet. Plasma tyrosine and CSF HVA concentrations increased significantly. Plasma phenylalanine levels remained high (>1200 μmol/L). Supplementation of a normal diet with tyrosine and tryptophan may prevent mental and neuropsychological dysfunction following diet discontinuation in PKU.

Journal of Inherited Metabolic Disease. ISSN 0141–8955. Printed in Great Britain by Titus Wilson & Son Ltd., Kendal.

Controversy persists regarding the possible effects of elevated phenylalanine on brain function in young adults with phenylketonuria (McKusick 26160) who commenced treatment early and whose development is nearly complete. Whether or not elevated concentrations of phenylalanine disturb central nervous system (CNS) functions in these patients is unknown. In 1980, Waisbren and colleagues reviewed 19 published studies on diet termination and psychological outcome. Almost half reported significant loss in IQ scores after termination and others reported no change or improvement in test scores.

Termination of a low phenylalanine regimen creates a situation in which the blood phenylalanine rises from more or less normal levels to levels characteristic of PKU. If this results in changes in personality and behaviour, then a new disease has been created, biochemically identical with PKU but clinically distinct. Juvenile forms of other inborn errors of metabolism have demonstrated that a chemical insult to the brain of a young adult will result in a clinical picture different from the effect of a similar insult to an infant. Several colleagues have observed that some of the previously well-adjusted PKU patients become moody, surly, withdrawn and uninterested in their work following diet discontinuation.

The interference by phenylalanine in more specialized aspects of tyrosine and tryptophan transport and metabolism may be of great significance in this context, as tyrosine and tryptophan are precursors of the CNS transmitters, dopamine, norepinephrine and serotonin.

This paper reviews the literature describing the relationship between phenylalanine levels, the synthesis of biogenic amines and performance of neuropsychological tests in patients with PKU.

BIOGENIC AMINES IN UNTREATED PKU

Serotonin

There is convincing evidence that the conversion of tryptophan to serotonin is impaired in untreated PKU. The first indication of this disturbance was the finding that the daily excretion of 5-HIAA is decreased in untreated PKU (Armstrong and Robinson, 1954). In addition, Paere and colleagues (1957) found that the blood concentration of serotonin is decreased in untreated PKU. They therefore proposed that tryptophan hydroxylase is impaired in untreated PKU (Paere *et al.*, 1957). Curtius and colleagues (1981) demonstrated that the excretion of serotonin decreases with increasing levels of blood phenylalanine in PKU. However, a consistent relationship between plasma phenylalanine and serotonin excretion was not found by Krause and colleagues (1985) in a study of 10 older, treated PKU patients using a triple-blind, cross-over design.

There is ample evidence to support the conclusion that high phenylalanine levels can decrease the tryptophan content in brain tissue (McKean, 1972). McKean (1972) and Butler and colleagues (1981) further demonstrated that a decreased accumulation of 5-HIAA in the CSF of PKU patients was largely corrected when the patients' plasma phenylalanine concentrations were reduced by dietary restriction of phenylalanine. These results complement the earlier ones of Paere and colleagues (1958) in that they show that the inhibition of serotonin synthesis that is seen in PKU can be corrected by a decrease in phenylalanine concentrations.

Dopamine and norepinephrine

High levels of phenylalanine also interfere with the conversion of tyrosine to the neurotransmitters, dopamine and norepinephrine. Weil-Malherbe (1955) found that the plasma levels of epinephrine and norepinephrine were lower in untreated PKU patients than in other mentally retarded individuals. These results were confirmed by Nadler and Hsia (1961), who also showed that untreated PKU patients excreted less dopamine, norepinephrine and epinephrine in their urine than did other controls or non-PKU patients. Furthermore, it was demonstrated that this decrease could be reversed when the patients were treated with a phenylalanine restricted diet.

Convincing evidence that the conversion of tyrosine to dopamine and norepinephrine is decreased by high blood concentrations of phenylalanine was obtained in experiments by Curtius and colleagues (1972, 1981), where deuterated L-tyrosine was given to PKU patients. It was found that the excretion of deuterated metabolites derived from dopamine and norepinephrine was decreased in patients with high blood phenylalanine levels (Curtius *et al.*, 1981).

THE EFFECT OF LOWERING BLOOD PHENYLALANINE LEVELS ON THE EXCRETION OF BIOGENIC AMINES IN PKU

Lowering phenylalanine blood concentrations to normal levels by dietary treatment increases dopamine and serotonin excretions to normal concentrations (Curtius *et al.*, 1981). It is interesting that at high blood phenylalanine concentrations, the reduced excretion of serotonin is more pronounced than the reduced excretion of dopamine. When blood phenylalanine concentrations were decreased to about 500 μmol/L, dopamine excretion was nearly normalized, but the excretion of serotonin was still depressed (Curtius *et al.*, 1981).

Krause and colleagues (1985) also observed an inverse relationship between dopamine excretion and plasma phenylalanine concentrations. However, a consistent relationship was not found between plasma phenylalanine and serotonin excretion in this study. The inconsistency between the studies of Curtius and colleagues (1981) and Krause and colleagues (1985) may be due to the fact that urinary serotonin and dopamine mainly reflect peripheral metabolism.

THE EFFECT OF BLOOD PHENYLALANINE LEVELS ON CNS TRANSMITTERS IN PKU

While these results show that the synthesis of biogenic amines is impaired in untreated PKU patients, they do not indicate whether the disturbance occurs in the periphery or within the central nervous system (CNS). Evidence that neurotransmitter synthesis in the CNS is in fact impaired by increased phenylalanine levels was presented by McKean (1972), who showed that the levels of serotonin, dopamine and norepinephrine in the brains of PKU patients, obtained at autopsy, was lower than that in the brains of control patients. McKean (1972) also showed that the accumulation in the CSF of the dopamine metabolite HVA is decreased in PKU patients.

The concentrations in CSF of the serotonin metabolite 5-HIAA and of the dopamine metabolite HVA are raised significantly by lowering blood phenylalanine concentrations (McKean, 1972; Butler *et al.*, 1981). These results support the conclusions that high levels of phenylalanine interfere with the biosynthesis in the CNS of serotonin, dopamine, and probably also of norepinephrine, and that this effect is reversible.

THE POSSIBLE MECHANISMS FOR INTERFERENCE BY PHENYLALANINE ON SYNTHESIS OF CNS TRANSMITTERS

The mechanism responsible for the decreased synthesis of dopamine, epinephrine and serotonin following discontinuation of diet in PKU is not known. Increased concentrations of blood phenylalanine could limit the transport of tyrosine and tryptophan across the blood–brain barrier and thus their availability to the brain cell-membrane for synthesis of these CNS transmitters (Pratt, 1982) (Figure 1). To explore the possibility that increased concentrations of phenylalanine might competitively inhibit tyrosine or tryptophan transport, Krause and colleagues (1985) quantified the renal tubular transport of these amino acids. Their data provided negative evidence for a significant effect of phenylalanine on tyrosine and tryptophan uptake in the proximal renal tubule at the same time that dopamine and serotonin was reduced. However, they note that the transport K_m of phenylalanine, tyrosine, and tryptophan in brain and kidney differ.

The branched chain amino acids, valine, isoleucine and leucine, share a common transport system with phenylalanine (Pratt, 1982). Berry and colleagues (1982) have demonstrated that a supplement of these amino acids administered orally to patients with PKU, either together with an unrestricted diet of natural protein or with a low phenylalanine diet, resulted in a significant reduction in CSF concentration of phenylalanine from 15–40% (mean 21%). They further found (McSwigan *et al.*, 1981) administration of the branched chain amino acids to be effective in preventing the increase in water-maze errors of hyperphenylalaninaemic rats compared to animals on the hyperphenylalaninaemic diet without branched chain amino acid supplementation.

The high CSF phenylalanine levels observed after discontinuation of diet in PKU (Lou *et al.*, unpublished) may reflect an increased concentration of CNS phenylalanine which may interfere with the synaptosomal uptake of tyrosine (Figure 1), and this with presynaptic availability of tyrosine for the synthesis of dopamine and norepinephrine (Peterson *et al.*, 1983).

It has been demonstrated that phenylalanine is a competitive inhibitor of tyrosine hydroxylase (Figure 1) which is the rate-limiting enzyme in the synthesis of dopa-

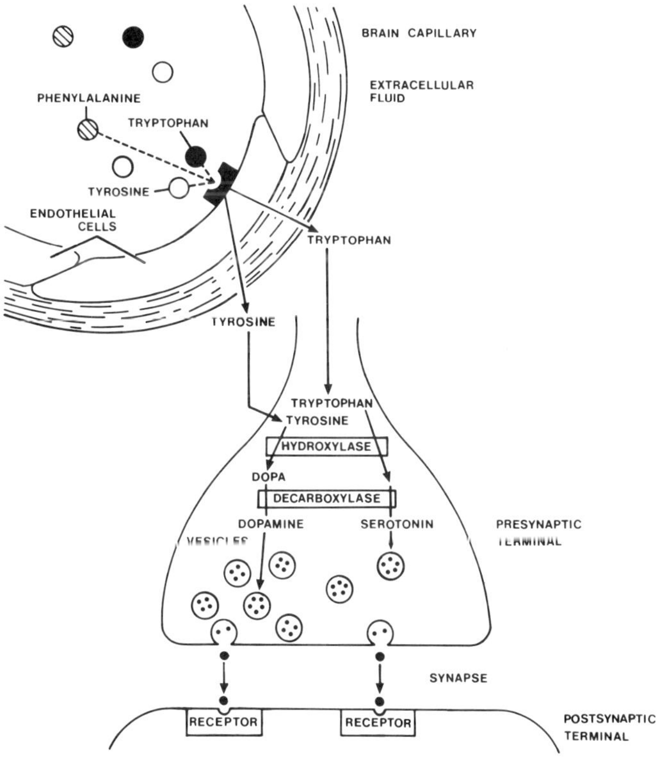

Figure 1 The possible mechanism for interference by phenylalanine on the synthesis of dopamine and serotonin. Increased concentrations of blood phenylalanine may limit the transport of tyrosine and tryptophan across the blood–brain barrier and may interfere with the synaptosomal uptake of tyrosine. Phenylalanine is a competitive inhibitor of tyrosine and tryptophan hydroxylase. The phenylalanine metabolites, phenylacetic acid and phenyllactic acid, are able to inhibit 5-hydroxytryptophan decarboxylase and dopa decarboxylase. To simplify the presentation, the dopaminergic and serotonergic mechanisms are illustrated in the same schematic presentation of the neuron

mine (Udenfriend, 1967; McKean, 1972). Phenylalanine has also been shown to be a competitive inhibitor of tryptophan hydroxylase (Figure 1), the rate-limiting enzyme in the synthesis of serotonin (Lovenberg *et al.*, 1968; Tong and Kaufman, 1975). Furthermore, Sandler and collaborators (1982) have demonstrated that certain phenolic acid metabolites of phenylalanine, particularly phenylacetic acid and phenyllactic acid, are able to inhibit 5-hydroxytryptophan decarboxylase (Figure 1) leading to decreased synthesis of serotonin (Paere *et al.*, 1958; Sandler, 1982).

The possible inhibitory actions of phenylalanine metabolites at two different enzyme steps in the biosynthesis of norepinephrine has recently been reviewed by Sandler (1982). Phenylpyruvic acid can, by a condensation reaction, form a pharmacologically active alkaloid with dopamine which inhibits dopamine β-hydroxylase, leading to decreased production of norepinephrine. Phenylacetic acid and phenyllactic acid inhibit dopadecarboxylase (Figure 1) and thus inhibit the biosynthesis of epinephrine.

In this context it should be mentioned that Sandler (1982), in his review on disturbances of central neurotransmission, with special reference to PKU, called attention to the observation that the metabolite of phenylalanine, phenylethylamine, possesses very similar pharmocological properties to amphetamine. Amphetamine psychosis is almost indistinguishable from paranoid schizophrenia. In accordance with a phenylethylamine hypothesis of schizophrenia, it is not surprising that a high proportion of untreated PKU persons manifest some of the stigmata of this disease, which can be attenuated by reduced phenylalanine intake.

Another metabolite of phenylalanine, phenylacetic acid, is not without toxic effect. Ingestion of relatively large amounts of phenylacetic acid results in an effect resembling alcoholic intoxication (Sandler, 1982). Finally, the substantial amounts of phenylpyruvic acid formed in untreated PKU are further metabolized in a number of different ways, one of which is conversion to *o*-hydroxyphenylacetic acid. This metabolite has a profound inhibitory effect on a wide range of prostaglandin-connected enzymes, including prostaglandin synthetase (Sandler, 1982).

THE EFFECT OF BLOOD PHENYLALANINE LEVELS ON THE SYNTHESIS OF CNS NEUROTRANSMITTERS AND PERFORMANCE ON NEUROPSYCHOLOGICAL TESTS IN TREATED PKU

Most of the studies mentioned above on the inhibition by excess phenylalanine of the metabolism of tyrosine and tryptophan in untreated PKU were performed in order to elucidate how hyperphenylalaninaemia leads to brain damage in PKU. Recently, however, several groups (Brunner *et al.*, 1983; Krause *et al.*, 1985: Lou *et al.*, 1985) have compared specific neuropsychological tests with changes in plasma phenylalanine and neurotransmitter synthesis in early treated young adults with PKU on and off diet using a cross-over design.

Brunner and colleagues (1983) examined 27 children with PKU who had undergone dietary restriction of phenylalanine since infancy. Neuropsychological status was assessed using age-appropriate variations of the Halstead and Reitan test batteries. These tests were developed for the particular purpose of being sensitive to brain damage or dysfunction. Motor performance was assessed using the manual accuracy speed test. The serum phenylalanine concentration on the day of testing was significantly negatively correlated with scores on several individual tests. Specifically, higher serum phenylalanine concentration on the day of testing was related to lower full-scale IQ, steadiness, concept formation and tactile-motor problem solution. Brunner and colleagues (1983) conclude that concurrent serum phenylalanine concentrations affect neuropsychological performance and that the practice of terminating dietary restriction therefore requires further scrutiny.

Krause and colleagues (1985) studied 10 older, treated phenylketonuric patients using a triple-blind, multiple-trials, cross-over design. The tests included a repetitive battery of neuropsychological tests, analyses of plasma amino acids and measurements of urine dopamine and serotonin. They found that blood phenylalanine levels above 1300 μmol/L impair performance on neuropsychological tests of higher integrative function and that this effect is reversible. Their data support the hypothesis that one probable mechanism of this reversible effect may involve impaired synthesis of the two biogenic amines, dopamine and serotonin.

In this context it is interesting that Berry and colleagues (1982) observed improvement in neuropsychological functioning during periods of supplementation with the branched chain amino acids, whereas no changes occurred during alternate periods without this supplementation to older PKU-children in whom there were behavioural or neurological changes.

Lou and colleagues (1985) studied four adolescent or young adults with PKU before and after discontinuation of diet. In this study reaction time and reaction time variability, calculated from continuous recording of reaction times, were measured to evaluate brain functions in PKU patients. CSF concentrations of the dopamine and serotonin metabolites HVA and 5-HIAA were measured. The reaction time variability increased with blood phenylalanine levels above 1200 μmol/L and the CSF concentrations of HVA and 5-HIAA decreased. The relationship between reaction time variability and the CSF 5-HIAA level could be presented as a linear function. However, it is concluded that a causal relationship is still unproven (Lou *et al.*, 1985).

These preliminary findings have recently been confirmed in 7 young adults with PKU treated early with on and off diet (Lou *et al.*, unpublished). It was observed that 3 patients performed well on free diet. Their reaction time variability was normal even on a free diet and no further improvement could be obtained when they returned to a 'relaxed' phenylalanine restricted diet. In the remaining 4 patients reaction time variability increased after discontinuation of diet and the patients complained of lack of power of concentration and emotional instability. When these patients returned to a partially phenylalanine restricted, tyrosine enriched diet the impaired neuropsychological and behavioural functions were restored. The improvements were associated with a significant increase in CSF concentrations of the neurotransmitter metabolites HVA and 5-HIAA (Lou *et al.*, unpublished). From this study, it seems possible to define a group of young adults with PKU who do not need continuous dietary treatment, and another group who will benefit from a restricted phenylalanine diet.

However, in some young adults it may be difficult to continue the highly artificial and unpalatable diet required for phenylalanine restriction. It is therefore interesting that supplementation of a free diet with tyrosine (approximately 150 mg/kg) restored personality, behaviour, reaction time and reaction time variability in patients who suffered from diet discontinuation. The improvement was associated with a signficant increase in plasma tyrosine and CSF HVA concentrations (Lou *et al.*, unpublished). It may be of great clinical significance that more recent observations on reaction time and reaction time variability, as well as the CSF concentrations of HVA and 5-HIAA, were normalized when young PKU adults off diet were treated with tyrosine (200 mg/kg) and tryptophan (100 mg/kg) (Lou, 1985).

ACKNOWLEDGEMENT

The authors are grateful for the skilled assistance of the personnel of the John F. Kennedy Institute. The Danish Medical Research Council, the P. Carl Petersen's Foundation and Privatbankens Foundation have supported the authors contributing to this review.

REFERENCES

Armstrong, M. D. and Robinson, K. S. On the excretion of indole derivatives in phenylketonuria. *Arch. Biochem.* 52 (1954) 287–288

Berry, H. K., Bofinger, M. K., Melanie, M. H., Philips, P. J. and Guilfoile, M. B. Reduction of cerebrospinal fluid phenylalanine after oral administration of valine, isoleucine, and leucine. *Pediatr. Res.* 16 (1982) 751–755

Brunner, R. L., Jordan, M. K. and Berry, H. K. Early treated phenylketonuria: neuropsychologic consequences. *J. Pediatr.* 102 (1983) 831–835

Butler, L. J., O'Flynn, M. E., Seifert, W. E. and Howell, R. R. Neurotransmitter defects and treatment of disorders of hyperphenylalaninemia. *J. Pediatr.* 98 (1981) 729–733

Curtius, H. C., Vollmin, J. A. and Baerlocher, K. The use of deuterated phenylalanine for the elucidation of the phenylalanine–tyrosine metabolism. *Clin. Chim. Acta* 37 (1972) 277–285

Curtius, H. C., Wiederwieser, A., Viscontini, M., Leimbacher, W., Wegman, H., Blehova, B, Rey, F., Schaut, J. and Schmidt, H. Serotonin and dopamine synthesis in phenylketonuria. *Adv. Exp. Med. Biol.* 133 (1981) 277–291

Katz, I., Lloyd, R. and Kaufman, S. Studies on phenylalanine and tyrosine hydroxylation by rat brain tyrosine hydroxylase. *Biochem. Biophys. Acta* 445 (1976) 567–578

Krause, W., Halminski, M., McDonald, L., Dembure, P., Salvo, R., Freides, D. and Elsas, L. Biochemical and neuropsychological effects of elevated plasma phenylalanine in patients with treated phenylketonuria. *J. Clin. Invest.* 75 (1985) 40–48

Lou, H. C. Large doses of tryptophan and tyrosine as potential therapeutical alternative to dietary phenylalanine restriction in phenylketonuria. *Lancet* 1 (1985) 151

Lou, H. C., Güttler, F., Lykkelund, C., Bruhn, P. and Neiderweiser. A. Decreased vigilance and neurotransmitter synthesis after discontinuation of dietary treatment for phenylketonuria in adolescents. *Eur. J. Pediatr.* 144 (1985) 17–20

Lovenberg, W., Jéquier, E. and Sjoerdsma, A. Tryptophan hydroxylation in mammalian systems. *Adv. Pharmacol.* 6A (1968) 21–35

McKean, C. M. The effects of high phenylalanine concentrations on serotonin and catecholamine metabolism in the human brain. *Brain Res.* 47 (1972) 469–476

McSwigan, J. D., Vorhees, C. V., Brunner, R. L., Butcher, R. E. and Berry, H. K. Amelioration of maze deficits from induced hyperphenylalaninemia in adult rats using valine, isoleucine, and leucine. *Behav. Neur. Biology* 33 (1981) 378–384

Nadler, H. L. and Hsia, D. Y. Y. Epinephrine metabolism in phenylketonuria. *Proc. Soc. Exp. Biol. Med.* 107 (1961) 721–722

Paere, C. M., Sandler, M. and Stacey, R. S. Decreased 5-hydroxytryptamine deficiency in phenylketonuria. *Lancet* 1 (1957) 551–553

Paere, C. M., Sandler, M. and Stacey, R. S. Decreased 5-hydroxytryptophan decarboxylase activity in phenylketonuria. *Lancet* 2 (1958) 1099–1101

Peterson, N. A., Shah, S. N., Raghupathy, E. and Riioads, R. Presynaptic tyrosine availability in the phenylketonuric brain: a hypothetical evaluation. *Brain Res.* 272 (1983) 189–193

Pratt, O. E. Transport inhibition in the pathology of phenylketonuria and other inherited metabolic diseases. *J. Inher. Metab. Dis.* 5 Suppl. 2 (1982) 75–81

Sandler, M. Inborn errors and disturbances of central neurotransmission (with special reference to phenylketonuria). *J. Inher. Metab. Dis.* 5 Suppl. 2 (1982) 65–70

Tong, J. H. and Kaufman, S. Tryptophan hydroxylase: purification and some properties of the enzyme from rabbit hindbrain. *J. Biol. Chem.* 250 (1975) 4152–4158

Udenfriend, S. The primary enzymatic defect in phenylketonuria and how it may influence the central nervous system. In Anderson, J. A. and Swaiman, K. F. (eds). *Phenylketonuria and Allied Metabolic Diseases*. Dept. of Health, Education and Welfare, Washington DC, 1967, pp. 1–8

Waisbren, S. E., Schnell, R. R. and Levy, H. L. Diet termination in children with PKU. A review of psychological assessments used to determine outcome. *J. Inher. Metab. Dis.* 3 (1980) 149–153

Weil-Malherbe. Blood adrenaline and intelligence. *J. Ment. Sci.* 101 (1955) 733–745

J. Inher. Metab. Dis. 9 Suppl. 2 (1986) 178–182

Diagnosis in Relationship to Treatment of Hyperphenylalaninaemia

M. E. Blaskovics
Southern California Permanente Medical Group, Kaiser Foundation Hospital, 9985 Sierra Avenue, Fontana, California 92335, and Childrens Hospital of Los Angeles, Los Angeles, California, USA

PKU is not a single simply defined entity. It is part of a spectrum of the hyperphenylalaninaemias. Natural protein loading studies with uniform Phe equivalents are simple, and they are an inexpensive and safe way to determine or catagorize the types of hyperphenylalaninaemias (excluding defects of biopterin). Evidence from the US PKU Collaborative Study indicates that all patients with PKU do not require indefinite or prolonged restrictive dietary therapy to maintain normal intellectual functioning. Although there are as yet no absolute criteria, it appears that the milder forms of PKU may need treatment for a shorter period of time.

Phenylketonuria (PKU) is a well known but still not well differentiated condition. Despite more than 50 years of research in trying to delineate PKU, we have not reached unanimous agreement in definition, diagnostic methods, or duration of treatment. I wish to comment briefly about each of the above.

A paper was written years ago summarizing the experiences at Childrens Hospital of Los Angeles, after the American PKU Collaborative Study was launched and well on its way, and after we had done a variety of studies in an attempt to clearly define the population we chose to call classical PKU (Blaskovics *et al*., 1971). It must be appreciated that for the study we arbitrarily chose the parameters for PKU. For example, a serum phenylalanine (Phe) level greater than 1200 μmol L^{-1} was agreed upon only after much debate. Newborn screening had been established in the United States for some time before the Collaborative Study started and many individuals participating in the study had already seen infants and siblings with mildly elevated blood Phe levels who did not follow the clinical course of children with classical PKU, that is, these children developed normally without treatment. We did not know what to call these infants and children, but recognized that they were of a unique type. They now fall into the rather loose category called 'Hyperphe'.

Because it was known that such patients could bias the outcome of the Collaborative Study, for an infant to be considered eligible for inclusion in the study, we suggested that the blood Phe levels should be 1200 μmol L^{-1} or greater, determined on 2 occasions at least 24 hours apart while on a normal diet. It must also be

Journal of Inherited Metabolic Disease. ISSN 0141–8955. Queen Square, Lancaster, UK. Printed in Great Britain by Titus Wilson & Son Ltd., Kendal.

appreciated that some treatment centres *still* consider PKU to be present whenever blood Phe is greater than 600 μmol L^{-1}, others 900 μmol L^{-1}. It was necessary to develop some means of recognizing these non-PKU patients early to prevent their inclusion in the study. In an attempt to identify the hyperphe patients, we first tried pure L-phe (100 mg/kg) single dose 4-hour loading studies as suggested by Hsia and colleagues (1958). These were of little help. We extended the duration of study to 24 and 36 hours and found a significant improvement in our ability to discriminate PKU from these other infants with hyperphenylalaninaemia. Our observations were reported in 1971 in Heidelberg and again in Tel Aviv (Blaskovics and Shaw, 1971a, b). It was only after studying more patients for an extended period that we recognized the fallibility of the pure L-phe studies. We then recommended instead the use of natural protein foods with a Phe equivalent of approximately 180 mg kg^{-1} day^{-1} for at least 72 hours. When the evaluation was done for a shorter period (less than 72 hours), errors in diagnoses were made.

In the Collaborative Study, approximately 15% of the patients admitted to the study were later excluded when restudied for confirmation of their tentative diagnosis utilizing this challenge procedure (O'Flynn *et al.*, 1980). One additional child was recognized not to have PKU after 8 to 10 years of dietary treatment. This was a child who was studied for less than 72 hours. PKU cannot be recognized intuitively. This point was convincingly made by the United States PKU Collaborative Study and more recently confirmed by the German Collaborative Study (Lutz *et al.*, 1982). One simply cannot accurately diagnose PKU from initial blood Phe levels obtained during the newborn period. A diagnostic protocol must be rigidly followed if we are to arrive at a probable diagnosis and avoid unnecessary treatment.

Some centres use 'tolerance to Phe', that is, the average Phe intake as a predictor of PKU. This writer knows of instances where misdiagnoses have been made because tolerances were based upon a usual Phe intake to keep a blood level in the range 240–360 μmol L^{-1}. Unless a maximum Phe intake is established as with the protein challenge, there is a reasonable likelihood that some patients will be misdiagnosed.

I believe that most large PKU centres no longer routinely measure urinary metabolites of PKU except to look for defects in biopterin synthesis. When analysed statistically in the US and German PKU Collaborative Studies, for diagnostic purposes the measurement of phenylpyruvic acid, orthohydroxyphenylacetic acid and other metabolites have added nothing over the blood values alone. Liver biopsies have given equivocal diagnostic results as have deuterated L-phe studies (Bickel, 1980; Dhondt and Farriaux, 1981). Until some newer methods are devised for diagnosing PKU, I would like to suggest that the natural protein challenge, which was used by both the US and German collaborative studies, be considered as an aid to diagnosis or at least for categorizing patients with elevated blood Phe levels (Lutz *et al.*, 1982).

The need to categorize patients brings me to a second concern or problem which requires solution. The results from the United States PKU Collaborative Study, in my opinion, have not clearly answered the question regarding the duration of treatment needed for all patients with significantly elevated blood Phe levels, that is, 1200 μmol L^{-1} or greater. When the data are reviewed and analysed collectively, it appears that 8 years of uninterrupted dietary therapy are better that 6 years of therapy; however, in individual instances some children demonstrated considerable improvement in intelligence test scores when dietary treatment was stopped after 6 years. 16% increased 10 points or more in IQ score between 6 and 8 years of age. Others had no change (62% remained within 10 points of baseline IQ) or worsened (22% decreased 10 or more IQ points). These patients have not been categorized as to type or severity of PKU. This may have relevance in light of DNA studies being done to identify haplotypes and hence patient populations.

The question of the need for treatment of the Hyperphe cases, if recognized, seems to be largely resolved. Even the most cautious amongst us seems to be satisfied that a patient with a blood Phe level persistently below 720 μmol L^{-1} on an ordinary diet, or better yet, when formally challenged with a measured protein intake, needs no dietary treatment to develop normally.

Which of the other categories of patients need treatment for 8 years or longer, and which, if any, needs less and for how long is still not clear. I suggest that perhaps the less severe forms of PKU correspond to those patients who did well when formal dietary treatment was ended after 6 years and that perhaps that group of atypical PKU patients needs even less treatment.

In both the United States and German PKU Collaborative Studies, patients were recognized whose blood Phe levels during the natural protein challenge rose to greater than 1200 μmol L^{-1} and then fluctuated around 1200 to 1500 μmol L^{-1} or decreased to slightly less than 1200 μmol L^{-1}. I call these Type III patients. I presume others call them childen with atypical PKU (Composite of types: Figure 1). Type I corresponds to severe PKU, Type II to milder PKU, Type III to atypical PKU and Types IV and V to Hyperphe cases. Figure 2 shows data provided by Dr R. Koch of Childrens Hospital of Los Angeles. These patients we determined were

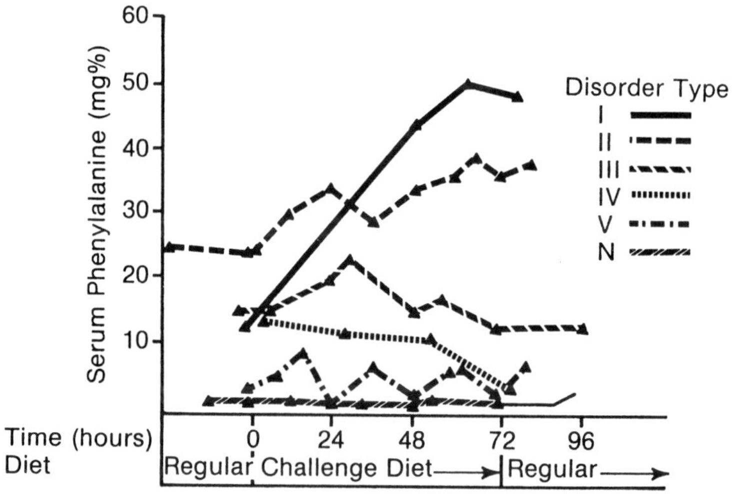

Figure 1 Responses to natural protein challenge with Phe equivalent of 180 mg kg^{-1} day^{-1}

Table 1 IQs off treatment: type III patients

Patient	*d.o.b.*	*Age Dx confirmed*	*Duration of Rx*	*Years off diet*	*Usual Phe level*	*Recent IQ*
J.M., m	1967	2 y	±2 y	14	9–21	124
R.D., m	1967	18 m	±1 y	16	12	94
S.W., f	1968	3 y	±3 y	14	13–21	123
H.H., f	1966	13 d	3 y	16	15	135
J.S., f	1966	NB	6 y	13	14–20	110
T.S., f	1962	5 y	±1 y	15	13–19	112
J. W., f	1963	NB	6 y	16	13–18	114
S.W., m	1955	6 y	None	30	12–23	128–132

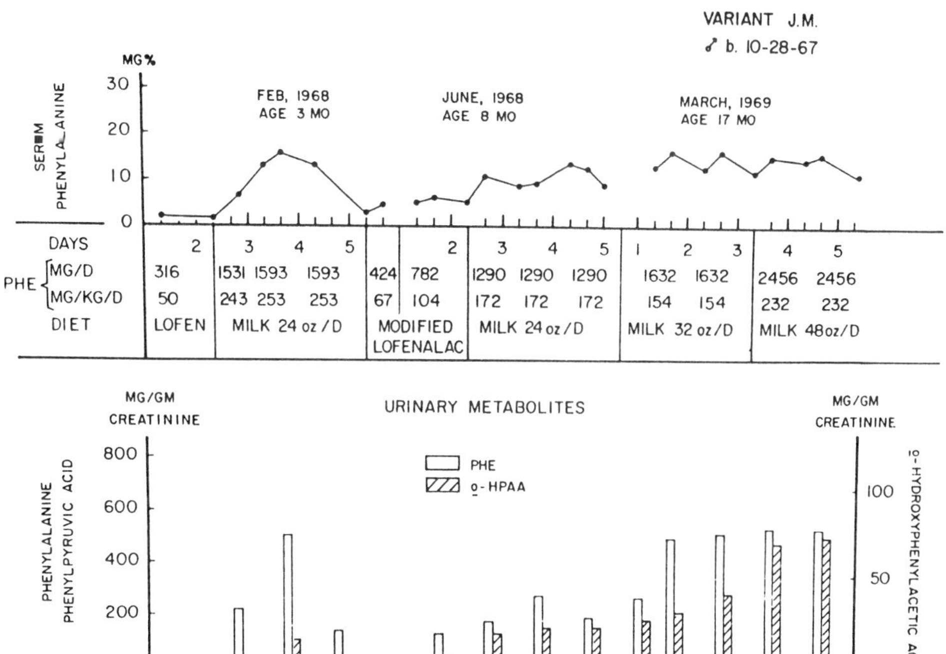

Figure 2 Milk tolerance tests on a variant patient, J.M.

Type III or atypical PKU, based upon protein challenges. The data illustrate the point that these patients fared quite well despite dietary treatment for very short periods and also after dietary treatment was discontinued. Patient J.M. (male) (Figures 2 and 3, see Table 1 also) illustrates responses to repeated studies and how he and other children fared after at least 13 years off dietary restrictions. Perhaps special neuro-psychological tests may define specific handicaps in these subjects, but on the whole it would be extremely difficult to identify these young people from the population at large.

We may someday be able to predict a diagnosis and whether or not a patient

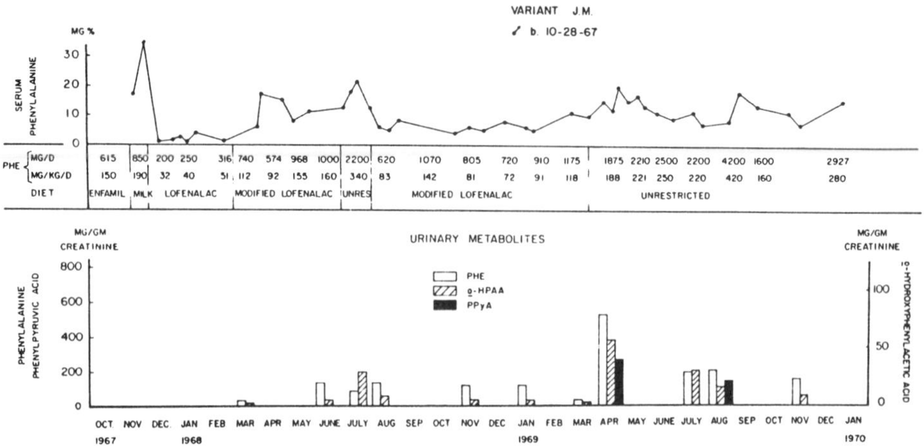

Figure 3 Course of treatment for a variant patient, J.M.

needs treatment and for how long because of his DNA haplotype; until then, however, decisions must be made on less than perfect tests.

REFERENCES

Bickel, H. Phenylketonuria: past, present, future. *J. Inherit. Metab. Dis.* 3 (1980) 123–132

Blaskovics, M. E., Schaeffler, G. and Hack, S. Phenylalaninemia, differential diagnosis. *Arch. Dis. Child* 49 (1974) 835–843

Blaskovics, M. E. and Shaw, K. N. F. Hyperphenylalaninemia: methods for differential diagnosis. In Bickel, H., Hudson, F. P. and Woolf, L. I. (eds.) *Phenylketonuria and some other Inborn Errors of Amino Acid Metabolism*, Georg Thieme Verlag, Stuttgart, 1971a, pp. 98–102

Blaskovics, M. E. and Shaw, K. N. F. Hyperphenylalaninemia. In Cohen, B. E., Robin, M. I. and Szeinberg, A. (eds.) *International Symposium on Phenylketonuria and Allied Disorders*, Tel Aviv, 1971b, pp. 218–219

Dhondt, J. L. and Farriaux, J. T. Hepatic phenylalanine hydroxylase activity in hyperphenylalaninemia. *J. Inher. Metab. Dis.* 4 (1981) 59–60

Hsia, D. Y.-Y., Driscoll, K., Troll, W. and Knox, W. E. Detection by phenylalanine tolerance tests of heretozygous carriers of phenylketonuria. *Nature* (London) 178 (1956) 1239–1240

Lutz, P., Schmidt, H., Frey, G. and Bickel, H. Standardized loading test with protein for the differentiation of phenylketonuria from hyperphenylalaninemia. *J. Inher. Metab. Dis.* 5 (1982) 29–35

O'Flynn, M. E., Holtzman, N. A., Blaskovics, M. E., Azen, C. and Williamson, M. L. The diagnosis of phenylketonuria. A report from the collaborative study of children treated for phenylketonuria. *Am. J. Dis. Child* 134 (1980) 769–774

J. Inher. Metab. Dis. 9 Suppl. 2 (1986) 183–201

Problems Related to Diet Management of Maternal Phenylketonuria

P. B. Acosta and S. Stepnick-Gropper
Department of Nutrition and Food Science, Florida State University, Tallahassee, Florida 32306–2033, USA

Provision of nutritionally complete elemental diets for pregnant women with PKU requires greater knowledge of 'conditionally' essential nutrient requirements than is presently available as well as application of known information. Formulation of elemental products needs to be improved to enhance aroma and taste and to decrease osmolality. Designers of the metal and vitamin components should keep in mind that a major portion (70–80%) of most of these nutrients must be obtained from the elemental products. Thus deletion of suspected essential minerals or vitamins could cause serious deficiencies. On the other hand, knowledge of appropriate ratios that make for improved trace metal absorption should be applied. Clinical nutritionists need to assist patients in selection of foods that are low in binding substances and provide 'conditionally' essential nutrients in adequate amounts. Closer cooperation between clinical nutritionists, nutrition scientists and food technologists should result in improved elemental products for care of pregnant women with PKU.

Innovations in technology have occurred and knowledge of human nutrient requirements has expanded during the 31 years since Bickel first employed an elemental diet to treat a child with phenylketonuria (PKU) (McKusick 26160) (Bickel, 1954). Elemental diets may result in normal growth (Holm *et al.*, 1979) and development (Dobson *et al.*, 1977) whilst creating a host of problems (Hanley *et al.*, 1970; Acosta *et al.*, 1982; Endres *et al.*, 1984). Elemental diets predispose to management problems and nutrient deficiencies and excesses in vulnerable patients for at least 6 reasons:

1. The role of taste and aroma in long-term consumption of elemental diets has not been adequately addressed. Taste and aroma of foods are of particular importance in nutritional support of maternal PKU since about 50% of pregnant women experience some nausea and vomiting (Baylis *et al.*, 1983).

2. Elemental diets, due to their chemically defined nature, consist of small molecules that often provide an osmolality greater than the physiological tolerance of the patient. Abdominal cramping, diarrhoea, distension, nausea and vomiting have resulted from use of hyperosmolar feeds (Cashel *et al.*, 1978). Aside from

Journal of Inherited Metabolic Disease. ISSN 0141–8955.

gastrointestinal distress, more serious consequences can occur such as hypertonic dehydration (Abrams *et al.*, 1975), hypovolaemia (Coodin *et al.*, 1971), hypernatraemia (Seegar and Chesney, 1977) and death (Endres *et al.*, 1984).

3. The physiological effects of liquid fats frequently used to supply nitrogen-free energy have not been considered. For example, an excess amount of one fatty acid may successfully compete for the activity of an enzyme required to desaturate several different fatty acids (Mohrhauer and Holman, 1963). Moreover, substitution of long chain polyunsaturated fatty acids (PUFAs) for saturated fatty acids may alter fluidity and permeability properties of membranes and affect ion transport and activity of membrane-bound enzymes (Mead, 1984).

4. While elemental products intended for infants are formulated based on the composition of human milk, bioavailability of nutrients from these chemical solutions is unknown.

5. Elemental products designed for use by infants are often fed to children and adults due to lack of acceptance or availability of more appropriately formulated diets. Use of products by age-specific populations for which they were not intended often precipitates nutrient deficiencies (Acosta *et al.*, 1982) and dietary excesses (Acosta *et al.*, 1977).

6. Clinicians who prescribe elemental products assume that all essential nutrients (a) are known and present in the product, (b) will be synthesized from a precursor in the product or (c) will be provided by the small quantities of natural foods ingested by the patient to supply the required amount of restricted essential amino acid(s) or nitrogen. Information from patients who require long-term use of total parenteral nutrition (TPN) has clearly demonstrated the essentiality of food constituents often considered to be contaminants (Chipponi *et al.*, 1982). The biosynthesis of ordinarily non-essential nutrients by patients with inherited disorders of metabolism may be compromised due to the enzyme defect(s). On the other hand, compounds essential to structure or function may not be synthesized by patients with inherited diseases of metabolism due to accumulated substrate(s) that inhibit activity of enzyme(s). Natural foods seldom supply more than 25% and often much less of the protein requirements of patients receiving elemental diets. Other nitrogen-free natural foods which provide energy are limited in their range of nutrients.

Diet management problems, nutrient deficiencies and dietary excesses that occur with the use of elemental products may be compounded in the pregnant woman with PKU who must obtain adequate nutrients for herself and her fetus if neither is to be compromised. The purposes of this paper are to discuss (1) physicochemical problems and (2) nutrition deficiencies that may be associated with use of elemental diets by pregnant PKU women.

PHYSICOCHEMICAL PROBLEMS

Physicochemical problems that occur with the use of elemental diets may result from solution osmolality and interactions of chemical nutrients in the intestinal lumen. Interactions of metals and non-nutritive substances, metals and metals, and lipids and metals will be discussed.

Osmolality of solutions

In our laboratory we have recently measured osmolalities of elemental products intended for therapy of pregnant women with PKU (Anderson *et al.*, unpublished data). Figure 1 describes osmolalities of 2 phenylalanine-free products in amounts

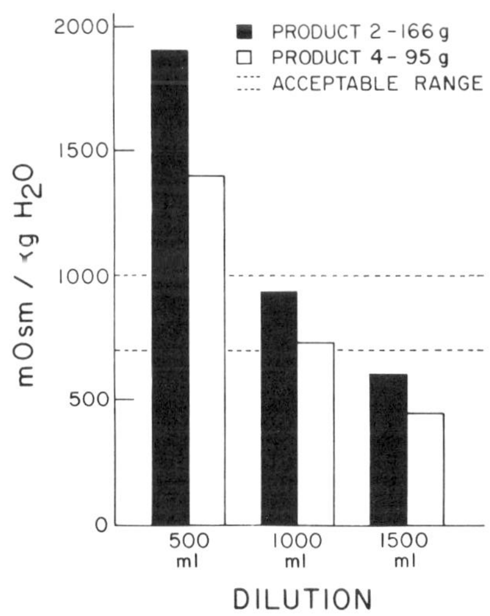

Figure 1 Osmolality of two elemental products intended for pregnant women with PKU

required to yield 65 g of protein. The addition of glucose polymers or sucrose to supply nitrogen-free energy contribute in ascending order to osmolality while fat, of itself, has no effect except to displace water and the osmolality contributed by carbohydrate (Figure 2). Relatively large amounts of water or fat must be added to decrease the osmolality to that recommended by Smith and Heymsfield (1983) for adults.

Hypertonic dehydration (Abrams *et al.*, 1975) and hypovolaemia (Coodin *et al.*, 1971) produced by hyperosmolar feeds may adversely affect required plasma volume expansion of pregnant PKU women. Plasma volume in the well-fed pregnant woman normally increases by about 40% to afford adequate blood flow to the placenta and is required to supply nutrients and oxygen in needed amounts to the fetus (Hytten, 1980). Not only may fetal growth be compromised by depressed nutrient supply occasioned by maternal dehydration but the fetus will share any dehydration suffered by the mother (Hytten, 1980).

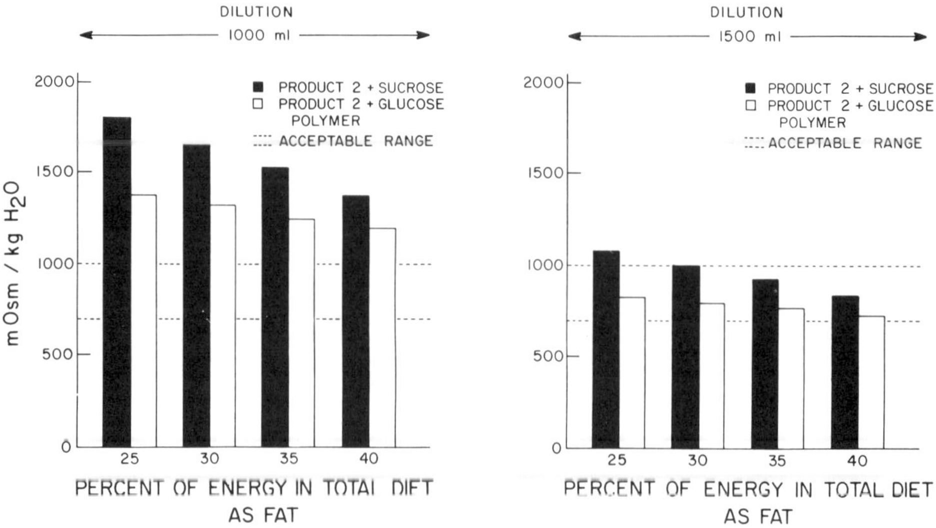

Figure 2 Effect of dilution, carbohydrate and fat on osmolality of elemental products

Nutrient interactions in the intestinal lumen

Lower than normal plasma concentrations of copper, iron, selenium and zinc in children undergoing therapy for PKU (Lombeck *et al.*, 1978; Acosta *et al.*, 1981; Hurry and Gibson, 1982) have led to a search for reasons for depressed plasma levels often in the face of apparently adequate intakes. Despite lack of knowledge of the clinical significance of the depressed plasma concentrations, trace metal deficiencies during pregnancy could have serious effects on fetal development (Hurley, 1981).

Inadequate dietary intake is likely to be a reason for the low plasma selenium concentrations since most elemental products contain little or no selenium and foods that may be eaten are low in selenium. Mechanisms that may be partially responsible for low plasma concentrations of copper, iron and zinc in patients undergoing therapy for PKU include: (1) depressed solubility, (2) competitive inhibition, (3) inadequate enhancing factors, (4) changes in intestinal membrane permeability and (5) greater than normal urinary loss.

Dietary factors that may influence *intestinal solubility* of metals include casein, fibre, oxalate, phytate and tannic acid. Casey and associates (1981) measured plasma zinc responses in humans for 3 hours following ingestion of 25 mg of zinc with human milk, 2% cows' milk or infant formulas, one of which was a low phenylalanine casein hydrolysate. After ingestion of the low phenylalanine casein hydrolysate with zinc, plasma zinc increased significantly less than after ingestion of zinc with human milk. Harzer and Kauer (1982) demonstrated that at slightly alkaline pH 1 mg of casein bound 8.4 μg of zinc and suggested that binding of zinc to casein and its phosphopeptides might explain, in part, the low zinc availability from some milk-based elemental products.

Dietary fibre, oxalate, phytate and tannic acid have all been reported to depress solubility of intestinal copper, iron and zinc. Mean daily fibre intake of 10 children with PKU who ingested an L-amino acid mix was 11.5 g (SD±4.6 g) while 12 children with PKU treated with a casein hydrolysate ingested 7.1 g (SD±5.7 g). Fibre in diets of treated children and adults with PKU is contributed primarily by fruit and vegetables. Fruit and vegetable fibre (24 g) (Kelsey *et al.*, 1979) or fruit fibre (15 g) (Lei *et al.*, 1980) produced fecal losses of copper and zinc that were significantly greater than when the fibre was not fed. Correlations between fibre intake of 10 children with PKU and plasma or whole blood concentrations of chromium, copper, iron, selenium and zinc were investigated by us. Selected

Table 1 Selected Pearson product moment correlation coefficients[a]

Correlation	*Coefficient (r)*	*Significance*
Dietary fibre intake *v* plasma copper	0.145	NS
Dietary fibre intake *v* plasma iron	0.171	NS
Dietary fibre intake *v* plasma zinc	−0.150	NS
Dietary $\frac{Ca+P}{Zn}$ *v* plasma Zn	−0.787	≤0.05
Dietary $\frac{Cu+Fe}{Zn}$ *v* plasma Zn	−0.486	NS
Dietary $\frac{Zn}{Cu}$ *v* plasma Cu	0.397	NS

[a] 10 children with PKU using product 3
NS = not significant

correlations are presented in Table 1. Dietary fibre did not appear to affect plasma concentrations of chromium, copper, iron, selenium or zinc.

Oxalic acid, present in large amounts in some foods and in smaller amounts in many foods (Pennington and Church, 1985), is reported to chelate calcium, iron and zinc depressing their solubility and absorption (Kelsey and Prather, 1981). Phytic acid, ubiquitous in grains and grain products, legumes and nuts (Pennington and Church, 1985), forms insoluble salts with minerals in the intestine. Pecoud and colleagues (1985) reported that 102 mg of phytic acid, with or without 500 mg of calcium, blunted the plasma response to an oral dose of 50 mg of zinc as zinc sulphate. Mills (1985) quantified interrelationships of calcium, phytate and zinc in human diets. He suggested that a molar ratio of calcium plus phytate to zinc exceeding 0.4 might significantly reduce the efficiency of zinc absorption, or if exceeding 3.0 might deplete tissue zinc.

Copper, magnesium and manganese also form complexes with phytate. However, both total amount of dietary protein as well as the pattern of amino acids in the protein may influence availability of copper, manganese and zinc from insoluble metal calcium or magnesium phytate complexes (Sandstrom *et al.*, 1980; Wise and Gilburt, 1982; Forbes *et al.*, 1983). Available evidence suggests that free histidine, cysteine and methionine readily desorb zinc from insoluble (metal calcium phytate) complexes. The yield of soluble copper, manganese or zinc from such complexes is directly proportional to the amino-N content of the intestinal soluble phase. The effectiveness of release of metals from their complexes with phytate was Cu>Mn>Zn (Wise and Gilburt, 1982).

Tannin, found in tea and in many vegetables and cereal foods, is a known inhibitor of trace metal absorption (Lynch and Morck, 1983). Tea decreases iron absorption by a factor of 4 when 1 cup is taken with a meal. This effect appears to be due to the formation of insoluble iron-tannate complexes.

Data are not yet available to determine whether oxalate, phytate and tannin are important in decreasing availability of trace metals to treated patients with PKU. Nor is it known whether these substances interact more readily with metals in solution than with metals in food.

Minerals with similar chemical properties often exhibit *biological competition* (Hill and Matrone, 1970). Such competitive inhibition has been reported between calcium and iron, calcium and zinc, copper and zinc, iron and zinc, phosphorus and iron, and phosphorus and zinc.

Adham and Song (1980) recently reported that zinc absorption from the mucosal to the serosal side of rat jejunal sacs was decreased by 40% in the presence of 25 mmol L^{-1} $CaCl_2$. However, no effect of copper on zinc absorption was found. Adversely, copper excretion and copper status are negatively influenced by minimal zinc supplements. Festa and coworkers (1985) fed 9 men 1.8 to 20.7 mg zinc and 2.63 mg copper daily. Faecal copper excretion increased when zinc intake reached 18.5 mg daily. The activity of erythrocyte Cu, Zn-superoxide dismutase is dependent on copper but not zinc status (Bettger *et al.*, 1979). Erythrocyte superoxide dismutase activity decreased significantly in 26 males after 6 weeks of daily supplementation with 50 mg zinc (Fischer *et al.*, 1984). Prasad and colleagues (1978) reported that 150 mg of zinc taken daily for 1–2 years produced iron deficiency anaemia due to copper deficiency. Fetal stores of copper may be compromised by high maternal zinc intake and may influence infant haemoglobin, haematocrit, organ copper stores and activity of Cytochrome c oxidase and lysyl oxidase for as long as 35 days after birth (Hill *et al.*, 1983).

Plasma zinc in humans decreased progressively as the iron/zinc ratio in solution increased from 0/1 to 3/1 while zinc remained constant at 25 mg (Solomons and Jacob, 1981). Valberg and coworkers (1984) showed that both inorganic iron and haeme iron inhibited zinc absorption from zinc chloride.

Effects of moderate (1 g) and high (2.5 g) phosphorus diets on faecal and urinary losses of copper, manganese and zinc by 8 adult males have been assessed (Greger and Snedeker, 1980). Copper and manganese retention were not affected by dietary phosphorus level: however, faecal zinc losses were significantly greater on high phosphorus than on low phosphorus diets.

Correlation coefficients were calculated by us for selected metals in the diets of 10 children with PKU and plasma copper, iron and zinc (Table 1). Clearly, as the ratio of dietary calcium plus phosphorus to zinc increased plasma zinc was significantly decreased. Ratios of selected metals in elemental products intended for pregnant women with PKU are given in Table 2.

A host of dietary factors are purported to *enhance* absorption of iron and zinc

Table 2 Ratios of selected metals in elemental products intended for pregnant women with PKU

Metals	*Product*			
	1	*2*	*3*	*4*
calcium/iron	69	69	58	87
calcium/zinc	243	80	117	90
iron/zinc	3.5	1.2	2.0	1.0
phosphorus/iron	67	89	75	87
phosphorus/zinc	236	104	151	90
zinc/copper	7	9	12	6

Table 3 Some dietary compounds that may enhance absorption of selected metals

Metal	*Compounds*	*Reference*
Iron	amino acids	Christensen *et al.*, 1984
	ascorbic acid	Lynch and Morck, 1983
	haem iron	Lynch and Morck, 1983
	maltodextrins	Monsen and Cook, 1979
Zinc	amino acids	Mills, 1985
	beef	Shah and Belonje, 1981
	citric acid	Lonnerdal *et al.*, 1980
	dipeptides	Steinhardt and Adibi, 1984
	lactose	Solomons, 1982
	picolinic acid	Evans and Johnson, 1980

(Table 3). Whether absorption of copper, iron and zinc by individuals with PKU could be significantly enhanced by the use of carbohydrates consisting of dextrimaltose, lactose and glucose polymers is unknown but should be evaluated. Carbohydrates present in products intended for treatment of pregnant women with PKU are listed in Table 4.

Table 4 Carbohydrate sources of elemental products intended for pregnant women with PKU

Product	*Carbohydrate source*	*% of energy*
1	corn syrup solids	52
	modified tapioca starch	
2	maltodextrins	46
3	sucrose	65
	corn syrup solids	
	modified tapioca starch	
4	sucrose	3

Intestinal membrane fluidity and permeability

Intestinal membrane fluidity and permeability, as influenced by fatty acids, may affect absorption of metals. Calcium (Hay *et al.*, 1980), iron and zinc (Lukaski *et al.*, 1982; Van Dokkum *et al.*, 1983) retention are affected by diets high in polyunsaturated fatty acids (PUFAs).

Specific reasons for decreased iron absorption and zinc retention on diets high in PUFAs are unknown. Change in fatty acid saturation of phospholipids in intestinal cell membranes is one possibility (Mead, 1984). PUFAs in erythrocyte membranes increase by 40% after 3 weeks of daily ingestion of 45 mL of sunflower seed oil (Ahmad and Leeds, 1983). Mitochondrial inner-membrane lipids in rat heart were maximally affected by 11 days after a change in composition of dietary fat (Innis and Clandinin, 1981).

Increased urinary loss

Metals in the blood may be free (ionic), bound to proteins (albumin and others) or complexed with amino acids. The metals complexed with amino acids are in equilibrium with albumin-bound metals and both fractions are in equilibrium with their ionic forms. The quantities of non-albumin-bound copper (Neumann and Sass-Kortsak, 1967) and zinc (Giroux and Henkin, 1972) vary with the concentration of free amino acids. This may be true for other trace metals as well. The amino acids histidine, glutamine, threonine and cystine at physiological concentrations compete with albumin for the binding of copper. Ligands of zinc form principally with cysteine, histidine, glutamine, cystine and glycine (Prasad and Oberleas, 1970; Giroux and Henkin, 1972). Amino acid bound metals may account for most of the urinary metals, as has been reported for zinc (Henkin *et al.*, 1972). Urinary copper losses of infants receiving free amino acid solutions intravenously have been reported to correlate positively with total excretion of α-amino nitrogen and the excretion of glycine, methionine, histidine and lysine (Tyrala *et al.*, 1982). Amino acid absorption may be more rapid from peptides and L-amino acid mixes than from whole proteins. Clearly, effects of hydrolysates and L-amino acid mixes on urinary metal loss should be evaluated.

NUTRITIONAL PROBLEMS

Some 'conditional' nutrients which may be essential for the pregnant woman with PKU and her fetus that will be addressed fall into 2 classes, lipids and nitrogen-containing compounds. Lipids that may be essential are α-linolenic acid and cholesterol. Nitrogen-containing compounds recently found to be significant are carnitine and taurine.

α-Linolenic acid

Two long chain polyunsaturated fatty acids are required by mammals. These are linoleic acid (C18 : 2W6; C18 : 2△9,12) and α-linolenic acid (C18 : 3W3; C18 : 3△9,12,15). By desaturation and elongation most mammalian systems can synthesize at least 8 different fatty acids from linoleic acid and 5 different fatty acids from α-linolenic acid. These elongated fatty acids contain 20–22 carbons and 3–5 double bonds.

Linoleic acid and its derivatives are of special importance in the structure of membrane lipid bilayers (Mead, 1984). Less well known but of equal importance is linoleate's role as a precursor of prostaglandins, thromboxanes, prostacyclin and leukotrienes (eicosanoids) (Marcus, 1984). Some 1–3% of energy as linoleate has been proposed as adequate to provide for synthesis of membrane bilayers and eicosanoids (Committee on Dietary Allowances, 1980). Most vegetable oils, such as corn, safflower and soy, contain abundant amounts of linoleate (Reeves and Weihrauch, 1979).

The attention of nutritionists was forcefully focused on α-linolenic acid in 1982 when Holman and coworkers ascribed numbness, paresthesia, weakness, inability to walk, pain in the legs and blurring vision in a 6-year-old girl to α-linolenate deficiency. The symptoms occurred after 5 months on a total parenteral nutrition preparation rich in linoleate but low in α-linolenate and were reversed by lowering the linoleate and increasing the α-linolenate.

Animal studies suggest that, in addition to its role in membrane lipid bilayers, α-linolenate has both structural and functional roles in the brain (Crawford *et al.*, 1976) and in the photoreceptor membrane of the eye (Anderson *et al.*, 1974; Neuringer *et al.*, 1984). Lipid accounts for some 50–60% of solid matter in the brain (Crawford *et al.*, 1981). Clandinin and associates (1981) evaluated the accretion of α-linolenate and its derivatives by the human fetus from 26 weeks to term. They reported daily brain accretion of about 3 mg and total body accretion of 67 mg

During pregnancy, when parent essential fatty acids are available, they are metabolized by the placenta into long chain derivatives that progressively increase from maternal liver, to placenta, to fetal liver and finally to fetal brain (Crawford *et al.*, 1981) in a process called 'biomagnification'. Parent essential fatty acids are not converted quantitatively to their long chain derivatives. In the developing rat pup only about 1 molecule in 30 of linoleic acid was converted to arachidonic acid (Crawford *et al.*, 1981).

High levels of linoleate in the diet of humans (Holman *et al.*, 1982) have been shown to suppress the tissue content of α-linolenate and its derivatives. A ratio of 6/1 linoleate to linolenate, however, did not suppress conversion of α-linolenate to its long chain derivatives when 44 mg of α-linolenate/kg (0.54% of energy) were fed to a 6-year-old.

Few vegetable oils other than soybean oil contain significant amounts of α-linolenate and the ratio of linoleate to α-linolenate is very high in corn oil and safflower oil (Reeves and Weihrauh, 1979). Amounts and ratios of essential fatty acids in elemental products intended for therapy of pregnant women with PKU that contain fat are given in Table 5. Not only are the amounts of α-linolenate low but the ratio of linoleate to α-linolenate is high. Energy modules available in the UK provide linoleate to α-linolenate ratios ranging from 28 to 56. Clearly, nutritionists who administer elemental products need to select with great care the type of fat to be added.

Table 5 Fat sources, percentages of energy from fat, essential fatty acid contents and essential fatty acid ratios of elemental products intended for use by pregnant women with PKU

Variable	Product	
	1	*3*
Fat source	corn oil	corn oil coconut oil
Fat (% of energy)	35	15
Linoleic acid (g/100 g)	10.44	2.76
α-linolenic acid (g/100 g)	0.13	0.03
Linoleate/linolenate	80	84

Cholesterol

Although often maligned due to its purported role in vascular disease, cholesterol has major structural and functional responsibilities in mammalian systems. As a precursor of steroid hormones (Winkel *et al.*, 1980), cholesterol is vitally important in the maintenance of pregnancy. In addition to its precursor role in steroid hormone synthesis, cholesterol is an essential component of plasma and intracellular membranes (Siperstein, 1984). A number of studies reviewed by Siperstein have demonstrated that cell proliferation cannot occur in the absence of structural cholesterol (1984). Mevalonate, an intermediate in cholesterol synthesis, is synthesized from

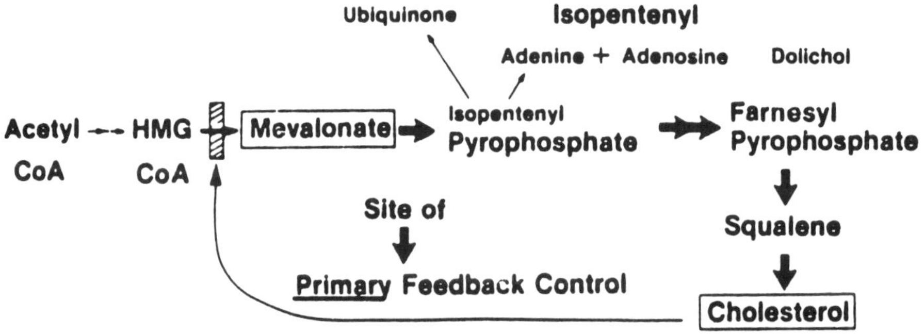

Figure 3 Cholesterol synthesis
By courtesy of M. D. Siperstein, *J. Lipid Res.*

HMG CoA, by HMG CoA reductase (Figure 3). HMG CoA reductase activity increases in cells at or just prior to each S-phase DNA replication. The cholesterol requirement is limited to the early and mid-G_1 phases whereas mevalonate is required at the late G_1–S interphase of the cell cycle (Quesney-Huneeus *et al.*, 1983). The proposed dual role of cholesterol and its precursor in cell growth and proliferation is shown in Figure 4.

Not only does maternal liver normally synthesize large amounts of cholesterol from acetate, but fetal liver, adrenal cortex, brain and other tissues utilize glucose for *de novo* cholesterol synthesis *in situ* (Figure 3) (Carr and Simpson, 1982). The

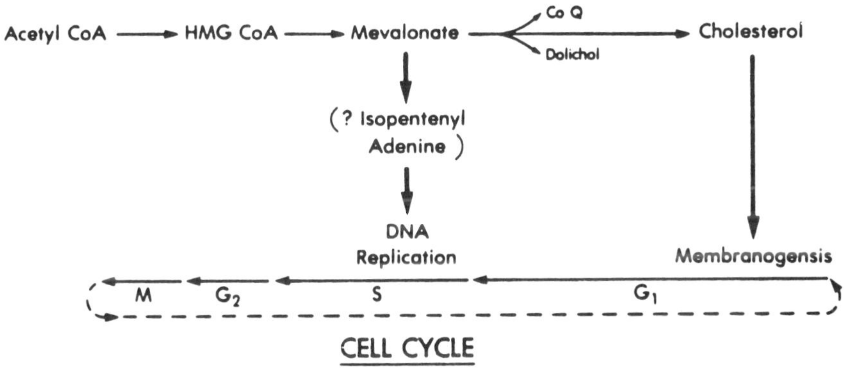

Figure 4 Role of cholesterogenesis in the cell cycle of DNA synthesis
By courtesy of M. D. Siperstein, *J. Lipid Res.*

fetus synthesizes the majority of its cholesterol since only about 20% is derived from maternal sources at 3 months gestation (Lin *et al.*, 1977).

The normal human brain at birth contains about 70% of its eventual number of cells (Winick, 1969). Svennerholm and Vanier reported that at term the cholesterol content of human brain was about 20 μmol/g^{-1} (1972). Active brain cholesterol synthesis occurs as early as 7 embryonic weeks (Plotz *et al.*, 1968) while fetal tissue cholesterol synthesis increases between 8 and 18 weeks gestation and then decreases somewhat (Carr and Simpson, 1982).

Should mevalonate and cholesterol synthesis or supply be curtailed for any reason, steroid hormone synthesis and cell proliferation and growth could be suppressed (Siperstein, 1984). Pregnant women with PKU often deliver prior to their expected date of confinement. Offspring of untreated women with PKU are microcephalic and undergrown at birth (Lenke and Levy, 1980) and catch-up growth does not occur. Observation of untreated children with PKU indicate that they fail to obtain their full growth potential. Studies of the cholesterol content of the brains from untreated patients with PKU have reported lower concentrations than found in normal brains (Crome *et al.*, 1962; Menkes, 1966; Gerstl *et al.*, 1967). Acosta and colleagues (1973) reported lower than normal plasma cholesterol concentrations in treated and untreated children with PKU. A relationship between plasma cholesterol concentration, often used to assess cholesterol synthesis or dietary supply, and reproductive outcome may exist in PKU women. Clearly this area requires further investigation.

Why should both treated and untreated patients with PKU have depressed plasma cholesterol concentrations? Lack of dietary cholesterol and enhanced biliary cholesterol excretion due to high intakes of PUFAs are 2 explanations (Table 6). However, lack of cholesterol intake and enhanced excretion are not acceptable reasons for low plasma cholesterol concentrations in untreated patients. As early as 1955, Goldstein demonstrated that phenylacetate or phenylpyruvate when present in relatively high concentration interfered with CoA-dependent reactions, in particular with biosynthesis of cholesterol (Gerstl *et al.*, 1967).

Table 6 Mean daily cholesterol, fat and unsaturated fat intakes of 10 treated children with PKU[a]

Nutrient	*Mean±SD*
Cholesterol (mg)	14± 9
Fat, total (g)	38±16
Unsaturated fat (g)	24±11
Unsaturated fat (% of total energy)	14

[a] Using product 3

Weber and colleagues (1970) evaluated activities of hexokinase and pyruvate kinase in human fetal brain tissue between 13 and 21 weeks of gestation. Activities were about 10% of activities found in adult human brain and were significantly depressed by L-phenylalanine and phenylpyruvate. Bowden and McArthur (1972) evaluated effects of 5 phenylalanine metabolites on pyruvate decarboxylation in rat liver and brain homogenates. Phenylpyruvic acid inhibited pyruvate decarboxylation in the brain by 50%. In addition to a decrease in available energy, Bowden and McArthur (1972) suggested that this inhibition of pyruvate decarboxylation would decrease the amount of acetyl-CoA available for the synthesis of cholesterol.

Effects of phenylalanine and phenylpyruvic acid on mevalonate and cholesterol synthesis by the placenta and fetal adrenal and liver have not been reported. With active transport of phenylalanine to the fetus (Lemons, 1979), this would seem an important area for investigation, particularly since elemental products intended for nutritional support of pregnant women with PKU contain no cholesterol. The complete diets as prescribed are devoid of or low in cholesterol and are often high in PUFAs.

Carnitine

First discovered in 1905, carnitine (gamma-trimethylamino-β-hydroxybutyrate) was not considered to be a 'conditionally' essential nutrient until the 1980s (Chipponi *et al.*, 1982). Carnitine functions to transport long chain fatty acids into the mitochondrial matrix, plays an important role in thermogenesis in brown adipose tissue and is involved in the initiation of ketogenesis. Carnitine is also suspected to function in the oxidation of the branched chain keto-acids derived from leucine and valine and in the regulation of gluconeogenesis (Borum, 1983).

Carnitine is normally made available to humans via diet and *de novo* synthesis. Meat and dairy products are the major dietary sources of carnitine (Borum, 1983). Even so, casein and casein hydrolysates contain only small amounts of carnitine (Borum *et al.*, 1979) and all L-amino acid mixes intended for use with patients with PKU have, until recently, been devoid of carnitine.

Lysine and methionine are utilized to synthesize gamma butyrobetaine in all human tissues examined. But gamma butyrobetaine is hydroxylated to form L-carnitine only in liver, kidney and brain (Rebouche, 1982). Carnitine biosynthesis is regulated by diet (lysine, methionine, ascorbate, niacin, vitamin B_6, iron), age and hormonal status. Dietary deficiencies of lysine, methionine or B_6, in particular, have led to depressed carnitine biosynthesis (Borum, 1983). In human infants, gamma butyrobetaine hydroxylase activity is about one-tenth of the normal adult mean (Rebouche, 1980). Neonates were unable to maintain normal plasma carnitine concentrations while receiving TPN (Schiff *et al.*, 1979).

Fatty acid oxidation by maternal tissues, particularly during the last trimester, is an important energy source since maternal peripheral tissues demonstrate insulin resistance and glucose is transferred to the fetus in large amounts. In fact, maternal fasting glucose concentrations are generally low. Free, total and acylcarnitine were measured in plasma of 21 women at term and compared to values obtained in 9 non-pregnant women and were found to be slightly less than one-third of normal values (Bargen-Lockner *et al.*, 1981). Amniotic fluid free carnitine decreased with gestational age from 10 to 40 weeks (Hahn *et al.*, 1977).

Plasma carnitine concentrations were measured in one woman with PKU (Koch, unpublished data) during the last trimester of pregnancy and were reported to be very low. If future studies find that plasma carnitine concentrations of treated pregnant women with PKU are lower than found in normal pregnant women, supplementation of all elemental diets with L-carnitine may be warranted.

Taurine

Taurine (2-aminoethane sulphonic acid) has been considered as an end product of sulphur amino acid metabolism with its only role that of conjugation with cholic acid (Hayes, 1981). These concepts began to change when Hayes and coworkers (1975) demonstrated that kittens fed a taurine-free diet became blind.

During the past 10 years intensive research has focused on taurine's functions and several volumes and reviews relating to this work have recently been published (Huxtable and Pasantes-Morales, 1982; Hayes, 1985; Oja *et al.*, 1985). In the retina and central nervous system taurine may serve a structural and functional role in stabilizing neural membranes. Taurine is believed to modulate calcium flux in muscle and platelets. In heart muscle, taurine increases the calcium available for contractions.

Sturman and associates (1984) raised 5 rhesus monkeys from birth to 26 months of age on a casein hydrolysate formula (Nutramigen®) which contains a trace of taurine ($1\,\mu mol\,L^{-1}$). A 2nd group of 5 monkeys were fed the same formula supplemented with $70\,\mu mol\,L^{-1}$ taurine. At 10 months of age the taurine deficient animals demonstrated 25–50% reductions in cone dominated electroretinogram (ERG) amplitudes in comparison to taurine supplemented animals. ERG changes were not present at 18 months. Electron microscopic examination of tissues from the eyes of taurine deficient animals at 26 months showed degeneration of the retinal cone photoreceptor cells.

Mean plasma taurine concentration was recently reported for 21 children who had been on TPN for 2–59 months ($\bar{x}$ 24 months) and was found to be less than half that of normal controls (Geggel *et al.*, 1985). ERGs were recorded for 8 children older than 1 year who had been on TPN more than 6 months. ERGs were abnormal in all of the 8 children examined. When taurine was added to the TPN solution, ERGs returned to normal within 12–14 weeks.

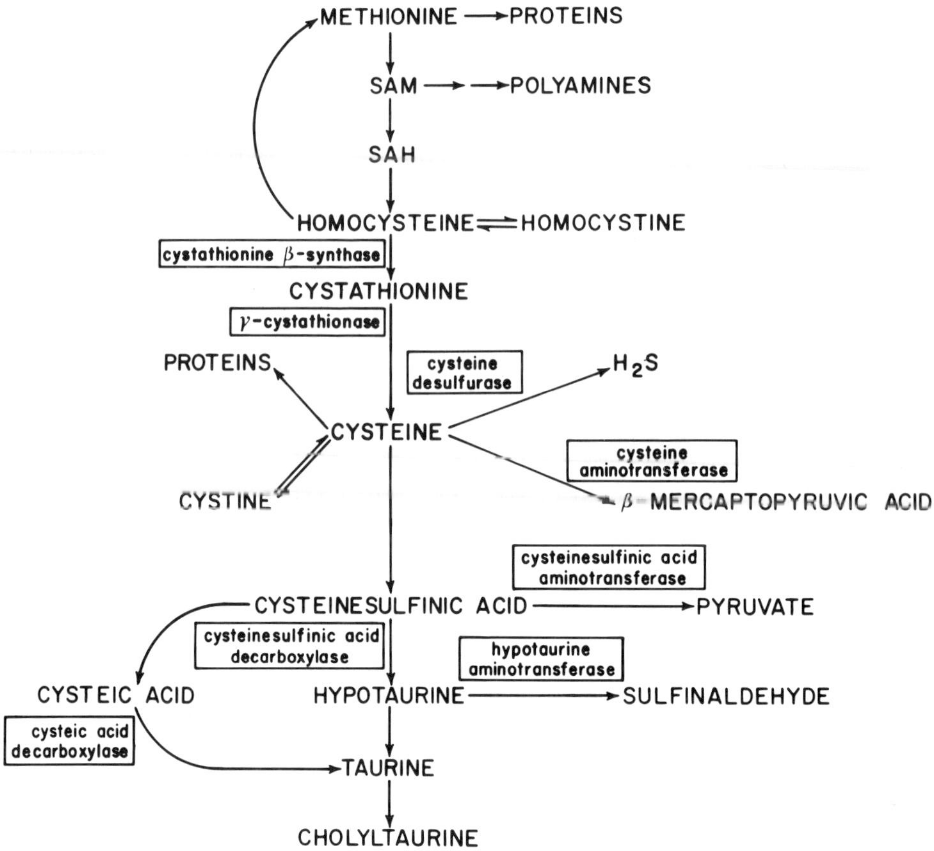

Figure 5 Taurine biosynthesis *By courtesy of* J. A. Sturman

Taurine is synthesized in mammalian cells from methionine (Figure 5) (Hayes, 1981). Gaull and coworkers (1977) reported very low activity of fetal and adult human hepatic cysteine sulphinic acid decarboxylase in comparison to activity in some other species. On the basis of these findings, Gaull and colleagues suggested that taurine may be essential at all ages.

Taurine has limited distribution in plants (Jacobsen and Smith, 1968). Consequently elemental products free of taurine and supplemented only with cereals, fruits and vegetables contain no taurine.

Taurine, as other amino acids, is actively transported to the fetus and maternal plasma concentrations decrease as pregnancy progresses (Table 7) (Hytten and Cheyne, 1972). Plasma taurine concentrations of treated pregnant women with PKU were approximately half the values of normal pregnant women (Koch, unpublished data). Whether taurine supplementation is required and of benefit to mother and fetus is unknown.

SUMMARY

Provision of nutritionally complete elemental diets for pregnant women with PKU requires greater knowledge of 'conditionally' essential nutrient requirements than

Table 7 Plasma taurine concentrations (μmol L^{-1}) of normal, pregnant women and pregnant women with PKU

Subjects	*Trimester*		
	1	*2*	*3*
Pregnant, normal[a]	80±34	75±26	62±15
Pregnant, PKU[b]	43± 6	47±18	36± 9

[a] Hytten and Cheyne, 1972
[b] Koch, R. Unpublished data (34 measures obtained on 3 women during 5 pregnancies).

is presently available as well as application of known information. Formulation of elemental products needs to be improved to enhance aroma and taste and to decrease osmolality. Designers of the metal and vitamin components should keep in mind that a major portion (70–80%) of most of these nutrients must be obtained from the elemental products. Thus, deletion of suspected essential minerals or vitamins could cause serious deficiencies. On the other hand, knowledge of appropriate ratios that make for improved trace metal absorption should be applied. Clinical nutritionists need to assist patients in selection of foods that are low in binding substances and provide 'conditionally' essential nutrients in adequate amounts. Closer cooperation between clinical nutritionists, nutrition scientists and food technologists should provide for improved elemental products for care of pregnant women with PKU.

REFERENCES

Abrams, C. A. L., Phillips, L. L., Berkowitz, C., Blackett, P. R. and Priebe, C. J. Hazards of overconcentrated milk formula. *J. Am. Med. Assoc.* 232 (1975) 1136–1140

Acosta, P. B., Alfin-Slater, R. B. and Koch, R. Serum lipids in children with phenylketonuria (PKU). *J. Am. Diet. Assoc.* 63 (1973) 631–635

Acosta, P. B., Fernhoff, P. M., Warshaw, H. S., Elsas, L. J., Hambidge, K. M. and McCabe, E. R. B. Zinc status and growth of children undergoing treatment for phenylketonuria. *J. Inher. Metab. Dis.* 5 (1982) 107–110

Acosta, P. B., Fernhoff, P. M., Warshaw, H. S., Hambidge, K. M., Ernest, A., McCabe, E. R. B. and Elsas, L. J. Zinc and copper status of treated children with phenylketonuria. *J. Parent. Ent. Nutr.* 5 (1981) 406–409

Acosta, P. B., Wenz, E. and Williamson, M. Nutrient intake of treated infants with phenylketonuria. *Am. J. Clin. Nutr.* 30 (1977) 198–208

Adham, N. F. and Song, M. K. Effect of calcium and copper on zinc absorption in the rat. *Nutr. Metab.* 24 (1980) 281–290

Ahmad, M. N. and Leeds, A. R. Oral sunflower seed oil and human erythrocyte fatty acid composition: a dose exposure–response study. *J. Plant Foods* 5 (1983) 221–223

Anderson, R. E., Benolken, R. M., Dudley, P. A., Landis, D. J. and Wheeler, T. G. Polyunsaturated fatty acids of photoreceptor membranes. *Exp. Eye Res.* 18 (1974) 205–213

Bargen-Lockner, C., Hahn, P. and Wittman, B. Plasma carnitine in pregnancy. *Am. J. Obstet. Gynecol.* 140 (1981) 412–414

Baylis, J., Leeds, A. R. and Challacombe, D. Persistent nausea and food aversions in pregnancy. *Clin. Aller.* 13 (1983) 263–269

Bickel, H. The effects of a phenylalanine-free and phenylalanine-poor diet in phenylpyruvic oligophrenia. *Exp. Med. Surg.* 12 (1954) 114–118

Borum, P. R. Carnitine. *Ann. Rev. Nutr.* 3 (1983) 233–259

Borum, P. R., York, C. M. and Broquist, H. P. Carnitine content of liquid formulas and special diets. *Am. J. Clin. Nutr.* 32 (1979) 2272–2276

Bowden, J. A. and McArthur, C. L. Possible biochemical model for phenylketonuria. *Nature* 235 (1972) 230

Carr, B. R. and Simpson, E. R. Cholesterol synthesis in human fetal tissue. *J. Clin. Endocrinol. Metab.* 55 (1982) 447–452

Casey, C. E., Walravens, P. A. and Hambidge, K. M. Availability of zinc: loading tests with human milk, cows' milk and infant formulas. *Pediatrics* 68 (1981) 394–396

Cashel, K. M., Thomas, M. P. and Pepperjohn, J. Hyperosmolar infant formulae: potential problems in clinical use. *J. Hum. Nutr.* 32 (1978) 264–269

Chipponi, J. X., Bleier, J. C., Santi, M. T. and Rudman, D. Deficiencies of essential and conditionally essential nutrients. *Am. J. Clin. Nutr.* 35 (1982) 1112–1116

Christensen, J. M., Ghannam, M. and Ayres, J. W. Effects of divalent amino acids on iron absorption. *J. Pharm. Sciences* 73 (1984) 1245–1248

Clandinin, M. T., Chappell, J. E., Heim, T., Swyer, P. R. and Chance, G. W. Fatty acid utilization in perinatal *de novo* synthesis of tissues. *Early Hum. Dev.* 5 (1981) 355–366

Committee on Dietary Allowances. *Food and Nutrition Board, Recommended Dietary Allowances*, 9th revised edn., National Academy of Sciences, 1980, pp. 31–38

Coodin, F. J., Gabrielson, I. W. and Addiego, J. E. Formula fatality. *Pediatrics* 47 (1971) 438–439

Crawford, M. A., Hassam, A. G. and Stevens, P. A. Essential fatty acid requirements in pregnancy and lactation with special reference to brain development. *Prog. Lipid Res.* 20 (1981) 31–40

Crawford, M. A., Hassam, A. G. and Williams, G. Essential fatty acids and fetal brain growth. *Lancet* 1 (1976) 452–453

Crome, L., Tymms, V. and Woolf, L. I. A chemical investigation of the defects of myelination in phenylketonuria. *J. Neurol. Neurosurg. Psychiat.* 25 (1962) 143–148

Dobson, J. C., Williamson, M. L., Azen, C. and Koch, R. Intellectual assessment of 111 four-year-old children with phenylketonuria. *Pediatrics* 60 (1977) 822–827

van Dokkum, W., Cloughley, F. A., Hulshof, K. F. A. M. and Oosterveen, L. A. M. Effect of variations in fat and linoleic acid intake on the calcium, magnesium and iron balance of young men. *Ann. Nutr. Metab.* 27 (1983) 361–369

Endres, W., Schaller, R. and Shin, Y. S. Diagnosis and treatment of argininaemia. Characteristics of arginase in human erythrocytes and tissues. *J. Inher. Metab. Dis.* 7 (1984) 8

Evans, G. W. and Johnson, P. E. Characterization and quantitation of a zinc binding ligand in human milk. *Pediatr. Res.* 14 (1980) 876–880

Festa, M. D., Anderson, H. L., Dowdy, R. P. and Ellersieck, M. R. Effect of zinc intake on copper excretion and retention in men. *Am. J. Clin. Nutr.* 41 (1985) 285–292

Fischer, P. W. F., Giroux, A. and Abbe, M. R. L. Effect of zinc supplementation on copper status in adult man. *Am. J. Clin. Nutr.* 40 (1984) 743–746

Forbes, R. M., Erdman, J. W., Parker, H. M., Kondo, H. and Ketelson, S. M. Bioavailability of zinc in coagulated soy protein (tofu) to rats and effect of dietary calcium at a constant phytate: zinc ratio. *J. Nutr.* 113 (1983) 205–210

Gaull, G. E., Rassin, D. K., Räihä, N. C. R. and Heinonen, K. Milk protein quantity and quality in low-birth-weight infants III. Effects on sulfur amino acids in plasma and urine. *J. Pediatr.* 90 (1977) 348–355

Geggel, H. S., Ament, M. A., Heckenlively, J. R., Martin, D. A. and Kopple, J. D.

Nutritional requirement for taurine in patients receiving long-term parenteral nutrition. *N. Engl. J. Med.* 312 (1985) 142–146

Gerstl, B., Malamud, N., Eng, L. F. and Hayman, R. B. Lipid alterations in human brains in phenylketonuria. *Neurol.* 17 (1967) 51–58

Giroux, E. L. and Henkin, R. I. Competition for zinc among serum albumin and amino acids. *Biochim. Biophys. Acta* 273 (1972) 64–72

Greger, J. L. and Snedeker, S. M. Effect of dietary protein and phosphorus levels on the utilization of zinc, copper and manganese by adult males. *J. Nutr.* 110 (1980) 2243–2253

Hahn, P., Skala, J. P., Seccombe, D. W., Frolich, J., Penn-Walker, D., Novak, M., Hynie, I. and Towell, M. E. Carnitine content of blood and amniotic fluid. *Pediatr. Res.* 11 (1977) 878–880

Hanley, W. B., Linsoa, L., Davidson, W. and Moes, C. A. F. Mulnutrition with early treatment of phenylketonuria. *Pediatr. Res.* 4 (1970) 318–327

Harzer, G. and Kauer, H. Binding of zinc to casein. *Am. J. Clin. Nutr.* 35 (1982) 981–987

Hay, A. W. M., Hassam, A. G., Crawford, M. A., Stevens, P. A., Mawer, E. B. and Jones, F. S. Essential fatty acid restriction inhibits vitamin D-dependent calcium absorption. *Lipids* 15 (1980) 251–254

Hayes, K. C. Taurine in metabolism. *Ann. Rev. Nutr.* 1 (1981) 401–425

Hayes, K. C. Taurine requirement in primates. *Nutr. Rev.* 43 (1985) 65–70

Hayes, K. C., Carey, R. E. and Schmidt, S. Y. Retinal degeneration associated with taurine deficiency in the cat. *Science* 188 (1975) 949–951

Henkin, R. I., Keiser, H. R. and Bronzert, D. *J. Clin. Invest.* 51 (1972) 44

Hill, G. M., Ku, P. K., Miller, E. R., Ullrey, D. E., Losty, T. A. and O'Dell, B. L. A copper deficiency in neonatal pigs induced by a high zinc maternal diet. *J. Nutr.* 113 (1983) 867–872

Hill, C. H. and Matrone, G. Chemical parameters in the study of *in vivo* and *in vitro* interactions of transition elements. *Fed. Proc.* 29 (1970) 1474–1481

Holm, V. A., Kronmal, R. A., Williamson, M. and Roche, A. F. Physical growth in phenylketonuria: II. Growth of treated children in the PKU collaborative study from birth to four years of age. *Pediatrics* 63 (1979) 700–707

Holman, R. T., Johnson, S. B. and Hatch, T. F. A case of human linolenic acid deficiency involving neurological abnormalities. *Am. J. Clin. Nutr.* 35 (1982) 617–623

Hurley, L. S. Trace metals in mammalian development. *Johns Hopkins Med. J.* 148 (1981) 1–10

Hurry, V. J. and Gibson, R. S. The zinc, copper and manganese status of children with malabsorption syndromes and inborn errors of metabolism. *Biol. Trace Elem. Res.* 4 (1982) 157–173

Huxtable, R. J. and Pasantes-Morales, P. *Taurine in Nutrition and Neurology,* Plenum, New York, 1982

Hytten, F. E. Placental transfer. In Hytten, F. E. and Chamberlain, G. (eds.) *Clinical Physiology in Obstetrics,* Blackwell Scientific, Oxford, 1980, pp. 470–490

Hytten, F. E. and Cheyne, G. A. The aminoaciduria of pregnancy. *J. Obstet. Gynaecol. Br. Commonw.* 79 (1972) 424–432

Innis, S. M. and Clandinin, M. T. Dynamic modulation of mitochondrial inner-membrane lipids in rat heart by dietary fat. *Biochem. J.* 193 (1981) 155–167

Jacobsen, J. G. and Smith, L. H. Biochemistry and physiology of taurine and taurine derivatives. *Physiol. Rev.* 48 (1968) 424–511

Kelsay, J. L., Jacobs, R. and Prather, E. S. Effect of fibre from fruits and vegetables on metabolic responses of human subjects. III. zinc, copper and phosphorus balances. *Am. J. Clin. Nutr.* 32 (1979) 2307–2311

Kelsay, J. L. and Prather, E. S. Effect of fiber and oxalic acid on mineral balance of adult human subjects. *Fed. Proc.* 40 (1981) 854

Lei, K. Y., Davis, M. W., Fang, M. M. and Young, L. C. Effect of pectin on zinc, copper and iron balances in humans. *Nutr. Repts. Int.* 22 (1980) 459–466

Lemons, J. A. Fetal–placental nitrogen metabolism. *Sem. Perinat.* 3 (1979) 177–190
Lenke, R. R. and Levy, H. L. Maternal phenylketonuria and hyperphenylalaninemia: an international survey of the outcome of untreated and treated pregnancies. *N. Engl. J. Med.* 303 (1980) 560–570
Lin, D. S., Pitkin, R. M. and Connor, W. E. Placental transfer of cholesterol into the human fetus. *Am. J. Obstet. Gynecol.* 128 (1977) 735–739
Lombeck, I., Kasperek, K., Feinendegen, L. E. and Bremer, H. J. Trace element disturbances in dietetically treated patients with phenylketonuria and maple syrup urine disease. *Hum. Genet.* 9 (1978) 114–117
Lönnerdal, B., Stanislowski, A. G. and Hurley, L. S. Isolation of a low molecular weight zinc-binding ligand from milk. *J. Inorg. Biochem.* 12 (1980) 71–78
Lukaski, H. C., Klevay, L. M., Bolonchuk, W. W., Mahalko, J. R., Milne, D. B., Johnson, L. K. and Sanstead, H. H. Influence of dietary lipids on iron, zinc and copper retention in trained athletes. *Fed. Proc.* 41 (1982) 275
Lynch, S. R. and Morck, T. A. Iron deficiency anemia. In Lindenbaum, J. (ed.) *Nutrition in Hematology,* Churchill–Livingstone, New York, 1983, pp. 143–165
Marcus, A. J. The eicosanoids in biology and medicine. *J. Lipid Res.* 25 (1984) 1511–1516
Mead, J. F. The non-eicosanoid functions of the essential fatty acids. *J. Lipid Res.* 25 (1984) 1517–1521
Menkes, J. H. Cerebral lipids in phenylketonuria. *Pediatrics* 37 (1966) 967–978
Mills, C. F. Dietary interactions involving the trace elements. *Ann. Rev. Nutr.* 5 (1985) 173–193
Mohrhauer, H. and Holman, R. T. Effect of linolenic acid upon the metabolism of linoleic acid. *J. Nutr.* 81 (1963) 67–74
Monsen, E. R. and Cook, J. D. Food iron absorption in human subjects V. Effects of the major dietary constituents of a semisynthetic meal. *Am. J. Clin. Nutr.* 32 (1979) 804–808
Neumann, P. Z. and Sass-Kortsak, A. The state of copper in human serum: evidence for an amino acid-bound fraction. *J. Clin. Invest.* 46 (1967) 646–658
Neuringer, M., Conner, W. E., Van Patten, C. and Barstad, L. Dietary omega-3 fatty acid deficiency and visual loss in infant rhesus monkeys. *J. Clin. Invest.* 73 (1984) 272–276
Oja, S. S., Ahtee, L., Kontro, P. and Paasonen, M. K. *Taurine. Biological Actions and Clinical Perspectives.* Alan R. Liss, New York, 1985
Pecoud, M. D., Donzel, P. and Schelling, J. L. Effects of foodstuffs on the absorption of zinc sulfate. *Clin. Pharm. Ther.* 17 (1975) 469–474
Pennington, J. A. T. and Nichols, H. N. *Bowes and Church's Food Values of Portions Commonly Used,* 14th edn., J. B. Lippincott, Philadelphia, 1985, pp. 232–233
Plotz, E. J., Kabara, J. J., Davis, M. E., LeRoy, G. V. and Gould, R. G. Studies on the synthesis of cholesterol in the brain of the human fetus. *Am. J. Obstet. Gynecol.* 101 (1968) 534–538
Prasad, A. S., Brewer, G. J., Schoomaker, E. B. and Rabbani, P. Hypocupremia induced by zinc therapy in adults. *J. Am. Med. Assoc.* 240 (1978) 2166–2168
Prasad, A. S. and Oberleas, D. Binding of zinc to amino acids and serum proteins *in vitro. J. Lab. Clin. Med.* 76 (1970) 416–425
Quesney-Huneeus, V., Galick, H. A., Siperstein, M. D., Erickson, S. A., Spencer, T. A. and Nelson, J. A. The dual role of mevalonate in the cell cycle. *J. Biol. Chem.* 258 (1983) 378–385
Rebouche, C. J. Comparative aspects of carnitine biosynthesis in microorganisms and mammals with attention to carnitine biosynthesis in man. In Frenkel, R. and McGarry, J. D. (eds.) *Carnitine Biosynthesis, Metabolism and Functions,* Academic Press, New York, 1980, pp. 57–72
Rebouche, C. J. Sites and regulation of carnitine biosynthesis in mammals. *Fed. Proc.* 41 (1982) 2848–2852
Reeves, J. B. and Weihrauch, J. L. *Composition of Foods. Fats and Oils: Raw, Processed, Prepared. Agriculture Handbook 8–4,* US Government Printing Office, Washington DC, 1979, pp. 15–142

Sandstrom, B., Arvidsson, B., Cederblad, A. and Bjorn-Rasmussen, E. Zinc absorption from composite meals. The significance of wheat extraction rate, zinc, calcium and protein content in meals based on bread. *Am. J. Clin. Nutr.* 33 (1980) 739–745

Schiff, D., Chan, G., Seccombe, D. and Hahn, P. Plasma carnitine levels during intravenous feeding of the neonate. *J. Pediatr.* 95 (1979) 1043–1046

Seegar, W. E. and Chesney, R. W. On certain physical–chemical properties of infant formulas. *Am. J. Dis. Child* 131 (1977) 137–138

Shah, B. G. and Belonje, B. Bioavailability of zinc with and without plant protein. *Fed. Proc.* 40 (1981) 855

Siperstein, M. D. Role of cholesterogenesis and isoprenoid synthesis in DNA replication and cell growth. *J. Lipid Res.* 25 (1984) 1462–1468

Smith, J. L. and Heymsfield, S. B. Enteral nutrition support. Formula preparation from modular ingredients. *J. Parent. Ent. Nutr.* 7 (1983) 280–288

Solomons, N. W. Biological availability of zinc in humans. *Am. J. Clin. Nutr.* 35 (1982) 1048–1075

Solomons, N. W. and Jacob, R. A. Studies on the bioavailability of zinc in man. IV. Effect of heme and nonheme iron on the absorption of zinc. *Am. J. Clin. Nutr.* 34 (1981) 475–481

Steinhardt, H. J. and Adibi, S. A. Interaction between transport of zinc and other solutes in human intestine. *Am. J. Physiol.* 247 (1984) G176–G182

Sturman, J. A., Wen, G. Y., Wisniewski, H. M. and Neuringer, M. D. Retinal degeneration in primates raised on a synthetic human infant formula. *Int. J. Devl. Neuroscience* 2 (1984) 121–129

Svennerholm, L. and Vanier, M. T. The distribution of lipids in the human nervous system. II. Lipid composition of human fetal and infant brain. *Brain Res.* 47 (1972) 457–468

Tyrala, E. E., Brodsky, N. L. and Auerbach, V. H. Urinary copper losses in infants receiving amino acid solutions. *Am. J. Clin. Nutr.* 35 (1982) 542–545

Valberg, L. S., Flanagan, P. R. and Chamberlain, M. J. Effects of iron, tin and copper on zinc absorption in humans. *Am. J. Clin. Nutr.* 40 (1984) 536–541

Weber, G., Glazer, R. I. and Ross, R. A. Regulation of human and rat brain metabolism: inhibitory action of phenylalanine and phenylpyruvate on glycolysis, protein, lipid, DNA and RNA metabolism. *Adv. Enzyme Regul.* 8 (1970) 13–36

Winick, M. Malnutrition and brain development. *J. Pediatr.* 74 (1969) 667–669

Winkel, C. A., Snyder, J. M., MacDonald, P. C. and Simpson, E. R. Regulation of cholesterol and progesterone synthesis in human placental cells in culture by serum lipoproteins. *Endocrinol.* 106 (1980) 1054–1060

Wise, A. and Gilburt, D. J. *In vitro* competition between calcium phytate and the soluble fraction of rat small intestine contents for cadmium, copper and zinc. *Toxicol. Lett.* 11 (1982) 49–54

J. Inher. Metab. Dis. 9 Suppl. 2 (1986) 203

Preface to Short Communications

This section is devoted to short communications based on oral and poster presentations at the free sessions of the Annual Meeting of the Society for the Study of Inborn Errors of Metabolism held in Liverpool, 3–6 September 1985. This year relatively few of the free communications were directly related to the main topic of the meeting, DNA analysis and inherited metabolic disease. More focussed around the clinical symposium on phenylketonuria, a disorder that continues to attract attention because of its high incidence and continuing problems in its effective management. Many other aspects of the study of inherited metabolic diseases were represented in the large display of posters which was an important feature of the meeting. Those presentations not reported elsewhere in this issue are listed below. Many of the short communications were submitted for the Noel Raine Award which commemorates the founding editor of the *Journal of Inherited Metabolic Disease*. This year the prize was awarded to R. J. A. Wanders, J. M. Tager, H. van den Bosch and R. H. B. Schutgens for their paper 'Pre- and postnatal diagnosis of the cerebro-hepato-renal (Zellweger) syndrome via a simple method directly demonstrating the presence or absence of peroxisomes in cultured fibroblasts, amniocytes or chorionic villi fibroblasts'.

With pressure on space in all scientific journals we hope that contributors and users will accept our suggestion that these papers be generated and used as short communications rather than as preliminary abstracts, at least in part. Even with the increased flexibility arising this year from the smaller page size we have been unable to accommodate all those offered and thus an element of appraisal is inherent in their selection. It is clear to the editors that some are preliminary communications which allow priority to be established. However, others are worthwhile additional records which are adequate in themselves as contributions to our accumulated experience and may not require additional recording.

R. A. Harkness
R. J. Pollitt
G. M. Addison

Journal of Inherited Metabolic Disease. ISSN 0141–8955.

Free Communications

Tetrahydrofurandicarboxylic aciduria resulting from the ingestion of castor oil. *L. Hegenfeldt and L. Blonqvist*

Detection of inherited adenylosuccinate lyase deficiency, a new inborn error of purine metabolism, by thin-layer chromatography. *S. K. Wadman, P. K. de Bree, H. Fabery de Jonge, G. van den Berghe, R. A. Holl, F. A. Beemer and M. Duran*

Mevalonic aciduria: a new inborn error of cholesterol; biosynthesis? *G. P. A. Smit, R. Berger, T. de Vries, H. Schierbeek, R. Bijsterveld, R. le Coultre and R. J. Vonk*

Studies on the degradation of dicarboxylic acids in rat liver mitochondria. *S. Kølvraa and N. Gregersen*

Screening and quantitative determination of urinary acyl carnitines in disorders of organic acid metabolism. *C. Charpentier, M. Coude, J. P. Harpey, J. L. Perignon and J. M. Saudubray*

Ethosuccimide (2-ethyl 2-methyl succinimide) administration in children: a pitfall in screening for organic acidurias. *B. Cartigny, G. Ricart, J. L. Dhondt and J. P. Farriaux*

Delayed diagnosis of methylmalonic aciduria. *H. R. Bhatt, M. J. Brueton and J. C. Linnell*

Prenatal diagnosis of a high-risk fetus of congenital lactic acidosis. *B. Merinero, F. Roman, C. Perez-Cerda, C. Hernande, B. Gutierrez, A. Jimenez, M. J. Garcia and M. Ugarte*

Prenatal diagnosis of medium chain acyl-CoA dehydrogenase deficiency. *M. J. Bennett, F. Allison, D. I. Johnston, R. G. F. Gray, G. Lowther, J. S. Fitzsimmons and R. J. Pollitt*

Transient multiple acyl-CoA dehydrogenase deficiency: an unexpected complication of total parenteral nutrition in very low birth weight infants. *B. Francois, L. Leyssens, A. Charon, A. Bachy and P. Gerard*

Heterogeneity associated with propionyl-CoA-carboxylase deficiency. *C. J. Reinecke and L. J. Mienie*

Crying baby syndrome: an autosomal or X-linked encephalo- and myopathy, with NADH–CoA reductase deficiency in muscle mitochondria. *H. R. Scholte, C. J. de Groot and I. E. M. Luyt-Houwen*

Atypical non-ketotic hyperglycinaemia. *C. Bachmann, M. Di Rocco, K. Tada, K. Hayasaka, R. Gatti and C. Borrone*

Clinical and biochemical studies on 24 cases of galactosialidosis. *Y. Suzuki, H. Sakuraba, K. Ohmura and E. Namba*

Uptake of α-mannosidase from fetal calf serum by mannosidosis fibroblasts. *C. Humphreys, A. Cooper, B. Fowler and I. B. Sardharwalla*

Purification of human iduronate 2-sulphate sulphatase from placenta, for the production of monoclonal and polyclonal antibodies. *W. Lissens, I. Decaluwe, A. Zenati and I. Liebaers*

Full expression of Hunter's disease in a female due to non-random inactivation of X-chromosome. *D. Broadhead, J. Kirk, A. Burt, V. Gupta, P. Ellis and G. Besley*

Aryl sulphatase isoenzymes of chorionic villi: implications for prenatal diagnosis. *L. Giles, A. Cooper, B. Fowler, I. B. Sardharwalla and P. Donnai*

DNA analysis in patients with hereditary fructose intolerance. *C. Besmond, C. Gregori, J. C. Dreyfus and A. Khan*

Cockayne syndrome – the boy with DNA-repair failure. *E. Pronicka and E. Wieczorek*

In vivo hormonal control of glycolytic enzyme gene transcript in the liver. *A. Munnich, H. Ogier, S. Vaulont, J. M. Saudubray and A. Khan*

Dietary and hormonal regulation of glycolytic enzyme gene expression in the small intestine. *H. Ogier, A. Munnich, S. Vaulont, J. M. Saudubray and A. Kahn*

Biotinidase deficiency: metabolites in CSF. *A. Fois, M. Cioni, P. Balestri, B. Gartalini, R. Baumgartner and C. Bachmann*

Abnormal cobalamin metabolism in familial glucocorticoid deficiency. *J. C. Linnell, H. R. Bhatt, D. B. Dunger, I. Smith and D. Grant*

In vivo studies of riboflavin deficient rats. *N. Gregersen and S. Kølvraa*

Uridine diphosphogalactose, galactose-1-phosphate and galactitol concentration in patients with classical galactosaemia. *Y. S. Shin, M. Rieth, S. Hoyer, W. Endres and C. Jakobs*

Glycerol-3-phosphate excretion in fructose-1,6-diphosphatase deficiency – a new observation. *S. Krywawych, S. Wyatt, G. Katz, A. M. Lawson and D. P. Brenton*

Fructose-1,6-diphosphatase deficiency presenting as Reye-like syndrome. *S. Mantagos, K. Frimas, B. Thanopoulos and N. Beratis*

Phosphate ester excretion in hypophosphatasia determined by ^{31}P nuclear magnetic resonance. *D. P. Brenton, P. Morris, R. Hardie, D. Griffiths, P. J. Garrod and S. Krywawych*

Diagnosis of type Ib glycogen storage disease. *R. Longhi, S. Paccanelli, C. Butte, A. Vittorelli, R. Valsasina, E. Riva and M. Giovannini*

Regional enteritis and glycogen storage disease type Ib. *T. Roe, D. Thomas, V. Gilsanz, H. Issacs and J. Atkinson*

Erythrocyte phosphorylase b kinase deficiency in families with glycogenosis type VIII. *G. Besley*

Ammonia measurements in small plasma volumes using a gas-sensing probe. *M. Haseler, S. Krywawych and D. P. Brenton*

Experience with interlaboratory surveys of screening tests for inherited metabolic diseases. *J. M. Rattenbury, J. C. Allen and E. Worthy*

Preliminary results of evaluation FT-NMR spectrometry for selective screening for metabolic disorders using native urine specimen. *W. Lehnert and D. Hunkler*

Selenium levels in milk and food prepared for metabolic disorders. *J. M. Fraga, J. A. Cocho, C. Parrado, C. Colon, J. R. Cervilla, C. Vidal and J. R. Alonso*

Prenatal diagnosis of phenylketonuria in a French family. *F. Rey, M. Berthelon, A. Munnich and J. Frezal*

Home monitoring with microcomputer in order to assist patients with phenylketonuria to adjust their daily phenylalanine intake. *R. Thijssen, J. Goven and B. Francois*

Plasma chromium and manganese levels in treated phenylketonuric patients. *A. Rottoli, E. Riva, G. Lista, L. Borgatti, M. T. Ortisi, R. Longhi and M. Giovannini*

Low levels of plasma immunoglobulins in hyperphenylalaninaemic children on a low phenylalanine diet. *E. Riva, C. Agostoni, R. Longhi, A. Rottoli, R. Valsasina and M. Giovannini*

Visual evoked potentials in phenylketonuria. *R. Longhi, R. Valsasina, A. Ducati, A. Landi, S. Paccanelli, C. Butte and M. Giovannini*

Effects of phenylalanine loading on protein synthesis in the fetal heart and brain of rat. *Y. Okano, I. Zen Chow, G. Issiki and T. Oura*

Increased vigilance and neurotransmitter biosynthesis in phenylketonuria induced by phenylalanine restriction or by supplementation of free diet with large amounts of tryosine and/or tryptophan. *C. Lykkelund, H. C. Lou, V. Rasmussen, A. M. Geredes, D. Bucher, E. Christensen and P. Bruhn*

A child with cystic fibrosis presenting with hepatomegaly and masquerading as a possible case of a glycogen storage disease. *R. G. F. Gray, M. A. Edwards, P. D. Griffiths, D. R. Carlton, J. Insley, M. Tarlow, T. Whitfield and A. Green*

Dihydropteridine reductase deficiency in a child with only mild hyperphenylalaninaemia. *A. Sahota, R. J. Leeming, J. A. Blair, A. Green and J. Hyanek*

The clinical specificity of succinylacetone excretion in the diagnosis of hereditary tyrosinaemia type I. *B. Pettit, L. Williams, J. V. Leonard and P. Clayton*

L-*allo*-Isoleucine: an inert marker of isoleucine metabolism in maple syrup urine disease. *U. Langenbeck, U. Wendel, H. Luthe and J. W. T. Seakins*

Protein-bound homocyst(e)ine: A possible risk factor for coronary artery disease. *S.-S. Kang and P. Wong*

Aspartylglycosaminuria in two Turkish brothers: clinical and biochemical aspects. *J. M. Boers, B. J. H. M. Poorthuis, R. J. A. Wanders and R. B. H. Schutgens*

Carnosinuria in a 4-month-old infant. *M. A. Edwards, J. C. Allen, S. H. Green and A. Green*

Combined xanthine and sulphite oxidase defect due to a deficiency of molybdenum cofactor. *R. A. Roesel, F. Bowyer, P. R. Blankenship and F. A. Hommes*

Tryptophanaemia: a study of tryptophan metabolites. *B. Fowler, A. K. Holmes, C. Whitehouse and I. B. Sardharwalla*

Joubert's syndrome associated with hyperpipecolic acidaemia in three siblings. *B. T. Poll-The, J. L. Perignon, P. Parvy, A. Lombes, J. Trybels, R. B. H. Schutgens, R. J. A. Wanders and J. M. Saudubray*

Diagnosis and family studies of several cases of urea cycle disorders. *P. Briones, A. Ribes, M. Rodes, M. A. Vilaseca and A. Maya*

Use of RFLP for carrier detection in ornithine transcarbamylase deficiency. *M. Schwartz, E. Christensen, N. Christensen, K. Davies and J. Old*

Neonatal screening for congenital adrenal hyperplasia in Scotland. *A. M. Wallace, G. H. Beastall, R. Kennedy and R. W. A. Girdwood*

Neonatal screening for congenital adrenal hyperplasia – what blood level constitutes a positive test? *I. C. T. Lyon, P. C. Dance, B. S. Knox and J. Johnson-Barrett*

Steroid sulphatase (ST-S) deficiency in patients with X-linked ichthyosis (XLI), hypogonadism and anosmia: Kallmann syndrome associated with XLI or a different mutation at the ST-S Locus? *A. Ballabio, G. Parenti, P. Tippett, D. Salvatore, E. Napolitano, A. Tenore, S. DiMaio and G. Andria*

The detection of carriers and pre-natal diagnosis of the Lesch–Nyhan syndrome using a restriction fragment length of DNA polymorphism closely linked to the HGPRT gene. *D. A. Gibbs, C. M. Headhouse-Benson, R. W. E. Watts*

J. Inher. Metab. Dis. 9 Suppl. 2 (1986) 206–208

Short Communication

Molecular Biology of Phenylalanine Hydroxylase

R. G. F. Cotton[1], H. H. M. Dahl[1], J. F. B. Mercer[1], I. Jennings[1], E. A. Haan[1], C. W. Chow[2], D. M. Danks[1] and F. J. Morgan[3]
[1]*Birth Defects Research Institute, Flemington Road, Parkville, Victoria, Australia 3052;* [2]*Department of Pathology, Royal Children's Hospital, Melbourne, Australia;* [3]*St. Vincent's Hospital, Melbourne, Australia*

Phenylalanine hydroxylase (PH; EC 1.14.16.1) is a complex enzyme with three substrates and three activators. Little is known about the structural features which are necessary for the function of this enzyme; only the phosphorylation site is known (Wretburn *et al.*, 1980). We have recently isolated rat and human cDNA clones for PH in order to obtain a deduced protein sequence for structure–function studies and to study the mutations in phenylketonuria (PKU) which would help define those areas in PH which are important for function.

METHODS

Rat phenylalanine hydroxylase was purified according to the method of Shiman and colleagues (1979). Antibody was produced in rabbits and purified by affinity chromatography on a PH reacti-gel (Pierce) column. This antibody was used to screen a rat liver cDNA library constructed in the expression vector λ gt11 (Howlett, unpublished). DNA from positive clones was sequenced to confirm their identity. The rat cDNA clones were used to screen a human cDNA library. Positive clones were characterized by restriction mapping and DNA sequence analysis.

The PH 8 monoclonal antibody was produced and used for immunohistochemical staining by standard methods.

HPLC purification of tryptic peptides was performed in two steps on an RP300 column: (a) 20 mmol l^{-1} ammonium bicarbonate pH 7.8, linear gradient, acetonitrile (8–60%); (b) 0.1% trifluoroacetic acid, linear gradient, acetonitrile (8–60%). The preparation of DNA and RNA from cells and tissues, respectively, and Northern and Southern blotting (Maniatis *et al.*, 1982) were by standard methods.

RESULTS AND DISCUSSION

A rat PH cDNA was isolated and sequenced (Dahl and Mercier, 1986). Authenticity of the clone was established by: (a) sequence agreement with partial rat clone sequence (Robson *et al.*, 1984); (b) high degree of sequence homology with human phenylalanine hydroxylase (Kwok *et al.*, 1985); (c) agreement with N-terminal

Journal of Inherited Metabolic Disease. ISSN 0141–8955.

sequence (Iwaki *et al.*, 1985; (d) agreement with phosphopeptide sequence. The rat PH amino acid sequence was compared with the human PH amino acid sequence and the homology was found to be 92%.

Because of the similarity of substrates and function of PH, tyrosine hydroxylase (TH) and tryptophan hydroxylase (TRPH), these aromatic hydroxylases are expected to be related in their sequence. A remarkable similarity is seen between the PH sequence and the TH sequence (Grima *et al.*, 1985) and this appears to be confined to the C-terminal three-quarters of the molecule.

This relationship had been earlier suggested by antibody studies. We isolated a monoclonal antibody (PH 8) to monkey liver phenylalanine hydroxylase which by immunoprecipitation was shown to react with tryptophan hydroxylase and by Elisa assay to react with tyrosine hydroxylase (Haan *et al.*, submitted). This immunoreactivity was confirmed by staining of rat and human brain sections. Thus regions of the brain containing tryptophan hydroxylase such as the raphe nucleus, and regions of the brain containing tyrosine hydroxylase such as the locus coeruleus stained with this antibody. As, in human autopsy brain, PH 8 stains the tryptophan hydroxylase-containing serotoninergic neurones, this allows for the first time the study of normal structure and pathology of these areas. The epitope recognised by PH 8 is obviously well conserved as this antibody reacts with PH of frog and fish.

The human cDNA probe was used to probe DNA and RNA from PKU patients. In 15 patients studied by Southern blots no alteration in gene structure was seen. In one patient studied by RNA blots analysis a substantial level of PH mRNA was present.

Allelic forms of rat PH protein have recently been described (Mercer *et al.*, 1984). This has explained earlier studies where two apparent molecular weight forms of this enzyme have been isolated in different laboratories. Peptide mapping studies have localized this difference to a single peptide. Two-dimensional electrophoretic analysis of monkey liver phenylalanine hydroxylase has indicated the presence of allelic forms (Smith *et al.*, 1985) but it cannot be assumed that the change is the same as that found in the rat.

REFERENCES

Dahl, H. H. M. and Mercier, J. F. B. Isolation and sequence of a cDNA clone which contains the complete coding region of rat phenylalanine hydroxylase. *J. Biol. Chem.* (1986) (in press)

Grima, B., Lamouroux, A., Blanot, F., Biguet, N. E. and Mallet, J. Complete coding sequence of rat tyrosine hydroxylase mRNA. *Proc.Natl.Acad.Sci. USA* 82 (1985) 617–621

Iwaki, M., Parniak, M. A. and Kaufman, S. Studies on the primary structure of rat liver phenylalanine hydroxylase. *Biochem.Biophys.Res.Commun.* 126 (1985) 922–932

Kwok, S. G. M., Ledley, F. D., Dilella, A. G., Robson, K. J. H. and Woo, S. L. C. Nucleotide sequence of a full length complementary DNA clone and amino acid sequence of human phenylalanine hydroxylase. *Biochemistry* 24 (1985) 556–561

Maniatis, T., Fritsch, E. F. and Sambrook, S. *Molecular cloning. A Laboratory Manual.* Cold Spring Harbor Laboratory, 1982

Mercer, J. F. B., Grimes, A., Jennings, I. and Cotton, R. G. H. Identification of two molecular mass forms of phenylalanine hydroxylase that segregate independently in rats. *Biochem. J.* 219 (1984) 891–898

Robson, K. J. H., Beattie, W., James, R. J., Cotton, R. G. H., Morgan, F. J. and Woo, S. L. C. Sequence comparison of rat liver phenylalanine bydroxylase and its cDNA clones. *Biochemistry* 23 (1984) 5671–5675

Shiman, R., Gray, D. W. and Pater, A. A simple purification of phenylalanine hydroxylase by substrate-induced hydrophilic chromatography. *J. Biol. Chem.* 254 (1979) 11300–11306

Smith, S. C., McAdam, W., Cotton, R. G. H. and Mercer, J. F. B. A novel two-dimensional gel pattern which may be due to allelic genes of phenylalanine hydroxylase in monkeys. *Biochem. J.* 231 (1985) 197–199

Wretburn, M., Humble, E., Ragnarsson, U. and Engstrom, L. Amino acid sequence of rat liver phenylalanine hydroxylase and phosphorylation of a corresponding synthetic peptide. *Biochem. Biophys. Res. Commun.* 93 (1980) 403–408

J. Inher. Metab. Dis. 9 Suppl. 2 (1986) 209–211

Short Communication

Hepatic Phenylalanine Hydroxylase and Dietary Tolerance in Hyperphenylalaninaemic Patients

C. Largilliere, J. L. Dhondt and J. P. Farriaux
Service de Génétique et Maladies Héréditaires du Métabolisme de l'Enfant, C.H.U., 59037 Lille Cédex, France

Since the development of neonatal screening for hyperphenylalaninaemic syndromes and of dietary management, heterogeneity of the disease has become evident. In most inborn errors of metabolism a direct enzyme assay is considered necessary to confirm the diagnosis. However, in hyperphenylalaninaemic syndromes this practice is not usual. Some authors have claimed that the measurement of liver phenylalanine hydroxylase activity (PAH) (EC 1.14.16.1) is necessary not only for a firm diagnosis of phenylketonuria (PKU) but also to provide information about the degree of dietary control which would be required for an optimum intellectual development (Berry *et al.*, 1982). On the other hand, other authors did not find an advantage in this practice (Danks and Cotton, 1983).

In the last ten years it has been observed that tetrahydrobiopterin deficiencies may also be responsible for hyperphenylalaninaemia. Consequently, we decided in 1979 to include PAH activity determination in the diagnostic procedure for hyperphenylalaninaemic syndromes.

The aim of this work was to determine (1) the correlation between the residual PAH activity and other parameters related to the *in vivo* metabolism of phenylalanine, and (2) the predictive value of such activity in regard to phenylalanine tolerance and the difficulty of dietary control.

PATIENTS AND METHODS

The study concerned 49 hyperphenylalaninaemic patients. Most of them ($n = 42$) were diagnosed by neonatal screening and the period of follow-up considered here was 4 years. Blood phenylalanine levels were determined using an automated fluorimetric method. Phenylalanine loading tests were usually performed at 6 months of age. Two protocols were carried out:

(1) a single oral load (18 patients) with 100 mg Phe kg^{-1} and blood phenylalanine level determination at 0, 1, 2, 4, 8 and 24 hours after load

(2) a 3-day challenge (27 patients) with 180 mg Phe $kg^{-1} d^{-1}$ and daily blood phenylalanine level determination.

Phenylalanine hydroxylase activity determinations were performed on liver needle biopsies according to Bartholome and colleagues (1975).

Journal of Inherited Metabolic Disease. ISSN 0141–8955.

RESULTS AND DISCUSSION

The 49 subjects were divided into two groups according to the presence or absence of residual PAH activity:

(1) PAH^-: 33 subjects with no detectable hepatic PAH activity. All of them needed a phenylalanine restricted diet.

(2) PAH^+: 16 subjects with a significant residual PAH activity (range: 1–37% of control value).

Table 1 Neonatal blood phenylalanine levels, dietary tolerance and individual course of blood phenylalanine levels (mean value and variance) according to the PAH residual activity

		PAH⁺			*PAH⁻*		
	n	*m±SD*	*Range*	*n*	*m±SD*	*Range*	
PAH residual activity	16		1–37%	33		0	
Neonatal Phe (mg/dL)							
5 days	15	9.5±6.3	3.5–25	27	19.6±10.6	5–56	$p \leqslant 0.001$
3 weeks	8	26.9±11.7	11–42	23	41.6±14	22–73	$p \leqslant 0.02$
Phenylalanine tolerance (mg/d)							
3 months	9	308±73	250–504	25	283±33	219–368	NS
6 months	9	354±112	256–520	26	288±39	213–380	NS
1 year	10	356±110	240–535	26	305±49	230–428	NS
18 months	9	384±110	248–597	24	325±56	234–465	NS
2 years	7	409±110	252–597	23	342±80	234–585	NS
3 years	7	433±132	265–597	17	367±91	228–560	NS
4 years	3		290–383	15	378±100	210–570	
Blood phenylalanine evolution							
0–6 months *mean* (mg/dL)	10	5.4±1.8	1.9–8.7	26	7.4±3.2	2.2–15.6	NS
variance (mg/dL)	10	16.7±29.5	1.4–9.9	26	22.6±16.9	2.8–85.8	NS
6–12 months *m*	9	6.5±2.9	2.1–9.8	24	6.4±3.0	1.5–13.3	NS
v	9	9.2±6.2	1.6–20.1	24	14.0±10.7	1.6–38	NS
1–2 years *m*	8	3.4±1.1	1.6–5.4	24	6.1±3.1	1.8–13.4	$p \leqslant 0.02$
v	8	4.7±3.9	1.1–10.8	24	10.3±8.5	1–35.9	NS
2–3 years *m*	7	3±1.1	1.6–4.7	18	6.5±3.1	2.7–13.8	$p \leqslant 0.01$
v	7	3.1±2.6	1.1–9	18	13.0±12.0	2.1–51	$p \leqslant 0.01$
3–4 years *m*	7	2.9±1.6	1.2–5.9	15	6.2±3.1	2.6–14	$p \leqslant 0.01$
v	7	2.9±2	0.6–5.8	15	8.1±5.4	2.1–20.9	$p \leqslant 0.02$

NS=not significant

In the latter group, only 2 patients did not require a phenylalanine restricted diet and in these PAH activities were 34 and 37% of normal values. One patient with 14% residual activity was put on a restricted diet at 1 year of age.

For the purpose of determining the correlation between PAH activity and parameters related to the metabolism of phenylalanine, the following criteria have been considered:

(1) blood phenylalanine level at the time of screening (5 days old), and at 3 weeks old after 3 days on a normal protein diet ($3\,g\,kg^{-1}d^{-1}$) (Table 1)

(2) maximum blood phenylalanine level, level at 24 hours, and area under the curve during the single oral phenylalanine load
(3) maximum blood phenylalanine level observed during the 3-day oral challenge
(4) dietary tolerance: daily phenylalanine intake which ensured a blood phenylalanine level between 5 and 8 mg/dL (Table 1).

Statistical comparison (Student or Mann–Whitney test) of the biochemical parameters of the two groups of patients revealed that only blood phenylalanine levels during the neonatal period allowed a relative prediction of the level of enzymatic deficiency (Table 1). However, even here an important overlap existed. Data from a single phenylalanine load or the 3-day challenge did not permit such a distinction (results not shown). Likewise, the dietary phenylalanine tolerance is not statistically different between the two groups (Table 1). Thus, the level of PAH activity did not permit a prediction of individual tolerance. For example, one patient with a residual PAH activity of 10% had a low phenylalanine tolerance (250 mg Phe d^{-1}). On the other hand another patient with a complete deficit had a good tolerance (350 then 590 mg Phe d^{-1}).

On analysing the individual courses of blood phenylalanine levels, it appears that the mean values were significantly lower in the group of patients with a residual PAH activity after 1 year of age. To investigate the dispersion of blood phenylalanine levels in individuals, the variance was considered. Lower values were observed in the PAH^+ group after 2 years old (Table 1). Thus it seems that these patients (PAH^+) are able to tolerate more easily the occasional dietary errors which cannot be avoided in such young patients.

In conclusion, besides the confirmation of enzyme defect, PAH activity determination may be of interest in a relative prediction of blood phenylalanine level evolution. Further investigations will be necessary to determine the relation between this evolution and the effectiveness of dietetic therapy in allowing normal intellectual development.

REFERENCES

Bartholome, K., Lutz, P. and Bickel, H. Determination of the phenylalanine hydroxylase activity in patients with phenylketonuria and hyperphenylalaninemia. *Pediatr. Res.* 9 (1975) 899–903

Berry, H. K., Hsieh, M. H., Bofinger, M. K. and Schubert, W. K. Diagnosis of phenylalanine hydroxylase deficiency (Phenylketonuria) *Am. J. Dis. Child.* 136 (1982) 111–114

Danks, D. M. and Cotton, R. G. H. Phenylalanine hydroxylase activity. *Am. J. Dis. Child.* 137 (1983) 409

J. Inher. Metab. Dis. 9 Suppl. 2 (1986) 212–214

Short Communication

Phenylalanine Metabolites in Treated Phenylketonuric Children

K. MICHALS,[1] M. LOPUS,[1] P. GASHKOFF[2] and R. MATALON[2]
Departments of Nutrition and Medical Dietetics[1] and Pediatrics[2], University of Illinois at Chicago, USA

Phenylketonuria (PKU, McKusick 26160) is an inborn error of metabolism caused by deficient activity of the enzyme phenylalanine hydroxylase. As a result of this enzyme deficiency, phenylalanine levels rise in the blood and other body fluids. The organic acid derivatives of phenylalanine – phenylacetate, phenyllactate, and phenylpyruvate – also increase due to the enzymatic block in the normal pathway of phenylalanine metabolism. The levels of phenylethylamine (PEA), which is an endogenous amine, increase because of this enzyme deficiency. In the treatment of PKU, blood phenylalanine is used as the only parameter to monitor compliance. The therapeutic range of blood phenylalanine has varied from 2 to 15 mg/dl, with some clinics allowing up to 20 mg/dl, although early phases of the national collaborative study for PKU in the United States recommended therapeutic levels of 2–10 mg/dl (Dobson *et al.*, 1977). More recently, reports of behavioural disorders (Michals *et al.*, 1985 and Waisbren *et al.*, 1980) and learning disabilities (Brunner *et al.*, 1983) have surfaced, requiring more careful evaluation of these standards of treatment. Therefore, this study was undertaken to examine whether the metabolites of phenylalanine can be used to further adjust the PKU diet and prevent these difficulties.

METHODS

Phenylalanine metabolites were assayed in freshly collected random urine samples. The organic acid derivatives of phenylalanine, including phenylacetic, phenyllactic, and phenylpyruvic, were solvent-extracted with ethyl acetate and diethyl ether, trimethylsilylated, and detected using a Perkin-Elmer gas chromatographic system (Goodman and Markey, 1981). Sample size included 71 urine specimens from 54 children diagnosed with PKU or hyperphenylalaninaemia under dietary treatment.

The PEA was determined by a modified method of the assay described by Brossat *et al.*, (1983) which utilizes a Waters high-performance liquid chromatography system. The method involves purification of the sample with a silica-gel Sep-Pak cartridge, pre-column derivatization and conversion to a dansylated intermediate. PEA is separated using a linear gradient of tetramethylammonium hydrochloride and is identified by fluorescence detection. Sample size was smaller, with urine specimens from six patients and three controls (non-PKU subjects).

Journal of Inherited Metabolic Disease. ISSN 0141–8955.

RESULTS

The excreted organic acid derivatives of phenylalanine were measured in 71 urine samples obtained from 54 children diagnosed with PKU or hyperphenylalaninaemia. These patients were divided into four groups based on their blood phenylalanine levels at the time of sample collection. The first group included those patients whose blood phenylalanine levels ranged from 1.1 to 5.0 mg/dl (mean = 2.98 mg/dl). Eleven of these 12 patients excreted one or more of the phenolic acids in the 15 urine samples assayed. The mean excretion of phenylacetate was 25.5, phenyllactate was 105.6, and phenylpyruvic was 96.4 mg/g creatinine (Table 1).

Table 1 Organic acids of phenylalanine in phenylketonuric children under dietary control

Blood phenylalanine range (mg/dl)	*Number of samples (patients)*	*Mean blood phenylalanine* (mg/dl) *(SD)*	*Urine metabolites* (mean, mg/g creat.) (SD)		
			Phenylacetic	*Phenyllactic*	*Phenylpyruvic*
1.1–5.0	15	2.98	25.5	105.6	96.4
	(12)	(1.2)	(55.7)	(145.9)	(86.7)
5.1–10.0	25	7.13	72.0	244.5	108.1
	(15)	(1.4)	(121.0)	(290.5)	(114.3)
10.1–15.0	11	12.04	93.0	471.2	144.2
	(9)	(1.0)	(117.0)	(571.4)	(210.5)
>15.1	20	20.87	104.6	1423.1	420.4
	(18)	(3.4)	(177.2)	(2197.0)	(842.5)

Group 2 included 15 subjects (25 samples) whose blood phenylalanine levels ranged from 5.1 to 10.0 mg/dl. One or more organic acids of phenylalanine were detected in each sample with mean excretion of phenylacetic equal to 72.0, phenyllactic – 244.5, phenylpyruvic – 108.1 mg/g creatinine.

Group 3 consisted of nine subjects (11 samples) with blood phenylalanine levels ranging from 10.1 to 15.0 (mean blood phenylalanine = 12.04 mg/dl. Mean excretion of phenylacetic was 93.0, phenyllactic was 471.2, and phenylpyruvic was 144.2 mg/g creatinine.

The final group was composed of 18 subjects (20 samples) whose blood phenylalanine levels ranged from 15.1 to 26.7 (mean blood phenylalanine = 20.87 mg/dl). Mean excretion of phenylacetic was 104.5, phenyllactic was 1423.1, and phenylpyruvic was 420.2 mg/g creatinine.

The PEA excretion was measured in urine samples from six patients and three normal individuals. The phenylalanine concentrations ranged from 2.9 to 18.3 mg/dl in the PKU patients. Excretion of PEA ranged from 2.55 to 53.81 ng/mg creatinine. The normal controls had blood phenylalanine levels ranging from 0.8 to 1.0 and excretion of PEA ranged from 0.6 to 0.13 ng/g creatinine.

DISCUSSION

The results presented indicate that organic acids of phenylalanine and PEA are elevated in patients with PKU and that these levels rise as the levels of blood phenylalanine increase. Since the organic acids of phenylalanine are not detected in normal individuals, it is striking to find that even at 'good' compliance levels of 5 mg/dl phenylalanine these compounds are excreted in excess. Because these metabolites are neurotoxic, these levels shold be minimized, especially in young children and pregnant PKU mothers. Whether these metabolites are responsible for behaviour and learning problems with PKU children remains to be seen.

The excretions of PEA in the six patients show similar trends to the organic acids of phenylalanine. Since this metabolite is an analogue of amphetamine it is tempting to relate hyperactivity to its increased level.

We suggest that the metabolites of phenylalanine should be monitored as part of the routine care for PKU children. Their levels should be lowered, irrespective of currently accepted ideas of 'safe' blood phenylalanine levels. Additional studies to monitor these metabolites need to be conducted in order to more fully examine the individual variation that occurs so that the optimal method of treatment for PKU is achieved.

ACKNOWLEDGEMENT

We acknowledge support by Grant No. 296 from the Campus Research Board, University of IL at Chicago.

REFERENCES

Brossat, B., Straczek, J., Belleville, F. and Nabet, P. Determination of free and total polyamines in human serum and urine by ion-pairing high performance liquid chromatography using a radial compression model. *J. Chomatogr.* 277 (1983) 87–89

Brunner, R., Jordan, M. and Berry, H. Early-treated phenylketonuria: neuropsychological consequences. *J. Pediatr.* 102 (1983) 821–835

Dobson, J., Williamson, M., Azen, C. and Koch, M. Intellectual assessment of 111 four year old children with phenylketonuria. *Pediatrics* 60 (1977) 822–827

Goodman, S. and Markey, S. *Diagnosis of Organic Acidemias by Gas Chromatography-Mass Spectrometry*. Alan R. Liss, New York, 1981, pp. 1–43

Michals, K., Dominik, M., Schuett, V., Brown, E. and Matalon, R. Return to diet therapy in patients with phenylketonuria. *J. Pediatr.* 106 (1985) 933–936

Waisbren, S., Schnell, R. and Levy, H. Diet termination in children with phenylketonuria: a review of psychological assessments used to determine outcome. *J. Inher. Metab. Dis.* 3 (1980) 149–153

J. Inher. Metab. Dis. 9 Suppl. 2 (1986) 215–217

Short Communication

Magnesium-Deficient Rickets in a Phenylketonuric Patient on Dietary Treatment

A. Rottoli, E. Riva, G. Zecchini, F. Magno, A. Fiocchi, R. Longhi and M. Giovannini
Clinica Pediatrica V dell' Università di Milano, Istituto di Scienze Biomediche, Ospedale San Paolo, Via A. di Rudinì 8, 20142 Milan, Italy

Absolute or relative vitamin D deficiency is the most frequent cause of rickets in children. Many reviews have shown that rickets may appear in association with environmental conditions, wrong dietary habits, gastrointestinal diseases and drug administration. Magnesium deficiency is also an uncommon cause of rickets. We report the case of a phenylketonuric (PKU) child with vitamin D-resistant rickets and magnesium deficiency.

CASE REPORT

Patient D.A., birth weight 3.750 kg, was diagnosed as having classical phenylketonuria by neonatal mass screening and began a low phenylalanine diet (Minafen and human milk) at 1 month. The dietary compliance was good and he showed normal psychomotory and physical development. At 11 months, stigmata of rickets (sabre-shaped bending of the tibiae and Harrison's groove) were noticed. An X-ray examination confirmed the diagnosis. Plasma calcium, phosphorus and alkaline phosphatase were within normal limits. Vitamin D_2 was given orally at a dosage of 2500 U d^{-1}. Three months later, in spite of the treatment, an aggravation of the bone lesions was noticed.

A magnesium deficiency syndrome (plasma Mg levels repeatedly $<1\,mg\,dl^{-1}$) was diagnosed and an oral 4% magnesium chloride–6% magnesium citrate solution ($3.2\,mEq\,kg^{-1}\,d^{-1}$ of Mg^{++}) was prescribed. Six months later the biochemical parameters were all normal and 1 year later a considerable improvement in all X-ray findings was noticed.

The biochemical data for our patient are summarized in Table 1. Ionized plasma calcium values have been calculated with Zeisler's simplified formula for total calcium correction (Zeisler, 1954). The ratio: maximum rate of renal tubular reabsorption of phosphate over glomerular filtrate rate ($TmPO_4$/GFR) has been calculated from the values of tubular reabsorption of phosphate (TRP) and of plasma phosphorus, utilizing Bijvoet's nomogram (Bijvoet and Walton, 1975). Plasma iPTH has been determined by a radioimmunological method (CEA-Sorin-Biomedica Kit).

Journal of Inherited Metabolic Disease. ISSN 0141–8955.

Table 1 Biochemical data of the phenylketonuric patient with rickets

Plasma creatinine ($mg\,dl^{-1}$)	0.48
Total plasma calcium ($mg\,dl^{-1}$)	9.2
Ionized plasma calcium ($mg\,dl^{-1}$)	4.39
Plasma magnesium ($mg\,dl^{-1}$)	1.0
Plasma phosphorus ($mg\,dl^{-1}$)	3.3
Alkaline phosphatase ($U\,l^{-1}$)	345
Plasma iPTH ($U\,l^{-1}$)	7.1
$TmPO_4$/GFR ($mg\,dl^{-1}$)	4.75
Urine calcium ($mg\,d^{-1}$)	74.7
Urine calcium ($mg\,(100ml\,GFR)^{-1}$)	0.341
Urine phosphorus ($mg\,d^{-1}$)	12.6

DISCUSSION

The pathogenesis of hypomagnesaemic rickets is not yet completely understood; probably a role is played by the concomitant hypercalciuria (Rapado *et al.*, 1975, Medalle *et al.*, 1976). The importance of magnesium in bone metabolism results also from its role in vitamin D activation, in the hydroxylation of $25(OH)D_3$ (Norman and Henry, 1974) and in the secretion of parathormone and calcitonin (Rojo-Ortega *et al.*, 1971).

Magnesium deficiency is not a rare occurrence in infancy. Besides the rare idiopathic form due to an intestinal absorption defect, low plasma magnesium levels can occur as a complication of numerous nutritional deficiencies (Rosen *et al.*, 1970). The alimentary restrictions of a low phenylalanine diet are probably not responsible *per se* for a symptomatic magnesium deficiency. This is more likely to be the result of a 'conditioned deficiency', a situation in which a normal intake does not fulfil the nutritional needs if particular concomitant factors are present. A similar condition was probably responsible for the clinical picture in our patient in whom, together with a magnesium intake at the lower limit of the normal range (100–150 $mg\,d^{-1}$), other factors certainly interfering with its absorption were present.

In man, intestinal magnesium absorption is influenced by many factors, among which are magnesium intake, quality of proteins and presence of phytates, calcium, phosphates and fatty acids (Alcock and MacIntyre, 1962). In the case of our patient, the following interfering factors were present: high intake of phytates, low intake of animal proteins (which favour magnesium absorption) and calcium supplementation.

In magnesium-dependent rickets, plasma calcium can be normal or low, but the urinary excretion of calcium is always high and the bone lesions are unresponsive to vitamin D therapy. Our patient, in fact, had both high urinary calcium excretion and vitamin D-resistant rickets.

The clinical and biochemical pictures of our patient are consistent with prolonged magnesium deficiency with normal parathyroid function. However, an oral supplementation with a magnesium salt solution brought about a normalization of the biochemical parameters first and of the rickety bone lesions later. In conclusion, this case report illustrates the importance of frequent clinical and biochemical control of patients on synthetic or semisynthetic restricted diets.

REFERENCES

Alcock, N. and MacIntyre, I. Inter-relation of calcium and magnesium absorption. *Clin. Sci.* 22 (1962) 185–193

Bijvoet, L. M. and Walton, R. J. Nomogram for derivation of renal threshold phosphate concentration. *Lancet* 1 (1975) 309–310

Medalle, R., Waterhouse, C. and Halm, R. J. Vitamin D resistance in magnesium deficiency. *Am. J. Clin. Nutr.* 29 (1976) 854–858

Norman, A. W. and Henry, H. 1,25-Dihydroxycholecalciferol. A hormonally active form of vitamin D. *Rec. Progr. Horm. Res.* 30 (1974) 431–480

Rapado, A., Castrillo, J. M., Arrayo, M., Traba, M. L. and Calle, M. Magnesium-deficient rickets. A clinical study. In Norman, A. W., Schaefer, K., Grigoleit, H. G., Herrat, D. V. and Ritz, E. (eds.) *Vitamin D and Problems Related to Uremic Bone Disease*. Walter de Gruyter, Berlin and New York, 1975, pp. 453–460

Rojo-Ortega, J. M., Brecht, H. M. and Genest, J. Effects of magnesium-deficient diet on the thyroid C cells and parathyroid gland of the dog. *Virchows Arch. Abt. B Zellpath.* 7 (1971) 81–89

Rosen, E. V., Campbell, P. G. and Mouse, G. M. Hypomagnesemia and magnesium therapy in protein-caloric malnutrition. *J. Pediatr.* 77 (1970) 709–714

Zeisler, E. B. Determination of diffusible serum calcium. *Am. J. Clin. Pathol.* 24 (1954) 588–592

J. Inher. Metab. Dis. 9 Suppl. 2 (1986) 218–222

Short Communication

Termination of Strict Diet in Phenylketonuria: Neurophysiological, Psychological and Biochemical Studies

A. W. BEHBEHANI[1*†], M. VOLLRATH[1], I. MATSCHKE[1] and U. LANGENBECK[2*]
[1]*Department of Pediatrics and* [2]*Institute of Human Genetics, University of Göttingen, D–3400 Göttingen, FRG*

While the positive effect of early dietary treatment on the intellectual development of patients with phenylketonuria (PKU) (McKusick 26160) has been clearly established, controversy exists regarding the termination of the phenylalanine-restricted diet in PKU-children. A strict dietetic scheme poses serious problems especially during school age and it may elicit psychosocial abnormalities in the children as well as in their families. This scheme should therefore be abandoned when development of recognizable CNS dysfunction is no longer to be expected.

PATIENTS

22 patients with PKU participated in the present study which extended over 10 years. 11 of them showed signs of cerebral damage with mental retardation of varying degrees. The other 11 patients were mentally normal. According to biochemical–diagnostic criteria, 21 have a classic type PKU (phenylalanine on loading well above 20 mg/dL, highly increased urinary levels of phenylalanine metabolites). One child has a hyperphenylalaninaemia (HPA). The mean age at termination of diet was 8.8 years in the retarded group and 8 years in the normal one.

The methods used are indicated in Table 1. In addition Frostig's developmental test of visual perception, evaluation of psychosocial aspects, estimation of the mean reaction time on optic and acoustic signals, evaluation of fine motor behaviour and computer-assisted frequency analysis were applied.

Psychometric examination of the patients was performed immediately before termination as well as at intervals of 4 months and 2–3 years after termination of strict diet therapy. The other examinations were performed every 6–12 months indefinitely. Parents were informed about controversy regarding the termination of diet therapy. Children were then allowed to choose their food freely. A recommendation, however, was given to avoid high protein intake so that the serum phenylalanine level would stay well below 20 mg/dL. There was and still is a regular control

* Supported by Deutsche Forschungsgemeinschaft SFB 33.
† Published in partial fulfilment of the postdoctoral thesis requirements.

Journal of Inherited Metabolic Disease. ISSN 0141–8955.

Table 1 IQ, motor development score, EEG and biochemical findings in PKU patients before and after termination of diet therapy

Case No.	Pat Age Diet-Init.	Dietary Control	Age Diet-Term.	IQ, T (HAWIK, CMMS-TBGB) before	IQ, T after	IQ, T cha.	Mot. Development LOS KF 18 (TN, TL, TG) before	Mot. Dev. after	Mot. Dev. cha.	Wake-EEG Visual Analysis before	Wake-EEG after	S.-Phe.-Levels (mg/dl) before	S.-Phe. after	U-PPA (μmol/mmol Cr.) before	U-PPA after
1	R.G. 15 M	satisf.	10 J	TG 51	TG 56 IQ 69	+ 5	—	—	—	P Dysrh. SHW	P Dysrh. SHW	12	28	—	824
2	S.S. 3.8 J	good	9.9 J	TG 55	TG 52 IQ 65	- 3	—	—	—	SHW	SHW	8	22	—	527
3	L.K. 2.6 J	exc.	10 J	TG 46	TG 53 IQ<70	+ 7	TL 44	TL 46	+ 2	norma	normal	3	27	10	181
4	Ch.M.	poor	9 J	T 33	TG 58 IQ 65		TL 43	TL 42	- 1	Interm.SW	Interm.SW FA ↑	17	24	212	447
5	K.T. 5 W	poor	8 J	TG 51	TG 49 IQ 66	- 2	TL 38	TL 45	+ 7	SA ↑	SA ↑	8	19	39	593
6	M.S. 10 W	poor	8 J	TG 45	TG 42 IQ 50-60	- 3	TG 31	TG 38	+ 7	Gen.Dys. abn. θ Rhy.	Gen.Dys. FA ↑	13	29	585	868
7	H.M. 18 M	exc.	8.6 J	TG 29	TG 29 IQ<50	—	TG 31	TG 37	+ 6	Gen.Dys. SHW	Gen.Dys. PDysrh.	2	20	ND	508
8	J.R. 17 M	satisf.	8.7 J	TG 42	TG 47 IQ 54	+ 5	TG 46	TG 52	+ 6	PDysrh SHW SW	PDysrh. SPW	12	21	377	512
9	D.L. 16 M	good	10 J	TG 28	TG 24 IQ<50	- 4	TG 32	TG 32	± 0	SA	SA	6	18	ND	698
10	J.B. 4 M	satisf.	8 J	TG 45	TG 46 IQ 65	+ 1	TL 38	TL 45	+ 7	Gen.Dys.	Gen.Dys. β A	9	16	261	368
11	A.S. 8 W	good	9.1 J	IQ 87	IQ 97	+10	TL 51	TL 50	- 1	normal	β A	8	21	97	466
12	D.O. 5 W	satisf.	8.2	89	102	+ 13	TN 31	TN 45	+ 14	Gen. Dys.	Gen.Dys. FA ↑	14	25	435	1206
13	A.S. 8 W	satisf.	8.5	T 53 IQ 104	T 45	- 8	TN 54	TN 47	- 7	PDysrh. SA	PDysrh. SA	8	15	165	336
14	M.B. 5 W	good	8	106	108	+ 2	TN 37	TN 60	+ 23	β A	β A	3	18	ND	572

15	S.M. 7W	good	8	T 55	T 56 IQ 107	+ 1	TN 58	TN 56 - 2	MDysrh.	MDysrh.	9	17	141	379
16	S.J. 4 W	good	8.2	95	93	- 2	TN 37	TN 50 + 13	MDysrh.	MDysrh.	8	23	147	738
17*	N.C. 4 W	good	8	109	116	+ 7	TN 51	TN 73 + 22	normal	normal	2	13	ND	277
18	U.L. 6 W	good	8.3	96	102	+ 6	TN 53	TN 56 + 3	normal	normal	7	23	55	365
19	R.G. 3 W	good	8	T 48 IQ 106	T 46.5	- 1.5	TN 40	TN 40 ± 0	β A	β A	4	25	ND	748
20	Ch.B. 4 W	good	8	127	123	- 4	TN 48	TN 60 + 12	Dysrh. β A	Dysrh. β A	9	23	55	418
21	M.Be. 5 W	good	8	126	132	+ 6	TN 56	TN 63 + 7	Dysrh. FA ↑	Dysrh. FA ↑ SA ↑	4	19	ND	839
22	I.M. 12 W	good	8	108	108	± 0	TN 51	TN 53 + 2	normal	normal	10	17	108	356

HAWIK	German adaption of the Wechsler-Intelligence-Scale for Children
CMMS	Columbia Mental Maturity Scale
T	T-Scale Score
TBGB	Test Battery for Mentally retarded Children
LOS	Lincoln Oseretzky Scale
TN	T-Score for normal Children
TL	T-Score for Children with Learning Impediment
TG	T-Score for retarded Children
Initiat.	Initiation
Termin.	Termination
MO	Month
W	Week
Y	Year
satisf.	Satisfactory
exc.	Excellent

P	Paroxysmal
Dys	Dysrhythmia
SHW	sharp-waves
SW	slow-waves
SpW	spike-waves
SA	Slow Activity
FA	Fast Activity
Rhy	Rhythm
βA	β-Activity
θ	θ-Activity
Interm.	Intermitent
Gen	Generalised
M	Moderate
Abn	Abnormal
Phe	Phenylalanine
PPA	Phenylpyruvic Acid
U	Urin
S	Serum
ND	Not detected

of the patients' somatic, nutritional, psychomotoric, neurological and biochemical status.

RESULTS

The neurophysiological, motor, psychometric, and biochemical results of the present study are summarized in Table 1. The phenylalanine values given are single determinations from the days of EEG registration.

In the group of patients with normal development there was no significant decline of general intelligence as calculated from verbal and performance IQ. With regard to reaction time and fine motor behaviour, no deterioration occurred in any of the children after diet termination. Evaluating the results on the Lincoln–Oseretzky scale showed no decrease of performance in any child.

Wake EEG: (a) Visual analysis: neither in the retarded nor in the normal group did pathological changes appear when compared to pre-termination patterns. Isolated sharp-waves were seen in three patients with psychomotor retardation (nos. 1, 2 and 8) before as well as after diet termination. (b) Computer spectral analysis: no important changes of α-peak amplitude were seen. In a few cases an increase of fast activity was observed. Also no significant changes of the sleep EEG were seen, either on visual or on spectral analysis (Behbehani, 1985).

DISCUSSION

An interpretation of the data from the literature is difficult because the studies comprise different and often rather small numbers of patients and because age at diet termination differs widely in the different studies, only one other group reporting on diet termination at 8 years (Smith *et al.*, 1978). The follow-up time after diet termination also differs considerably. In half of the studies a decline of intellectual performance was observed whereas in the other studies no change was seen (Waisbren *et al.*, 1980).

In a 4- to 6-year follow-up study (Cabalska *et al.*, 1977) a decrease of IQ was found in children with classical PKU who had been treated for periods ranging from $2^{4}/_{12}$ to $4^{8}/_{12}$ years. A large proportion of patients treated early, whose diet was terminated before 5 years, had EEG anomalies. Within the US Collaborative Study diet was terminated at 6 years of age in a group of 62 children. Only subtle changes in cerebral function seemed to be present at an age of 8 years when compared to the group of 53 continuers (Koch *et al.*, 1982). Seashore and colleagues (1985) reported loss of intellectual function in children with PKU after discontinuation of phenylalanine-restricted diet between the ages of 5 and 6 years. Two children have had a change in EEG from normal to abnormal.

The results of our study which comprised neurophysiological and psychological parameters indicate that generous termination of strict diet at an age of 8 to 10 years may not measurably harm the CNS of children with PKU. However, further follow-up studies are indicated to delineate the long-term prognosis of these patients. Some of our patients have now been 10 years off the strict dietetic therapy without impairment of psychosocial adjustment and EEG.

REFERENCES

Behbehani, A. W. Termination of strict diet therapy in phenylketonuria. *Neuropediatrics* 16 (1985) 92–97

Cabalska, B., Duczynska, N., Borzymowska, J., Zorska, K., Koslacz-Folga, A. and Bozkowa, K. Termination of dietary treatment in phenylketonuria. *Eur. J. Pediatr.* 126 (1977) 253–262

Koch, R., Azen, C., Friedman, E. G. and Williamson, M. L. Preliminary report on the effect of diet discontinuation in PKU. *J. Pediatr.* 100 (1982) 870–875

Seashore, M. R., Friedman, E. G., Novelly, R. A. and Bapat, V. Loss of intellectual function in children with phenylketonuria after relaxation of dietary phenylalanine restriction. *Pediatrics* 75 (1985) 226–232

Smith, I., Lobascher, M. E., Stevenson, J. E., Wolff, O. H., Schmidt, H., Grubel-Kaiser, S. and Bickel, H. Effect of stopping low-phenylalanine diet on intellectual progress of children with phenylketonuria. *Br. Med. J.* 2 (1978) 723

Waisbren, S. E., Schnell, R. R. and Levy, H. L. Diet termination in children with phenylketonuria: a review of psychological assessments used to determine outcome. *J. Inher. Metab. Dis.* 3 (1980) 149–153

J. Inher. Metab. Dis. 9 *Suppl.* 2 *(1986) 223–224*

Short Communication

Effects of Stopping Phenylalanine-Restricted Diet on Intellectual Progress of Children with Phenylketonuria

R. CERONE, S. SCALISI, M. C. SCHIAFFINO and C. ROMANO
University Department of Pediatrics 'R', G. Gaslini Institute, Via 5 Maggio 39, 16148 Genova, Italy

In spite of more than 30 years' experience with the treatment of phenylketonuria (PKU) we still do not know the age at which the diet can safely be stopped. Some studies (Smith *et al.*, 1978) report that complete withdrawal of the low-phenylalanine diet during childhood leads to a fall in intellectual progress in many patients. Other reports (Holtzman *et al.*, 1975; Koff *et al.*, 1979) have revealed no significant differences in intellectual functioning before and after diet termination.

The purpose of the present study is to determine the effects of termination of the phenylalanine-restricted diet in 22 PKU subjects (out of a total of 141 patients) after two years of follow-up

METHODS

In 22 PKU patients the low-phenylalanine diet was stopped between the ages of 9 and 10 years. The 22 children with PKU included in the present analysis were divided in two groups. Group 1 (12/22) were patients treated early (diagnosis by neonatal screening, and diet started soon after birth). Group 2 (10/22) were patients treated late (diagnosis on clinical symptoms, diet started after 12 months of age). The diagnosis of phenylketonuria was confirmed in each child by the presence of elevated serum phenylalanine (above 20 mg/dL) and urinary metabolites characteristic of phenylketonuria.

All the children were tested with the Wechsler Intelligence Scale for Children (WISC). The last IQ on diet was compared with the last IQ measured 2 years after diet termination.

RESULTS AND DISCUSSION

WISC tests results are shown in Table 1. No differences were found between the mean scores of any of the tests at diet termination and two years later. These results suggest that complete withdrawal of low-phenylalanine diet between 9 and 10 years of age does not lead to a fall in intellectual progress. However, our policy is that every decision concerning diet termination must be made in the context of the family situation and the biochemical data; moreover it is very important that

Journal of Inherited Metabolic Disease. ISSN 0141–8955.

Table 1 Comparison between last IQ on diet and IQ measured after diet change in groups 1 and 2

	On diet termination		*After diet change*	
	mean	*range*	*mean*	*range*
Group 1	106	91–121	105	91–119
Group 2	71	59–83	72	56–88

every child whose diet is terminated should be followed strictly. Any changes in behaviour, intellectual development or school performance must lead to a reinstitution of diet.

REFERENCES

Holtzman, N. A., Welcher, D. W. and Mellits, E. D. Termination of restricted diet in children with phenylketonuria: a randomized controlled study. *N. Engl. J. Med.* 293 (1975) 1121–1124

Koff, E., Kammerer, B., Boyle, P. and Pueschel, S. M. Intelligence and phenylketonuria: effects on diet termination. *J. Pediatr.* 94 (1979) 534–537

Smith, I., Lobascher, M. E., Stevenson, J. E., Wolff, O. H., Schmidt, H., Gruber-Kaiser, S. and Bickel, H. Effect of stopping low phenylalanine diet on intellectual progress of children with phenylketonuria. *Br. Med. J.* 2 (1978) 723–726

J. Inher. Metab. Dis. 9 Suppl. 2 (1986) 225–226

Short Communication

Maternal Hyperphenylalaninaemia: Dietary Treatment during Pregnancy

C. ROMANO[1], R. CERONE[1], C. BORRONE[2], S. SCALISI[1], U. CARUSO[1] and S. GATTI[1]

[1]*University Department of Pediatrics 'R' and* [2]*3rd Pediatric Division, G. Gaslini Institute, Via 5 Maggio 39, 16148 Genova, Italy*

Pregnancies in hyperphenylalaninaemic women indicate a high frequency of prenatal and postnatal growth retardation, microcephaly, mental retardation and congenital anomalies (Fisch *et al.*, 1966). Fetal abnormalities are less frequent in women with plasma phenylalanine (Phe) levels in the range between 240–600 μmol/L (Lenke and Levy, 1980). Dietary treatment during pregnancy appears to reduce the frequency of damaged offspring (Lenke and Levy, 1982). We report the results of treatment during pregnancy in a woman with hyperphenylalaninaemia.

CASE REPORT

A 31-year-old woman came to our clinic in the 13th week of her pregnancy, because of hyperphenylalaninaemia and three previous unfortunate pregnancies (newborns exitus on the 2nd, 3rd and 17th days after the birth, respectively). At admission there were no abnormal physical and neurological findings; laboratory findings were within the normal range but the plasma Phe level was 640 μmol/L.

The diet was revised to provide 2500 Cal and 77 g of protein per day (natural foods and PKU 3®). The total daily Phe and tyrosine (Tyr) intakes were 850 mg and 6 g respectively. The diet was well tolerated and the fetal growth was adequate (ultrasound measurements were in the normal range). The protocol for treatment at the 16th, 26th and 38th weeks consisted of measurement of red blood cells, haemoglobin, haematocrit, ferritin, zinc, copper, iron, magnesium, folic acid, vitamin B_{12}, total protein and plasma amino acids. The plasma Phe was determined weekly and remained between 181 and 302 μmol/L (Figure 1).

A boy was delivered: weight 3200 g; head circumference 35 cm; physical and nutritional conditions good. Cord blood Phe and Tyr levels were 244 and 51 μmol/L respectively; plasma Phe and Tyr were 87 and 102 μmol/L.

On the 2nd day from birth hyperammonaemia developed and brought the child to death a month later. The diagnosis was carbamyl phosphate synthetase deficiency: CPS activity in liver biopsy was absent.

DISCUSSION

The outcome of the previous pregnancies in our patient does not appear referable to maternal hyperphenylalaninaemia; on the other hand dietetic treatment of this

Journal of Inherited Metabolic Disease. ISSN 0141–8955.

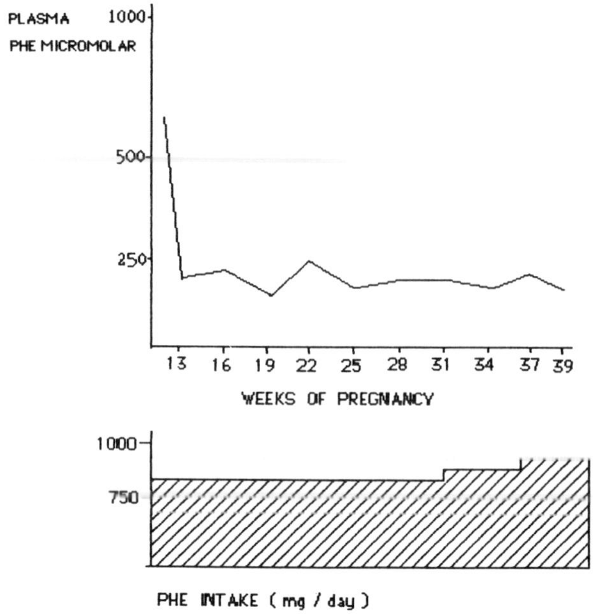

Figure 1 Plasma phenylalanine levels and phenylalanine intake

pregnant woman seemed unquestionable. Dietary management in our patient can be considered successful in controlling the mother's plasma Phe levels during pregnancy, and in maintaining the mother's good health and fetal growth.

Obviously the exitus of newborns in this family must be related to carbamyl phosphate synthetase deficiency, not to maternal hyperphenylalaninaemia.

REFERENCES

Fisch, R. O., Walker, W. A. and Anderson, J. A. Prenatal and postnatal developmental consequences of maternal phenylketonuria. *Pediatrics* 37 (1966) 979–986

Lenke, R. R. and Levy, H. L. Maternal phenylketonuria and hyperphenylalaninaemia. *N. Engl. J. Med.* 20 (1980) 1202–1208

Lenke, R. R. and Levy, H. L. Maternal phenylketonuria: results of dietary therapy. *Am. J. Obstet. Gynecol.* 142 (1982) 548–553

J. Inher. Metab. Dis. 9 Suppl. 2 (1986) 227–230

Short Communication

Maternal Hyperphenylalaninaemia in Israel

B. E. COHEN[1], A. SZEINBERG[2], Y. ZARFIN[1], M. NORMAND[1], I. PELED[2], Y. BLONDER[2], A. ELITZUR[1], R. HADAR[1] and S. MASHIACH[3]
[1]*Weinberg Child Development Institute, Department of Pediatrics;* [2]*Department of Chemical Pathology and* [3]*Department of Obstetrics and Gynaecology, The Chaim Sheba Medical Center, Tel Hashomer, Israel*

During the 21 years of national newborn screening for phenylketonuria (PKU) in Israel, originally supported by grants from the NIH, Washington (HEW–WA/CB–Israel–9, 1964–1967) and subsequently taken up by the Israeli Ministry of Health (Cohen *et al.*, 1966) an average of over 95% coverage was achieved by 1979, revealing 85 cases of classical PKU, 20 of variant or atypical PKU, and 2 cases of malignant PKU with a biopterin synthetase deficiency (Cohen *et al.*, 1985). In addition, there were 18 cases of high hyperphenylalaninaemia (HPA) with blood phenylalanine levels of 12–16 mg/dL who had never been on diet and 132 mild persistent HPA with blood phenylalanine below 12 mg/dL. No cases of classical PKU have been found amongst 'pure' Ashkenazi families whereas atypical and mild HPA are frequently found. Thus, the two classical PKU cases in mixed Ashkenazi families may be due to a double heterozygote effect for the PKU and HPA gene (Cohen *et al.*, 1978).

Of 33 girls with classical PKU born before 1970, many are so seriously retarded that they are not candidates for maternity. 5 moderately retarded girls and 6 with normal intelligence from our screening programme are undergoing a programme of education and/or diet. Of our 34 male PKUs none have married or fathered children.

Three mothers with classical PKU delivered 5 children without dietary treatment during pregnancy (Table 1). Only one (N.M.) had any dietary treatment during infancy and in her case, biochemical and dietary control were inadequate. Note the high incidence of spontaneous abortion, one during a period of inadequate dietary control. In only one case was data available on cord and maternal blood phenylalanine levels, and only a slightly increased cord blood level was noted. This information, incomplete where available, was not helpful even amongst our high HPAs.

The treated maternal PKU (A.R.) was identified at 12 years as the sibling of a severely retarded PKU. Although not treated and showing evidence of brain damage, she was only minimally affected with borderline retardation and had excellent social adaptation. In spite of counselling at 18 years and later, she married and was three months pregnant before coming to our attention. A therapeutic abortion was recommended and agreed upon. After 6 months of dietary control she again became pregnant. Her initial dietary control was inadequate however,

Table 1 Biochemical and clinical data on mothers and offspring with phenylketonuria and hyperphenylalaninaemia

Type	*Name and IQ*	*Blood Phe (mg/dL)*	*Urinary phenyl-ketones*	*Blood Tyr (mg/dL)*	*Previous abortions*	*Cord blood Phe (mg/dL)*	*Maternal Blood Phe at birth*	*Mother's no. of children*	*Head circumference at birth (cm)*	*Birth weight*	*Congenital heart disease*	*Other congenital abnormalities*	*Age at last visit*	*IQ*
PKU untreated	D.M. 72	25.6	+	–	–	–	–	1	31	2700	–	–	2.6	60
	N.M. 75	30.6	+	1.4	1	–	–	1	28.9	2200	–	–	1.2	25
	S.B. 55	20–30	+	–	3	–	–	3	30	2790	–	–	6.6	48
									29	2700	–	S.D.[a]	4.9	32
									28	2200	–	Crypt[b] E.A.[c]	1.1	25
PKU treated	A.R. V–95 P–75	19–23	+	1.3–1.7	2 (1 therapeutic)	13.9	10.0	1	35	3300	–	–	0.6	N[d]
High HPA	S.N.(Z) 65	6–14	–	1.0–3.4	–	1–	–	3	35.5	2980	–	–	4.6	93
						2–9.2	5.4		31.5	3130	–		2.6	76
						3–	–		34.0	3580	–	–	0.7	N
	Z.N.(S)	8–12	–	1.2	–	–	–	2	31.3	2090	–	–	0.7	N
									32.3	2280	–	–	0.7	N

[a]Spastic diplegia; [b]Cryptorchidism; [c]Oesophageal atony; [d]Within normal limits

with blood phenylalanine levels of 11–15 mg/dL and at 3 months she aborted spontaneously. Subsequent dietary control during a 3rd pregnancy was satisfactory, with 34 levels below 10 mg/dL (average 5.5), and she finally delivered at full-term after an uneventful pregnancy. During the last 2 months of her pregnancy her phenylalanine tolerance increased so that dietary readjustments had to be continually made. After delivery she was kept on the same diet and during the 4 postpartum days there was a steady rise in her phenylalanine levels up to 15.9 mg/dL suggesting that the fetal phenylalanine hydroxylase had assisted in the utilization of her phenylalanine.

The data on the offspring of these classical PKU mothers (Table 1) confirm the results quoted in the literature (Lenke and Levy, 1982; Levy and Waisbren, 1983). All the untreated infants showed microcephaly, birth weight below 3000 g and mental retardation on follow-up, with IQs ranging from 25–60. No congenital heart lesions were found, but other congenital anomalies were seen, e.g. spastic diplegia, cryptorchidism and oesophageal atony. The treated child, however, showed normal birth weight, a head circumference of 35 cm and no evidence of congenital anomalies. Development at 1 year was normal.

We can also confirm a recent suggestion from Australia (Lipson *et al.*, 1984) that the offspring of untreated PKU women showed many of the features of the fetal alcohol syndrome (FAS). We observe the microcephaly, thin vermillion of the upper lip, long undeveloped philtrum, micrognathism, small button nose and hypoplastic maxilla described in the classic FAS.

The last 2 cases are sisters diagnosed at 12 and 14 years as high HPA with blood phenylalanine levels of 12–14 mg/dL on normal diet, both with borderline intelligence. The younger (Z.N.) had an IQ of 91 when last tested, whereas her sister (S.N.) had an IQ of 65, but functioned much above this socially. Their urines were generally negative for phenylpyruvic acid.

The elder sister was first seen at the 8th week of her first pregnancy. A low protein diet without Lofenalac maintained her blood levels below 10 mg/dL (22 examinations) with an average of 7 mg/dL. Delivery of a normal boy was uneventful and follow-up after 4½ years shows normal development. Her subsequent pregnancy, again revealed to us at 8 weeks, showed rather higher phenylalanine levels (15–18 mg/dL). She refused Lofenalac after a trial of 2–3 days and in the next 5 months only 3 blood specimens were received showing blood levels of 10–15 mg/dL. Subsequent blood samples (16) were all below 10 mg/dL, with an average of 7.8 mg/dL. Cord blood showed 9.2 mg/dL but the nearest maternal phenylalanine level 13 days previously had been 4.2 mg/dL. The infant girl, microcephalic at birth, has borderline development at 2½ years (IQ 75), some evidence of attention deficit disorder, and a head circumference now at the 3rd percentile, whilst her height and weight are at the 25th and 50th percentiles respectively. A third pregnancy, notified at 20 weeks, showed phenylalanine levels below 10 mg/dL (average of 8.3 mg/dL) and the female infant also has a head circumference on a lower percentile than the rest of her measurements. At 8 months she is functioning at a normal level.

The younger sister was seen in the 8th week of her pregnency with a blood phenylalanine level of 10.5 mg/dL and tyrosine of 1.2 mg/dL, with urine negative for phenylpyruvic acid. Protein restriction without Lofenalac maintained 9 subsequent blood levels below 10 mg/dL (average 7.4 mg/dL). Twin infants, normal on ultrasound examination during pregnancy, were delivered and they too are functioning normally at 8 months.

Our results confirm those in the literature: untreated maternal PKU resulted in low birth weight, microcephaly and mental retardation, in addition to a high incidence of abortion. Hyperphenylalaninaemia above 10 mg/dL may cause fetal damage. We need information on cord and maternal blood levels at birth as well as detailed follow-up of the offspring.

REFERENCES

Cohen, B. E., Szeinberg, A., Peled, I., Szeinberg, B. and Bar-or, R. Screening program for early detection of phenylketonuria in newborn in Israel. *Isr. J. Med. Sci.* 2 (1966) 156–164

Cohen, B. E., Szeinberg, A., Quint, J., Normand, M., Blonder, J. and Peled, I. Malignant phenylketonuria due to defective synthesis of dehydrobiopterin. *Isr. J. Med. Sci.* 21 (1985) 520–525

Cohen, B. E., Szeinberg, A., Levine, Y., Peled, I., Pollack, S., Crispin, M. and Normand, M. Phenylketonuria in Israel. *Human Genet.* 9 (1978) 95–101

Lenke, R. R. and Levy, H. L. Maternal phenylketonuria: results of dietary therapy. *Am. J. Obstet. Gynecol.* 142 (1982) 548–553

Levy, H. L. and Waisbren, S. Effects of untreated phenylketonuria and hyperphenylalaninemia on the fetus. *N. Engl. J. Med.* 309 (1983) 1269–1274

Lipson, A., Beuhler, B., Bartley, J., Walsh, D., Yu, J., O'Halloran, M. and Webster, W. Maternal hyperphenylalaninemia fetal effects. *J. Pediatr.* 104 (1984) 216–220

Koch, R. and Blascovics, M. Four cases of hyperphenylalaninaemia: studies during pregnancy and of the offspring produced. *J. Inher. Metab. Dis.* 5 (1982) 11–15

J. Inher. Metab. Dis. 9 Suppl. 2 (1986) 231–233

Short Communication

Maternal Phenylketonuria with Increased Tyrosine Supplements

O. SHEIL[1], N. DUIGNAN[1], I. P. SAUL[2] and E. R. NAUGHTEN[2]
[1]*The Department of Obstetrics, Coombe Lying-In Hospital, Dublin 8, and* [2]*The Metabolic Unit, The Children's Hospital, Temple Steet, Dublin 1, Eire*

The outcome in maternal phenylketonuria (PKU) is variable (Lenke and Levy, 1980; Murphy *et al.*, 1985). It is generally accepted that pre-conception treatment is essential (Nielson *et al.*, 1979; Lenke and Levy, 1982). The optimal management has yet to be established. High serum phenylalanine (Phe) and low serum tyrosine (Tyr) have been implicated in the teratogenesis. The tyrosine requirements of the growing fetus are unknown and varying supplements have been used (Lenke *et al.*, 1983). We describe here the pregnancy of a woman with classical phenylketonuria on a diet with high tyrosine supplements.

MATERIALS AND METHODS

Amino acids were measured using the Locarte amino acid analyser. Blood levels were monitored twice weekly. We aimed to keep the serum phenylalanine between 200–600 μmol/L (Koch and Blasovics, 1982; Lipson *et al.*, 1984) and serum tyrosine between 20–90 μmol/L. Maternal weight was measured twice weekly. Fetal biparietal diameter was measured monthly.

DIET AND MANAGEMENT

Although the mother was on diet before conception, initial control was erratic (serum Phe 727–1103 μmol/L). Compliance improved following confirmation of the pregnancy at 6 weeks. The prescribed phenylalanine intake was $6\,mg\,kg^{-1}\,d^{-1}$ but the actual intake at conception was higher as indicated by the serum levels. The intake increased to $18\,mg\,kg^{-1}\,d^{-1}$ at term. Serum Phe ranged from 121–873 μmol/L throughout the rest of the pregnancy. The tyrosine intake increased from $62–326\,mg\,kg^{-1}\,d^{-1}$. This included supplements of 5 g/d commencing at 20 weeks and increasing to 20 g/d at 35 weeks (Figure 1). The serum tyrosine levels ranged from 19–133 μmol/L.

The calorie : nitrogen ratio, calculated retrospectively, was low. Maternal weight increased from 83–88.7 kg during the pregnancy (Figure 1). Serial biparietal diameter measurements were within normal limits. The diet was adjusted as pregnancy progressed. The Phe and Tyr varied with the serum levels and the other nutrients altered in accordance with the recommended dietary allowances. (Food Advisory Committee, 1983).

Journal of Inherited Metabolic Disease. ISSN 0141–8955.

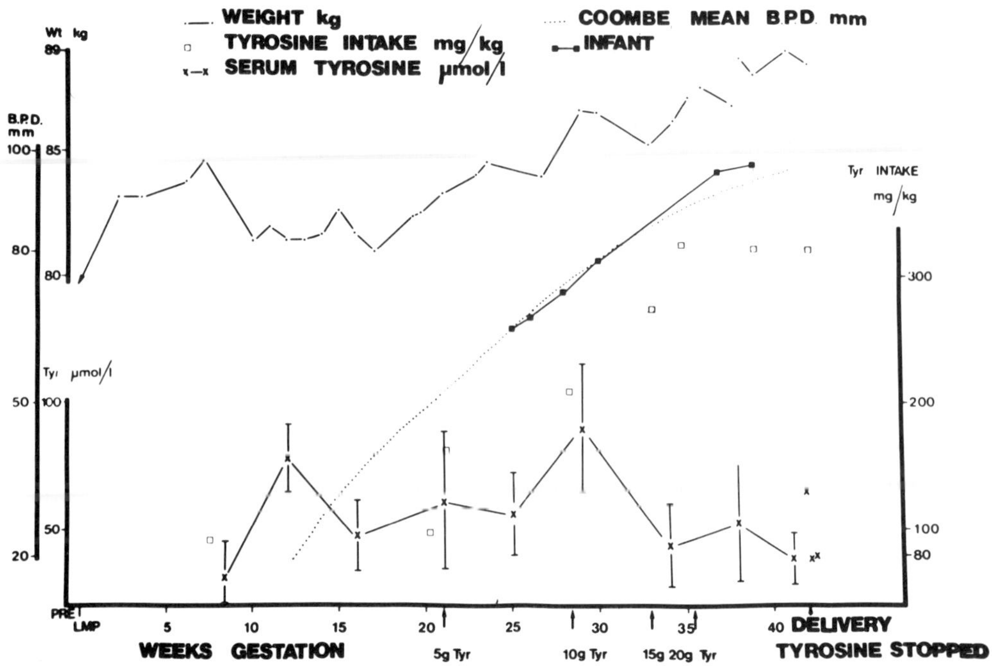

Figure 1 Maternal weight, fetal biparietal diameter and tyrosine levels during the pregnancy

The diet comprised:

Protein	Synthetic: phenylalanine-free amino acid mix (Maxamum XP SHS and Aminogran food mix) to a total of 1 g protein $kg^{-1} d^{-1}$ Natural: 50 mg Phe exchanges (6–18 mg/d) L-Tyrosine supplements
Fat (allowed freely)	Synthetic: arachis oil emulsion (Prosparol) Natural: butter or margarine or vegetable oil
Carbohydrate (allowed freely)	Synthetic: low protein bread, biscuits, pasta Natural: sugars, sweetened drinks, fruit, vegetables
Minerals Trace elements Vitamins	included in the formulation of Maxamum XP to recommended intake

The daily calorie intake increased from 2200–3200 (27–36 cal/kg). The total protein intake increased from 68–119 g/d (Natural: 0.06–0.34 $g\,kg^{-1} d^{-1}$; synthetic: 1.0 $g\,kg^{-1} d^{-1}$).

OUTCOME

A healthy non-phenylketonuric female infant was delivered at 42 weeks: head circumference 35.9 cm (>50th centile), weight 3.9 kg (>50th centile), length 52 cm (50th centile). Cord phenylalanine and tyrosine were 327 and 119 μmol/L respectively and were within normal levels at 24 hours. At 1 year she is developmentally normal.

DISCUSSION

This was an unplanned pregnancy during a period of erratic control in a woman on a phenylalanine restricted diet. She was receiving 62 mg $kg^{-1} d^{-1}$ of tyrosine at the time of conception as part of her synthetic amino acid mixture. The tyrosine was increased initially in accordance with the recommended supplements of 5 g at 20 weeks. Thereafter, because there was a tendency to lower serum levels and because weight gain seemed to parallel tyrosine increases, further supplements were given. These had no obvious adverse effect.

The nutrition of a normal pregnant woman and growing fetus is little understood. The roles of protein, calories and their ratio are unknown. The calorie : nitrogen ratio, when calculated retrospectively, was low in this patient because of the very large protein intake necessary as a result of her weight.

The apparently normal neonate may be the result of either biological variation or the biochemical manoeuvres. Neurological development will be followed closely. The increased tyrosine supplements, in our opinion, contributed to growth. It may be possible that tyrosine also protects against the teratogenic effect of raised phenylalanine at the time of conception in women with phenylketonuria.

REFERENCES

Food Advisory Committee. *Recommended Dietary Allowances*, Dept. of Health (Ireland), Public Health Education Bureau, 1983

Koch, R. and Blasovics, M. 4 cases of hyperphenylalaninaemia: studies during pregnancy and of the offspring produced. *J. Inher. Metab. Dis.* 5 (1982) 11–15

Lenke, R. R. and Levy, H. L. Maternal phenylketonuria and hyperphenylalaninemia. *N. Engl. J. Med.* 303 (1980) 1202–1208

Lenke, R. R. and Levy, H. L. Maternal phenylketonuria – results of dietary therapy. *Am. J. Obstet. Gynaecol.* 142 (1982) 548–553

Lenke, R. R., Koch, R., Fishler, K. and Platt, L. D. Tyrosine supplementation during pregnancy in a woman with classical phenylketonuria. *J. Reprod. Med.* 28 (1983) 411–414

Lipson, A., Beuhler, B., Bartley, J., Walsh, D., Yu, J., O'Halloran, M. and Webster, W. Maternal hyperphenylalaninemia fetal effects. *J. Pediatr.* 104 (1984) 216–220

Murphy, D., Saul, I. and Kirby, M. Maternal phenylketonuria and phenylalanine restricted diet. *I.J.M.S.* 154 (1985) 66 70

Nielson, K. B., Wamberg, E. and Weber, J. Successful outcome of pregnancy in a phenylketonuric woman after low-phenylalanine diet introduced before conception. *Lancet* 1 (1979) 1245

J. Inher. Metab. Dis. 9 Suppl. 2 (1986) 234–236

Short Communication

Screening for Phenylketonuria in Yugoslavia (SR Croatia) 1979–1984

D. Mardešić[1], G. Gjurić[1], J. Jančiković[2], P. Granić[2] and A. Stavljenić[2]

[1]*Department of Paediatrics and* [2]*Institute of Clinical Laboratory Diagnostics, University Hospital Rebro, 41000 Zagreb, Yugoslavia*

In 1979 a screening programme for phenylketonuria (PKU) was started in SR Croatia by the Department of Paediatrics, University Hospital Rebro, Zagreb. This is one of three regional programmes now running in Yugoslavia (Mardešić *et al.*, 1983); the other two are covering SR Slovenia and SR Serbia with a common screening laboratory organized at the Institute for Mother and Child Health in Belgrade (Nadaški-Basta, 1969; Vulović *et al.*, 1979; Pintar, 1983).

ORGANIZATION

SR Croatia is one of the six federal republics of Yugoslavia with a population of 4.63 million and a birth rate of 14.3 per 1000. In Yugoslavia there is no legislation enforcing neonatal screening for PKU. The programme therefore depends upon voluntary participation of each maternity hospital (99.2% of all infants in SR Croatia are born in hospitals), and upon financial coverage by the local (communal) public health insurance funds. The cost of the programme amounts to 68.00 din (£0.17) per newborn infant. The screening laboratory, the laboratory for diagnostic work-up of infants with a positive Guthrie test and the clinical facilities for long-term treatment and follow-up of the children amenable to treatment are affiliated to the University Department of Paediatrics at the University Hospital Rebro, Zagreb, and staffed by members of the University.

The coverage of the newborn population of SR Croatia by the programme in 1984 is shown by the following data:

Total number of infants born in 1984	65 242
Number of hospitals participating	28
Number of infants born in participating hospitals	48 944
Percentage of newborn infants covered by the programme	74.8
Number of Guthrie tests performed in 1984	45 294
Percentage of newborn infants covered by the programme who were tested	92.5

The most important task in the future will be to include in the programme the non-participating hospitals where 25% of the infants are born.

Journal of Inherited Metabolic Disease. ISSN 0141–8955.

The screening laboratory performing the Guthrie tests participates regularly in the periodic international quality control programme organized by the University Children's Hospital in Heidelberg, West Germany (Dr Mathias).

DIAGNOSTIC WORK-UP

Every child with a positive Guthrie test (phenylalanine $4.0\,mg\,dl^{-1}$ or higher) has a plasma phenylalanine and tyrosine determination by fluorometry and/or column chromatography, and a measurement of urinary pterins. Infants with a phenylalanine level of less than $10.0\,mg\,dl^{-1}$ have no dietary restriction, but only periodic phenylalanine measurements. All infants with a phenylalanine level greater than $15.0\,mg\,dl^{-1}$ are put on a phenylalanine-restricted diet. Infants with levels of 10.0–$14.9\,mg\,dl^{-1}$ have a restricted protein intake with regular phenylalanine measurements (Schmidt, 1983).

A phenylalanine challenge is performed to all children on a phenylalanine-restricted diet at 6 or 12 months of age by the method of Blaskovics *et al.* (1971) for the exclusion of transient forms of PKU.

RESULTS

The cumulative results of screening for PKU in SR Croatia from 1979 to 1984 are given in Table 1.

The incidence of classical phenylketonuria was about 1:14 500 newborn infants with a male/female ratio of 1.2:1 and a classical PKU to non-PKU hyperphenylalaninaemia ratio of 3.1:1.

Table 1 Cumulative results of screening for phenylketonuria in SR Croatia from 1979 to 1984

	No. of tests performed	*No. of positive results*	*No. of classical PKU cases*	*No. of non-PKU hyperphenyl-alaninemia cases*
Females		11	9	2
Males		14	10	4
Total	274 881	25	19	6

The age at which blood samples were drawn was as follows: 3% of samples were drawn on the second day of life, 76% on the third and fourth days, and 21% after the fourth day.

Treatment of infants started before the 21st day of life in only 3 (out of 22 treated) children, in 11 children between the 21st and the 30th day of life, in 7 children between the 31st and the 40th day of life, and in one child after the 41st but before the 50th day of life.

The main improvements in our screening programme can be achieved by (1) including the still non-participating hospitals in the programme; (2) increasing the number of infants tested in hospitals already participating and (3) starting treatment of PKU infants at an earlier age through organizational improvements.

We thank Prof. Otto Thalhammer (Universitäts Kinderklinik, Vienna) for his help and advice in the organization of the PKU screening laboratory in Zagreb.

The excellent collaboration of the physicians and nurses in the maternity hospitals participating in the programme and the technical and administrative skills of Mrs. Ljiljana Kulik from the PKU screening laboratory in Zagreb are highly appreciated.

Part of this work was supported by the Self-managing Interest Association for Science of the Socialist Republic of Croatia.

REFERENCES

Blaskovics, M. E. and Shaw, K. N. F. Hyperphenylalaninemia: Methods for differential diagnosis. In Bickel, H., Hudson, F. P. and Woolf, L. I. (eds.) *Phenylketonuria and some other Inborn Errors of Amino Acid Metabolism.* Thieme, Stuttgart, 1971, pp. 98–102

Mardešić, D., Gjurić, G., Kulik, L., Dumić, M., Jančiković, J., Žanić, T., Radica, A., Vlatković, M. and Gregurić, N. The newborn screening programme for phenylketonuria and congenital hypothyroidism in Socialistic Republic Croatia. *Jug. Pedijat.* 26 (1983) 91–97

Nadaški-Basta, L. Incidence of phenylketonuria in Yugoslavia. *Nar. Zdrav.* 25 (1969) 403–405

Pintar, L. Results of the early detection of phenylketonuria in Slovenia. *Zdrav. Vestn.* 52 (1983) 595–562

Schmidt, H. Praktisches Vorgehen zur Differentialdiagnose von Hyperphenylalaninämien. In Bickel, H. and Wachtel, U. (eds.) *Neugeborenen-Screening auf hereditäre Stoffwechselstörungen.* Thieme, Stuttgart, 1983

Vulović, D., Vilhar, N., Banićević, M., Šićević, S., Hajduković, R. and Subotić, Z. Genetic screening of newborn infants. *Srp. Arh.* 107 (1979) 269–281

J. Inher. Metab. Dis. 9 *Suppl.* 2 *(1986) 237–239*

Short Communication

Incidence of Phenylketonuria and Hyperphenylalaninaemia in a Sample of the Turkish Newborn Population

I. ÖZALP[1], T. COŞKUN[1], M. CEYHAN[1], S. TOKOL[1], O. ORAN[2], G. ERDEM[2], G. TEKINALP[2], Z. DURMUŞ[3] and Y. TARIKAHYA[3]
[1]*Department of Metabolism and* [2]*Department of Neonatology, Institute of Child Health, Hacettepe University, Hacettepe, Ankara, Turkey;* [3]*General Maternity Hospital, Ankara, Turkey*

The incidence of hereditary aminoacidopathies has been determined and nationwide programmes focussed on the most common diseases have been set up in the USA and most of the European countries. Specifically, the programme for phenylketonuria (PKU, McKusick 26160) has been successful and has served as a model for the detection and preventive treatment of genetic diseases.

In Turkey, consanguineous marriages are quite frequent (21% between first degree relatives) and therefore the incidence of some hereditary aminoacidopathies would be expected to be high. In fact, the prevalence of PKU was found to be as high as 1 in 18 (5.4%) in 3500 children with mental-motor retardation who are systematically screened (Özalp *et al.*, 1983).

A survey has been carried out to determine the incidence of PKU in order to assess the magnitude of the problem in Turkey. In this communication, we report the preliminary results which give a picture of the situation in the developing, partly Asian and partly European countries.

MATERIALS AND METHODS

The survey has been carried out on 20979 newborn babies in the General Maternity Hospital in Ankara during the period of July 1983 to May 1985. Blood samples were obtained from the newborn by heel prick into standard 'S and S' filter paper just before discharge, regardless of how young the infant was. They were, however, retested if the initial sample had been obtained before the infant was 24 h old. After being air dried the samples were sent to the Metabolic Unit of Hacettepe Institute of Child Health where a screening test, the 'Guthrie' inhibition assay (Guthrie and Susi, 1963) was applied. A blood phenylalanine level $\geqslant$4 mg dl^{-1} was accepted as a positive result. Every infant with a positive test was followed up until a definitive diagnosis was reached.

Infants with a serum phenylalanine level exceeding 20 mg dl^{-1} by the fluorometric method and with urine giving a positive reaction with ferric chloride, either initially or at the time of a protein challenge later in infancy, were regarded as having

Journal of Inherited Metabolic Disease. ISSN 0141–8955.

classical PKU. Infants whose serum phenylalanine levels were persistently higher than 8–10 mg dl^{-1}, but who did not meet the above mentioned criteria were classified as having hyperphenylalaninaemia.

RESULTS

The results of the screening are presented in Table 1. Twelve cases with persistent hyperphenylalaninaemia were detected. In 8 out of 12 cases, confirmatory tests were compatible with typical PKU. Blood phenylalanine levels have been found to be persistently between 8–12 mg dl^{-1} on a normal dietary intake in the other 4 cases.

Table 1 Incidence of phenylketonuria and hyperphenylalaninaemia among 20979 newborn screened by the Guthrie test

	No. of cases detected	*Incidence*
Typical phenylketonuria	8	1:2622
Hyperphenylalaninaemia	4	1:5243
Total	12	1:1747

DISCUSSION

There is no doubt that since their serum phenylalanine levels exceeded 20 mg dl^{-1} and their ferric chloride tests were positive, either before dietary therapy was begun or on the protein challenge, 8 cases have classical PKU (1 in 2622 newborns). A tetrahydrobiopterin loading test was performed and urinary neopterin and biopterin excretions were determined in two of these infants and found to be not compatible with a defect in BH_4 metabolism. In the other 6 cases developing normally on a diet restricted in phenylalanine, the above mentioned variants were not considered.

The results of this preliminary study indicate that the incidence of PKU is strikingly high in Turkey. The population of the capital city of Ankara has increased recently due to migration from almost all provinces of Turkey. We therefore believe that this study carried out in Ankara may represent the whole country.

As far as reported surveys are concerned, Ireland has the highest incidence of PKU in the world (Bickel *et al.*, 1975; Woolf, 1978). It seems that in Turkey the incidence of PKU is almost twice that in Ireland.

Since serum phenylalanine concentrations have never exceeded 10 mg dl^{-1} on 2–2.5 g protein kg^{-1} d^{-1} and serum phenylalanine returned to preloading levels within 24 h in 4 infants with an initial positive Guthrie test, they were classified as having mild persistent hyperphenylalaninaemia. Consequently, a diet restricted in phenylalanine has not been started in any of these infants.

In children with a defect in BH_4 metabolism, serum phenylalanine level is generally not expected to be as high as in typical PKU (Dhondt, 1984). Since the infants with persistent hyperphenylalaninaemia who were older than 6 months were free of the symptoms, we did not think that any of them had a defect in BH_4 metabolism either. However, the diagnosis of partial or peripheral forms of dihydrobiopterin synthetase deficiency (McKusick 26164, 26169) cannot be excluded unless specific tests are performed (Dhondt, 1984).

When the cases with PKU and the cases with hyperphenylalaninaemia in the survey are considered together, the incidence of hyperphenylalaninaemia goes up to 1 in 1747 (Table 1). This could be the result of the high prevalence of consanguineous marriages in Turkey (Say *et al.*, 1973).

In conclusion, it seems that in Turkey the incidence of PKU and hyperphenylalaninaemia is higher than in many other countries. A programme of routine screening for PKU can easily be justified by the preliminary data presented here.

REFERENCES

Bickel, H., Brandon, G. R., Cabalska, B. *et al.* Frequency of inborn errors of metabolism, especially PKU in some representative newborn screening centers around the world. A collaborative study. *Humangenetik* 30 (1975) 273–286

Dhondt, J. L. Tetrahydrobiopterin deficiencies. Preliminary analysis from an international survey. *J. Pediatr.* 104 (1984) 501–508

Guthrie, R. and Susi, A. A simple phenylalanine method for detecting phenylketonuria in large populations of newborn infants. *Pediatrics* 32 (1963) 328–343

Özalp, I., Tanzer, F., Hasanoğlu, A., Tuncer, M., Durmuş, Z. and Say, B. Türk Çocuklarında kalıtsal amino asit metabolizması bozukluklarının görülme sıklığı. *Doğa Bilim Dergisi* 7 (1983) 289–292

Say, B., Tunçbilek, E., Balcı, S., *et al.* Incidence of congenital malformations in a sample of Turkish population. *Hum. Hered.* 23 (1973) 434–441

Woolf, L. I. The high frequency of phenylketonuria in Ireland and Western Scotland. *J. Inher. Metab. Dis.* 1 (1978) 101–103

J. Inher. Metab. Dis. 9 Suppl. 2 (1986) 240-243

Short Communication

Atypical Phenylketonuria with Mild Mental Retardation Caused by Tetrahydrobiopterin Deficiency in a Chinese Family

K.-J. Hsiao[1], P.-C. Chiu[2], W.-H. Cheng[3] and S.-L. Chao[3]
Departments of [1]Medical Research and [2]Pediatrics, Veterans General Hospital; [3]Cheng Hsin Rehabilitation and Medical Center; Taipei, Taiwan 11217, Republic of China

Tetrahydrobiopterin (BH_4) is the cofactor for aromatic amino acid hydroxylases, including phenylalanine hydroxylase (EC 1.14.16.1) which is deficient in classical phenylketonuria (PKU, McKusick 26160). Most atypical PKU due to defects in biopterin metabolism have been reported to be very severe (Smith *et al.*, 1975) and have been described as 'malignant hyperphenylalaninaemia' (Danks *et al.*, 1979). The BH_4 deficiencies may be caused by deficient activity of dihydropteridine reductase (DHPR; EC 1.6.99.7; McKusick 26163), GTP cyclohydrolase I (EC 3.5.4.16), or 'dihydrobiopterin synthetase' (DHBS; McKusick 26164 and 26169) (Niederwieser *et al.*, 1982). Autosomal recessive inheritance is proved in DHPR deficiency, but is only suspected in DHBS deficiency (Dhondt, 1984). The incidence of BH_4 deficiency among hyperphenylalaninaemic babies was estimated to be 1.5–2% in the Caucasian population (Niederwieser *et al.*, 1982; Dhondt, 1984). Very few cases of PKU of Chinese origins have been reported (Hsiao *et al.*, 1984) and no case of BH_4 deficiency has been published.

We recently found two hyperphenylalaninaemic brothers, Y.S. (4.7 years old) and Y.C. (6.7 years old), from a Chinese family presenting with mild mental retardation (I.Q.: 53 and 65, respectively). They were both full-term normal spontaneously delivered well babies at birth, but delayed milestones were found gradually. They could not walk until 4 years old. Seizures began at about 1 year old. Although anticonvulsant drugs have been given since then, seizure activity persisted. They were referred to our special clinic for evaluation of their growth and psychomotor retardation. Neurological examination revealed decreased muscle tone, deep tendon reflex, and slurred speech. EEG revealed diffuse cerebral dysfunction. The parents have no consanguinity and their third boy is normal. We report here the clinical observations and biochemical evidence that these two patients have atypical PKU caused by defective synthesis of biopterin.

MATERIALS AND METHODS

The dry blood spot phenylalanine (Phe) was determined by the Guthrie test. The same specimen was used to assay the activity of DHPR by measuring the pterin-

Journal of Inherited Metabolic Disease. ISSN 0141–8955.

dependent reduction of NADH, by a method modified from Firgaira *et al.* (1979). Plasma Phe (Tocci, 1982) and tyrosine (Tyr) (Ambrose, 1977) were determined by fluorometric methods and by a LKB Alpha amino acid analyser. The urinary organic acids were analysed by gas chromatography (Hewlett Packard 5793A) according to Tanaka *et al.* (1980).

The BH_4 tablets (10 mg), neopterin, biopterin and other pteridines were obtained from Dr B. Schircks' Laboratories (Jona, Switzerland). Urinary pterins were analysed quantitatively by a reverse phase (C_{18}) high-performance liquid chromatographic (Shimadzu LC-3A) method (Niederwieser *et al.*, 1982). The oral BH_4 loading test (7.3–7.6 mg/kg body weight) was performed according to Niederwieser *et al.* (1982) after oral loading of Phe for 3 days. Blood was collected at 0.5, 1, 2, 4, 6, 8, 24 and 48 hours and urine at 4, 6, 24 and 48 hours after oral BH_4 intake.

RESULTS AND DISCUSSION

The results of the first blood spot Phe screening test performed in March 1984 were 10.8 mg/dl (Y.S.) and 9.0 mg/dl (Y.C.). Hyperphenylalaninaemia was confirmed by serum amino acid analysis (Phe 9.6 and 6.9 mg/dl), Tyr 1.1 and 1.3 mg/dl for Y.S. and Y.C., respectively). Although the results of urinary ferric chloride and 2,4-dinitrophenylhydrazine (DNPH) tests were negative or weakly positive, the diagnostic metabolites, phenylpyruvate (PPA), *o*-hydroxyphenylacetate (HPAA), phenylacetate, and phenyllactate (PLA), were demonstrated in the urine by gas chromatography. With oral loading of Phe (2200 mg/day; 140 mg/kg) for 3 days, the patients' blood Phe increased from 4.7–5.5 mg/dl to 13–18 mg/dl and acute clinical symptoms (drowsiness, drooling, muscle weakness, hypotonia, unable to stand up and slurred speech) appeared simultaneously. The blood Phe returned to 3–6 mg/dl 2 days after they went back to their normal diet (1100 mg Phe/day), and the clinical symptoms also disappeared. They were then diagnosed as a variant form of hyperphenylalaninaemia with relatively high biochemical tolerance and low clinical tolerance to Phe intake.

Following the diagnosis of the first case of malignant PKU caused by BH_4 deficiency in Taiwan (not yet published) and the establishment of BH_4 loading test and urinary pterin analysis, these patients were recalled for further evaluation in March 1985. Urinary pterin analysis showed that they had high neopterin (5000–18 900 μmol/mol creatinine), low biopterin (136–293 μmol/mol creatinine), and a low total biopterin ratio (biopterin/(biopterin+neopterin): 1.3–2.5%). They were orally loaded with Phe (1600–1700 mg/day; 90–100 mg/kg/day) for 4 days. On the morning of the 4th day their blood Phe values were 16.8 mg/dl (Y.S.) and 6.0 mg/dl (Y.C.) (Table 1), and the same acute clinical symptoms appeared again. Their blood Phe decreased drastically to normal (<2 mg/dl), the Phe/Tyr ratio was inverted (Table 1), and the clinical symptoms disappeared after oral intake of BH_4 (7.3–7.6 mg/kg) which was given to them on the morning of the 4th day. The uptake of BH_4 was confirmed by urinary pterin analysis (Table 1). DHPR deficiency was ruled out by the normal DHPR activities, 5.73 U/g haemoglobin (Y.S.) and

Table 1 Results of oral Phe and BH_4 loading tests for cases Y.S. and Y.C.

Tests	*Case Y.S.*			*Case Y.C.*			*Normal reference range (without loading)*
	Before Phe loading	*Before BH_4 loading**	*After BH_4 loading†*	*Before Phe loading*	*Before BH_4 loading**	*After BH_4 loading†*	
Plasma Phe (mg/dl)	4.4	16.8	1.1	6.8	6.0	1.0	0.6–2.2
Plasma Tyr (mg/dl)	1.2	1.5	2.9	1.3	1.1	1.6	1.4–3.4
Urinary analysis							
$FeCl_3$ test	–	+	–	–	–	–	–
DNPH test	–	+	–	–	±	–	–
Gas chromatography	–	HPAA, PLA, PPA	HPAA, PPA	–	–	–	–
Neopterin (μmol/mol creatinine)	5340	18 939	14 526	18 902	13 285	5276	377–2045
Biopterin (μmol/mol creatinine)	136	293	6988	252	308	2900	549–1837
Total biopterin ratio (%)	2.5	1.5	32.5	1.3	2.3	35.5	43–76

* Oral Phe intake 1600–1700 mg/day for 4 days, and the BH_4 (7.3–7.6 mg/kg) were loaded orally on the morning of the 4th day.
† Four hours after BH_4 loading.

5.52 U/g haemoglobin (Y.C.) (reference range: 2.78–8.70), found in the dry blood spots. Because of objection from the parents, their CSF was not sampled.

After establishing the diagnosis of biopterin synthesis deficiency, both patients were put on a low-Phe diet (Phe 50–53 mg/kg/day, protein 30–40 g/day, and 1500 kcal/day), using 'Lofenalac' and normal local food. Since the diet alone could not keep their blood Phe below 2 mg/dl, we gave them BH_4 tablets, 10 mg/day (0.5–0.6 mg/kg/day) for supplementation. Their blood Phe has thus been controlled within the normal range. Three months later, physical examination revealed the same growth percentile, but neurological improvement was observed by normalized muscle tone and the seizures could be controlled by anticonvulsant drugs. The long-term effect of the limited–controlled diet with small supplement doses of BH_4 remains to be established.

The data indicate that these are cases of atypical PKU due to defective synthesis of biopterin. Further study is needed to reveal which enzyme is defective in the 'DHBS' system. There was a relatively high tolerance of serum Phe in response to Phe intake, but a low clinical tolerance of serum Phe level. This suggests that the boys may have a partial deficient form of defective synthesis of the cofactor as described by Dhondt (1984). It also indicates that the atypical PKU is not always 'malignant', the atypical PKU may be even milder than classical ones (Dhondt, 1984; Hoganson *et al.*, 1984). The low clinical tolerance of serum Phe level is worth further study, which may elucidate the neurological effect of hyperphenylalaninaemia and its interaction with BH_4 metabolism and other neurotransmitters.

Our experience with classical and atypical PKU demonstrates that PKU in China may be not as rare as we thought (Hsiao *et al.*, 1984) and the incidence of atypical

PKU in hyperphenylalaninaemic patients may be higher than that in Caucasians. A nationwide neonatal screening program with proper differential diagnosis for early detection and treatment of PKU to prevent mental retardation and to understand its prevalence in the Chinese population is highly indicated.

ACKNOWLEDGEMENTS

We wish to thank Ms. S.-J. Wu, T.-T. Liu and L. Wang for their technical assistance and Ms. S.-L. Yeh for the dietary management. This work is supported in part by National Science Council (NSC–74–0412–B075–24), and a grant from the Department of Health, Executive Yuan, Republic of China.

REFERENCES

Ambrose, J. A. Fluorometric measurement of tyrosine in serum and plasma. In Cooper, G. R. (ed.) *Selected Methods of Clinical Chemistry*, Vol. 8, American Association for Clinical Chemistry, Washington DC, 1977, pp. 183–188

Danks, D. M., Schlesinger, P., Firgaira, F., Cotton, R. G. H., Watson, B. M., Rembold, H. and Hennings, G. Malignant hyperphenylalaninaemia – Clinical features, biochemical findings, and experience with administration of biopterins. *Pediatr. Res.* 13 (1979) 1150–1155

Dhondt, J.-L. Tetrahydrobiopterin deficiencies: preliminary analysis from an international survey. *J. Pediatr.* 104 (1984) 501–508

Firgaira, F. A., Cotton, R. G. H. and Danks, D. M. Human dihydropteridine reductase. A method for the measurement of activity in cultured cells, and its application to malignant hyperphenylalaninaemia. *Clin. Chim. Acta* 95 (1979) 47–59

Hoganson, G., Berlow, S., Kaufman, S., Milstein, S., Schuett, V., Matalon, R., Naylor, E. and Seifert, W. Biopterin synthesis defects: Problems in diagnosis. *Pediatrics* 74 (1984) 1004–1011

Hsiao, K.-J., Wuu, K.-D., Sheen, F.-M., Feng, W.-C. and Ting, W.-K. Congenital metabolic diseases in mentally retarded Chinese children: screening for congenital hypothyroidism, phenylketonuria, galactosemia, maple syrup urine disease and homocystinuria. *Chin. Med. J.* 34 (1984) 31–32

Niederwieser, A., Matasovic, A., Staudenmann, W., Wang, M. and Curtius, H.-C. Screening for tetrahydrobiopterin deficiency. In Wachter, H., Curtius, H.-C. and Pfleiderer, W. (eds.) *Biochemical and Clinical Aspects of Pterins*. Vol. 1, Walter de Gruyter, Berlin, 1982, pp. 293–306

Smith, I., Clayton, B. E. and Wolff, O. H. New variant of phenylketonuria with progressive neurological illness unresponsive to phenylalanine restriction. *Lancet* 1 (1975) 1108–1111

Tanaka, K., Hine, D. G. and West-Dull, A. Gas chromatographic method of analysis for urinary organic acids. Retention indices of 155 metabolically important compounds. *Clin. Chem.* 26 (1980) 1839–1846

Tocci, P. M. Phenylalanine, fluorometric methods. In Faulkner, W. R. and Meites, S. (eds.) *Selected Methods of Clinical Chemistry*, Vol. 9, American Association for Clinical Chemistry, Washington DC, 1982, pp. 305–311

J. Inher. Metab. Dis. 9 Suppl. 2 (1986) 244–246

Short Communication

Dihydropteridine Reductase Deficiency: Clinical, Biochemical and Therapeutic Aspects

R. Cerone, S. Scalisi, M. Cotellessa, M. C. Schiaffino, U. Caruso and C. Romano
University Department of Pediatrics 'R', G. Gaslini Institute, Via 5 Maggio, 39, Genova, Italy

Inborn errors of biopterin metabolism are detected in 1–3% of patients with hyperphenylalaninaemia and appear to result from a deficiency of dihydropteridine reductase (DHPR, EC 1.6.99.7) (Kaufmann *et al.*, 1975) or dihydrobiopterin synthetase (Bartholomè *et al.*, 1977) or GPT-cyclohydrolase (EC 3.5.4.16) (Niederwieser *et al.*, 1982). In addition to hyperphenylalaninaemia, most infants and children with congenital defects of biopterin metabolism have decreased levels of neurotransmitter metabolites in CSF.

The clinical, biochemical and therapeutic aspects of an Italian patient with DHPR deficiency are reported.

CASE REPORT

The patient (S.F.), a male infant born at term after uncomplicated pregnancy, is the third child of healthy and unrelated parents. The first child, a female, is well; the second child died at 6 months with neurologic complications. The patient was admitted to our division at the age of 13 months. Slowing of developmental milestones and episodes of eye rolling and disturbance of consciousness were reported by the parents from 4 months. Neurological examination revealed severe psychomotory retardation, (IQ 48) and hypotonia.

Table 1 Biochemical findings in patient S.F.*

	Plasma Phe	*Urine* (mmol/mol of creatinine)			*CSF* (nmol/1)			
	(μmol/1)	*N*	*B*	*BNCR*	*HVA*	*5-HIAA*	*B*	*N*
Patient	845	2.15	10.7	889	117	12.1	42	9.11
Controls	42–74	0.51	1.1	13–66	250–880	110–360	10–34	9–20

* Abbreviations used are: N, neopterin; B, biopterin; BNCR, biopterin-neopterin ratio ($[B/C]\cdot[B/(B+N)]\cdot 10^{-5}$); HVA, homovanillic acid; 5–HIAA, 5–hydroxyindoleacetic acid.

Journal of Inherited Metabolic Disease. ISSN 0141–8955.

Biochemical findings are shown in Table 1. Urinary biopterins excretion was found to be very high. DHPR activity was extremely low in liver biopsy and absent in dried blood spots. Homovanillic acid (HVA) and 5-hydroxyindoleacetic acid (5-HIAA) levels were very low in CSF. No significant decrease in serum phenylalanine was observed after tetrahydrobiopterin (BH_4) load.

MATERIALS AND METHODS

Plasma amino acids were determined by ion exchange chromatography. Tetrahydrobiopterin loading tests were performed by oral administration of 7.5 mg of BH_4 per kg body weight after overnight fasting, with measurement of plasma phenylalanine and tyrosine at zero, 4 and 8 h after the load. Total pterins in urine and HVA and 5–HIAA in CSF were analysed by high-performance liquid chromatography (we thank Dr A. Niederwieser, Zurich). DHPR activity was measured in liver biopsy (we thank Dr K. Bartholomè, Bochum) and in dried blood spots according to Arai *et al.* (1982).

RESULTS AND DISCUSSION

Despite good control of plasma phenylalanine level on the restricted diet (700 mg of phenylalanine per day) there was no clinical improvement. Thereafter dietary treatment with neurotransmitter therapy was started (Dopa 9 mg/kg^{-1} day^{-1}; Carbidopa 1 mg kg^{-1} day^{-1} 5-hydroxytryptophan 7 mg kg^{-1}day^{-1}). Under this therapy, 8 months later, muscular tone had improved considerably and IQ was 60. HVA and 5-HIAA levels in CSF were normalized.

Improvement of neurological signs with neurotransmitter replacement therapy is known, but still not discussed (Danks *et al.*, 1978; Fukuda *et al.*, 1985). In our patient such therapy did not produce adverse effects. Monitoring of neurotransmitter levels in CSF during treatment with neurotransmitter precursors is of paramount importance.

REFERENCES

Arai, N., Narisawa, K., Hayakawa, H. and Tada, K. Hyperphenylalaninemia due to dihydropteridine reductase deficiency; diagnosis by enzyme assay on dried blood spots. *Pediatrics* 98 (1982) 426–430

Bartholomè, K., Byrd, D. J., Kaufmann, S. and Milstein, S. Atypical phenylketonuria with normal phenylalanine hydroxylase and dihydropteridinereductase activity in vitro. *Pediatrics* 59 (1977) 757–761

Danks, D. M., Bartholomè, K., Clayton, B. E., Curtius, H., Grobe, H. and Rey, F. Malignant hyperphenylalaninaemia-Current status (June, 1977). *J. Inher. Metab. Dis.* 1 (1978) 49–53

Fukuda, K., Tanaka, T., Hyodo, S., Kobayashi, Y. and Usui, T. Hyperphenylalaninaemia due to impaired dihydrobiopterin biosynthesis: leukocyte function and effect of tetrahydrobiopterin therapy. *J. Inher. Metab. Dis.* 8 (1985) 49–52

Kaufmann, S., Holtzmann, N. A., Milstein, S., Butler, I. J. and Krumholz, A. Phenylketonuria due to a deficiency of dihydropteridine reductase. *N. Engl. J. Med.* 293 (1975) 785–790

Niederwieser, A., Staudenmam, W., Wang, M., Curtius, H., Atares, M. and Crdesa-Garcia, J. Hyperphenylalaninemia with neopterin deficiency. A new enzyme defect presumably of GPT-cyclohydrolase. *Eur. J. Pediatr.* 138 (1982) 97

J. Inher. Metab. Dis. 9 Suppl. 2 (1986) 247–249

Short Communication

Partial Dihydropteridine Reductase Deficiency and Mental Retardation

A. SAHOTA[1], R. J. LEEMING[2], J. A. BLAIR[1], R. A. ARMSTRONG[1], A. GREEN[3] and B. E. COHEN[4]
[1]*University of Aston, Birmingham B4 7ET, UK;* [2]*General Hospital, Birmingham, UK;* [3]*Children's Hospital, Birmingham, UK;* [4]*Chaim Sheba Medical Centre, Tel-Hashomer, Israel*

A complete deficiency of dihydropteridine reductase (DHPR, EC 1.6.99.7) leads to severe mental retardation, hyperphenylalaninaemia, and depletion of cellular tetrahydrobiopterin in childhood (McKusick 26163). It is not clear at present whether a partial deficiency of this enzyme is associated with any degree of mental retardation. As part of a study on tetrahydrobiopterin metabolism in mental disease, we have measured DHPR activity in blood from children with a variety of neurological and mental disorders. Our findings are presented here.

PATIENTS AND METHODS

The patients, aged up to 12 years, were under the care of one of us (BEC). The nature of mental retardation and the number of children in each group are given in Table 1. Children in groups 1–6 had normal levels of blood phenylalanine. Group 7 contained children with hyperphenylalaninaemia; the vast majority of these were cases of classical PKU on a low protein diet. The siblings and parents

Table 1 Comparison of DHPR activity in blood from control children and children with a variety of mental disorders

Group	*DHPR* (nmol NADH min^{-1}(ml blood)$^{-1}$)				
	No.	*Range*	*Mean*	*SD*	*t test*
1 Control	17	61–278	184	52	—
2 IMR	12	70–197	128	43	Significant at 1%
3 FMR	11	89–301	185	71	Not significant at 5%
4 UNS	12	31–234	127	69	Significant at 5%
5 MBD	5	74–154	123	34	Significant at 5%
6 Autism	7	38–181	119	48	Significant at 1%
7 HPA	33	43–323	132	59	Significant at 1%

IMR Idiopathic mental retardation; FMR Familial mental retardation;
UNS Unusual neurological syndromes; MBD Minimal brain dysfunction;
HPA Hyperphenylalaninaemia

Journal of Inherited Metabolic Disease. ISSN 0141–8955.

of some of these children, as well as eight adult obligate heterozygotes for DHPR deficiency, were also examined. DHPR activity was measured in dried blood spots as previously described (Sahota *et al.*, 1985).

RESULTS

Enzyme activity in the various patient groups is compared with control children in Table 1. The mean activity was significantly reduced (Student's *t* test) in: idiopathic mental retardation (1%); unusual neurological syndromes (5%); minimal brain dysfunction (5%); autism (1%); and hyperphenylalaninaemia (1%). There was no significant reduction in activity in familial mental retardation.

Enzyme activity was abnormally low (31 nmol $min^{-1} ml^{-1}$) in an 8.5-year-old girl (OE) with an unusual neurological syndrome comprising ataxia, mild mental retardation and cataract. A mildly affected 2.5-year-old brother (BZE), but without cataract, and a 4.5-year-old normal sibling (SE) had activities (56 and 60 nmol $min^{-1} ml^{-1}$ respectively) at the lower end of the normal range for children. Enzyme activity in the parents (father 92 and mother 89 nmol $min^{-1} ml^{-1}$) was also towards the lower end of the normal range for adults (155±41 nmol $min^{-1} ml^{-1}$, n=110). Enzyme activity was also low (38 nmol $min^{-1} ml^{-1}$) in a 2.7-year-old child with autism (AZE), and again the parents had activities (father 91 and mother 85 nmol $min^{-1} ml^{-1}$) towards the lower end of the normal adult range. DHPR activity in eight adult obligate heterozygotes was 71±25 nmol $min^{-1} ml^{-1}$ (range 20–97).

DISCUSSION

DHPR activity was significantly reduced in some neurological and mental disorders compared with control subjects. Enzyme activity was markedly low in a child with an unusual neurological syndrome and in another with autism. We have previously observed low DHPR activity in three children with varying degrees of neurological and mental deficiency (RW, RK and SH; 39, 63, and 61 nmol $min^{-1} ml^{-1}$, respectively) (unpublished observations). A partial reduction in DHPR activity has also been reported in two children with hyperphenylalaninaemia and progressive mental deterioration (Grobe *et al.*, 1978; Nakabayashi *et al.*, 1984).

The enzyme activity values in our five patients were similar to those in the eight heterozygotes for DHPR deficiency. However, the finding of partial DHPR deficiency with associated mental retardation suggests that there might be a possible link between these two conditions. Some support for this is provided by the finding of abnormally low levels of the serotonin metabolite, 5-hydroxyindole-3-acetic acid, in the cerebrospinal fluid from patients OE and BZE (Dr K. Hyland, London, personal communication). Further investigations are required to ascertain the relationship between partial DHPR deficiency and mental retardation.

This work was supported by a grant from the Medical Research Council.

REFERENCES

Grobe, K., Bartholome, K., Milstien, S. and Kaufman, S. Hyperphenylalaninaemia due to dihydropteridine reductase deficiency. *Eur. J. Pediatr.* 129 (1978) 93–98

Nakabayashi, H., Owada, M., Yoshida, Y., Sakiyama, T. and Kitagawa, T. Clinical and biochemical study of mild dihydropteridine reductase deficiency (abstract). *22nd Annual SSIEM Symposium* (1984), Newcastle, UK

Sahota, A., Blair, J. A., Barford, P. A., Leeming, R. J., Green, A. and Pollitt, R. J. Neonatal screening for dihydropteridine reductase deficiency. *J. Inher. Metab. Dis.* 8 Suppl. 2 (1985) 99–100

J. Inher. Metab. Dis. 9 Suppl. 2 (1986) 250–253

Short Communication

Urine Amino Acid Analysis by HPLC in the Investigation of Inborn Errors of Metabolism

J. M. LEAH[1], T. PALMER[1], M. GRIFFIN[1], C. J. WINGAD[1], A. BRIDDON[2] and V. G. OBERHOLZER[2]
[1]*Department of Life Sciences, Trent Polytechnic, Nottingham NG11 8NS, UK;*
[2]*Clinical Chemistry Department, Queen Elizabeth Hospital for Children, London E2 8PS, UK*

Reversed-phase high performance liquid chromatography (HPLC) of *o*-phthalaldehyde (OPA) derivatives provides a technique that is readily applicable to the estimation of free amino acids (Turnell and Cooper, 1982; Griffin *et al.*, 1982; Price *et al.*, 1984; Palmer, 1985). It has the advantage over classical ion-exchange chromatography of rapidity, increased sensitivity and the ability to handle small sample sizes, utilizing apparatus which is not dedicated to one technique. In previous reports we have described the application of the procedure to amino acid analysis of plasma specimens from normal individuals (Griffin *et al.*, 1982) and from patients with inborn errors of metabolism (Palmer, 1985). Here we describe its application to the screening of urine samples for suspected amino acid disorders.

PATIENTS AND METHODS

All patients with inborn errors of metabolism had previously been diagnosed by other procedures, including thin layer and/or ion exchange chromatography.

The HPLC system was essentially that described by Griffin *et al.* (1982). A Zorbax C_8 column was employed using a linear gradient from 20% to 90% methanol. Gradients were formed from two solvents: potassium acetate buffer (0.02 mol/l, pH 5.5) and methanol. Both solvents contained 1% (v/v) tetrahydrofuran. A flow-rate of 1.8 ml/min was employed, eluting most amino acids within 25 min.

The derivatization procedure was that described by Price *et al.* (1984), which gives greater sensitivity than that previously employed. Immediately before use, 250 μl of OPA reagent (60 mg/10 ml methanol) was added to 250 μl 0.4 mol/l boric acid buffer, pH 9.4, and 25 μl 2-mercaptoethanol; 250 μl of this mixture was vortex-mixed with 25 μl prepared sample for 2 min, and then a 10 μl aliquot removed and applied to the column. For urine amino acid analysis, 70–170 μl urine was mixed with 1 ml of methanol and centrifuged; 25 μl supernatant was then treated with reagent as described above.

RESULTS AND DISCUSSION

It was found that the technique which had been used for plasma amino acid analysis could be applied without modification for the analysis of amino acids in urine.

Journal of Inherited Metabolic Disease. ISSN 0141-8955. Queen Square, Lancaster, UK. Printed in Great Britain by Titus Wilson & Son Ltd., Kendal.

Ammonia may first be removed from the urine, if required, by rotary evaporation or vacuum desiccation after the specimen has been made slightly alkaline with NaOH. However, the ammonia peak does not interfere with the analysis of any amino acid normally present in urine so that prior removal of ammonia is not essential; for simplicity this step was not incorporated into the procedure used here. The total analysis time, including derivatization, was less than 30 min even with the inclusion of two isocratic stages in the linear solvent gradient. These isocratic stages could be removed with only a slight deterioration in performance.

A series of urine specimens from patients with known disorders of amino acid metabolism all gave clearly abnormal results when analysed by this procedure. A specimen from a patient with argininosuccinic aciduria (ASAuria) (McKusick 20790) gave a large peak in the ASA position, retention time approximately 4 min, where no significant peak occurs in a normal urine (Figure 1). Urine from a patient with α-amino-adipic aciduria (McKusick 24513) had an equally conspicuous peak in the α-amino-adipic acid position, retention time about 6 min. The abnormal ornithine peak in a specimen from a patient who had hyperornithinaemia with gyrate atrophy (McKusick 25887) was not in itself so conspicuous, but the ornithine/lysine ratio was clearly far in excess of normal. A δ-lactam is present in the urine of patients with hyperornithinaemia, but this co-elutes with ammonia, so it is not easily detectable by this technique, especially since the procedure which may be used to remove ammonia also removes the δ-lactam.

A urine specimen from a patient with aspartylglycosaminuria (McKusick 20840) gave a conspicuous peak with a retention time of approximately 5 min, presumably *N*-acetylglucosaminyl-asparagine. The abnormalities in a specimen from a patient with hyperargininaemia (McKusick 20780) were not conspicuous, since the arginine concentrations found in this disorder are not particularly high in absolute terms, and arginine elutes in a crowded portion of the chromatogram. Nevertheless, a distinct arginine peak was detectable between threonine and taurine, and the glutamine and lysine peaks were relatively high in comparison to the other peaks.

Two urine specimens from patients with other disorders were also investigated. One from a patient with fumaric aciduria showed no obvious amino acid abnormalities; one from a patient who had xanthinuria with sulphite oxidase deficiency gave a conspicuous peak in the taurine position and another in the leucine region.

The value of this technique in screening for amino acid disorders is clearly apparent. It has a big advantage over paper or thin-layer chromatography in that it is fully quantitative, and its only significant disadvantage when compared to conventional ion exchange chromatography is its inability to detect the amino acids proline and hydroxyproline. Our preliminary studies suggested that the reagent might react with urea (Griffin *et al*., 1982), but we have now established that this is not the case. It detects only substances with primary amino groups, so is more selective than conventional amino acid analysis, and may be complementary to this technique.

REFERENCES

Griffin, M., Price, S. J. and Palmer, T. A rapid and sensitive procedure for the quantitative determination of plasma amino acids. *Clin. Chim. Acta* 125 (1982) 89–95

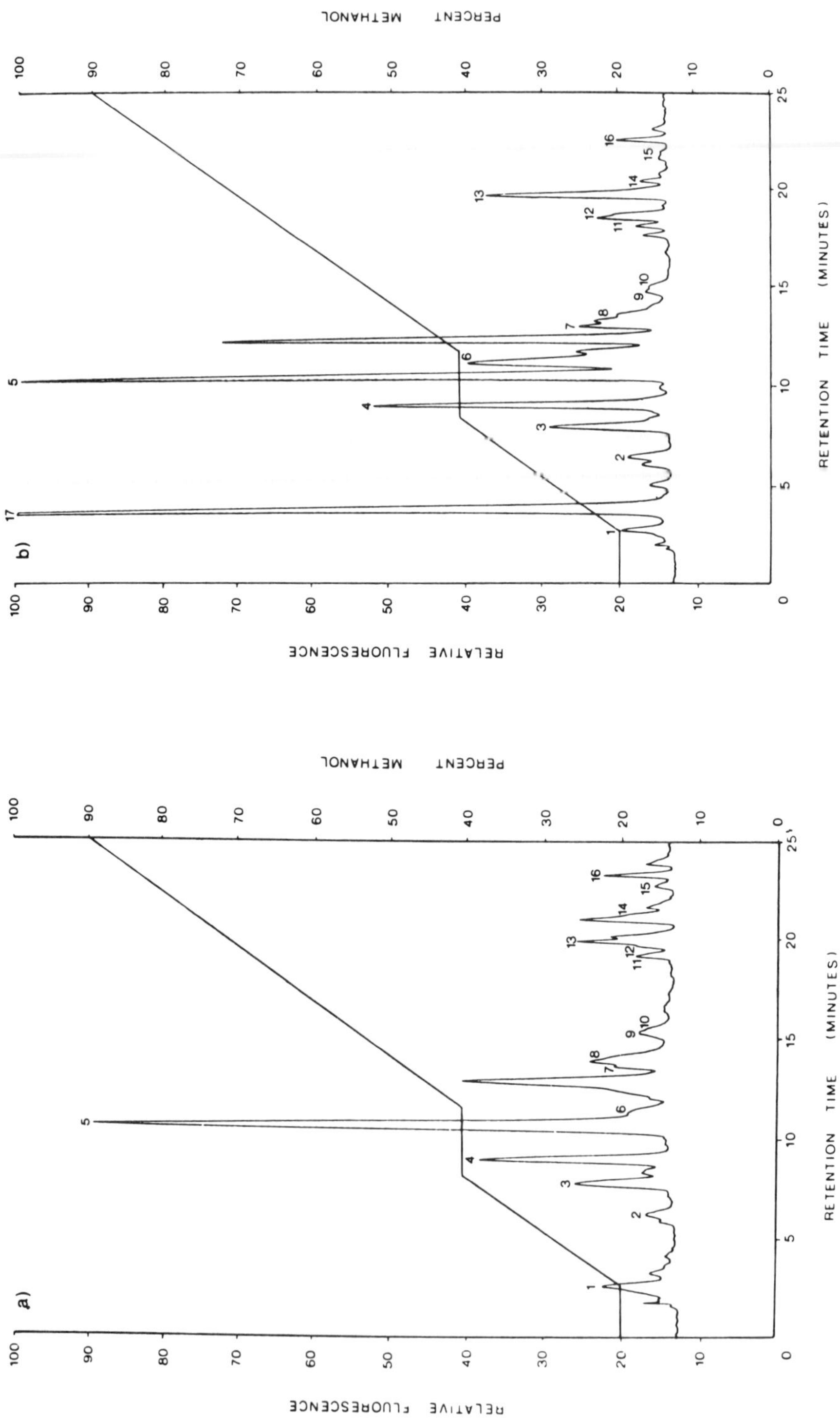

Figure 1 HPLC amino acid chromatograms, obtained using the method described in the text, from (a) a normal urine and (b) a urine specimen from a patient with ASAuria. Peak 1, aspartate; 2, asparagine; 3, serine; 4, glutamine; 5, glycine; 6, threonine; 7, alanine; 8, tyrosine; 9, β-amino-isobutyrate; 10, α-amino-*n*-butyrate; 11, valine; 12, phenylalanine; 13, ammonia; 14, leucine; 15, ornithine; 16, lysine; 17, argininosuccinate. The main peak between threonine and alanine is taurine.

Palmer, T. Amino acid analysis: reversed-phase HPLC compared to other techniques. *Chromatog. Internat.* 6 (1985) 5–6

Price, S. J., Palmer, T. and Griffin, M. High-speed assay of amino acids using reversed-phase liquid chromatography. *Chromatographia* 18 (1984) 62–64

Turnell, D. C. and Cooper, J. D. H. Rapid assay for amino acids in serum or urine by pre-column derivatisation and reversed-phase liquid chromatography. *Clin. Chem.* 28 (1982) 527–531

J. Inher. Metab. Dis. 9 Suppl. 2 (1986) 254–256

Short Communication

Plasma Amino Acid Patterns in Critically Ill Children

A. BRIDDON and V. G. OBERHOLZER
Department of Clinical Biochemistry, The Queen Elizabeth Hospital for Children, Hackney Road, London E2 8PS

The usefulness of plasma amino acid levels as an indicator of suspected metabolic disease in the critically ill infant may be diminished as a result of physiological changes occurring in the preterminal state. Early studies have shown that blood amino nitrogen is increased in the premortal phase (Kirk, 1968) and increases in individual plasma amino acids have been reported in patients with traumatic shock (Labrosse *et al.*, 1967). However, guidelines on the interpretation of such results in infants with suspected metabolic disease are lacking in the literature.

Amino acid levels were measured in plasma from seven infants in a premortal state and in four postmortem specimens. Clinical and biochemical evidence did not indicate any specific metabolic defect in these patients. The results have been compared with those obtained from severely ill infants with confirmed amino acid disorders. Analyses were carried out on a Locarte analyser using sodium buffers (Palmer *et al.*, 1973) and the data are summarized in Table 1.

RESULTS AND DISCUSSION

There is a marked similarity between the amino acid pattern of the premortal and postmortem groups, although individual levels fall within a wide range. In every case the glutamine and alanine levels are significantly raised and other amino acids, proline, methionine, lysine, aminobutyrate and tyrosine are frequently elevated. The branched chain amino acids and citrulline and arginine, were generally within normal limits.

The similarity between these two groups suggests that the abnormal patterns found in the premortal cases are the result of secondary changes taking place. The terminal elevation of plasma amino acids has been attributed to autolysis and leakage from cells (Labrosse *et al.*, 1967). That these changes can occur rapidly was shown in case 2 (premortal group), where blood was taken 20 min after sudden collapse and immediate resuscitation. All amino acid levels had returned to normal 24 h later.

The results obtained from seven patients with Reye syndrome (Table 1), which confirm those reported by others (Romshe *et al.*, 1981), also show a close resemblance to those found in the premortal phase. It is probable that the raised aminobutyrate thought to be a good indicator of Reye syndrome may be the result of secondary changes occurring *in extremis*.

Journal of Inherited Metabolic Disease. ISSN 0141–8955.

Table 1 Plasma amino acid concentrations ($\mu mol\,l^{-1}$)

	Premortal		*Postmortem*		*Moribund citrullinaemia*	*Reye syndrome*		*Concentrations in relevant disorder*
	Mean	*(Range)*	*Mean*	*(Range)*		*Mean*	*(Range)*	
Tau	318	(51–829)	330	(129–524)	180	371	(24–1195)	
Thr	299	(156–612)	232	(74–379)	177	161	(35–327)	
Ser	208	(110–439)	233	(110–312)	310	161	(45–285)	
Gln	1285	(909–2240)	1318	(681–1640)	2889	1219	(487–2250)	
Glu	129	(40–252)	424	(236–853)	176	427	(99–840)	
Pro	855	(391–1645)	521	(395–670)	384	404	(35–806)	
Cit	25	(14–47)	8	(trace–20)	1807	34	(23–61)	1807–2171[a]
Gly	571	(328–1140)	712	(427–1228)	602	420	(218–709)	
Ala	1568	(890–3179)	1269	(938–1595)	1979	1075	(535–1995)	
Abu	73	(30–112)	27	(9–50)	100	58	(20–100)	
Val	429	(393–506)	385	(322–444)	199	303	(157–557)	378–975[b]
Met	88	(60–172)	90	(58–145)	98	65	(39–91)	577–872[c]
Ile	123	(100–156)	141	(118–160)	61	100	(51–161)	328–495[b]
Leu	277	(188–372)	299	(236–366)	132	246	(104–499)	678–1943[b]
Tyr	286	(121–601)	180	(98–277)	255	175	(95–283)	1271–1713[c]
Phe	219	(106–293)	182	(93–286)	57	210	(83–351)	
His	163	(91–335)	170	(121–218)	129	169	(73–425)	
Orn	154	(71–263)	319	(220–384)	31	166	(48–279)	
Lys	436	(251–642)	673	(436–946)	664	632	(238–1202)	
Arg	89	(ND–148)	16	(ND–50)	41	53	(5–106)	

Premortal: Case 1–pneumonia, 30 min before death; Case 2–bronchiolitis and cardiac failure, recovered; Case 3–collapse, shock ? cause; Case 4–acidosis, shock ? cause; Case 5–grey baby syndrome, recovered; Case 6–malrotation, cardiac arrest, perished; Case 7–TOF, perished
Postmortem: Case 1–cot death; Case 2–trisomy 13; Case 3–pulmonary haemorrhage; Case 4–undiagnosed
Reye syndrome cases: 7 patients including 5 histologically proven
[a] Citrullinaemia; [b] maple syrup urine disease; [c] tyrosinaemia
ND; not detectable

The problem exists of distinguishing the effects of secondary changes following poor circulation, hypoxia and tissue breakdown (Haan and Danks, 1981) from those due to genetic disorders of metabolism. Grossly increased levels of methionine, tyrosine, lysine and especially glutamine and alanine may suggest to the unwary a primary metabolic disorder and in particular one of the urea cycle. The ammonia levels were measured in four out of the seven premortal cases studied and were only moderately raised (100–300 $\mu mol\,l^{-1}$), whereas a case of haemophilia in hypovolaemic shock, in whom amino acid levels were not quantitated, had a plasma ammonia of 900 $\mu mol\,l^{-1}$. Ammonia estimation alone in the collapsed child may therefore be misleading. In patients prior to death, elevated glutamine, alanine and ammonia levels as part of a generally abnormal amino acid pattern do not provide sufficient evidence for a diagnosis of ornithine transcarbamylase deficiency (McKusick 31125) or carbamoyl phosphate synthetase deficiency (McKusick 23730).

Certain amino acidopathies may be more confidently diagnosed despite distortion of the plasma amino acid pattern due to terminal secondary changes. This is well illustrated by a case of citrullinaemia (McKusick 21570), (Table 1 and Bennett *et al.*, 1984).

Other metabolic disorders which may also be distinguishable are tyrosinaemia Type I (McKusick 27670), maple syrup urine disease (McKusick 24860) (Table 1), and possibly argininosuccinic aciduria (McKusick 20790), by a significantly increased citrulline level; and hyperornithinaemia (McKusick 23897). These conditions may be diagnosed on blood taken in a life-threatening situation and postmortem.

We would like to thank Dr Martin Bellman for providing plasma from some of the cases of Reye syndrome.

REFERENCES

Bennett, M. J., Dear, P. R. F., McGinlay, J. M. and Gray, R. G. F. Acute neonatal citrullinaemia. *J. Inher. Metab. Dis.* 7 (1984) 85

Haan, E. A. and Danks, D. M. Clinical investigation of suspected metabolic disease. In Barson, A. J. (ed.) *Laboratory Investigation of Fetal Disease*. J. Wright, Bristol, 1981, pp. 410–428

Kirk, J. E. Premortal clinical biochemical changes. In Bodansky, O. and Stewart, C. P. (eds.) *Advances in Clinical Chemistry*, Vol. 11. Academic Press, London, 1968, pp. 175–212

Labrosse, E. H., Beech, J. A., McLaughlin, J. S., Mansberger, A. R., Keene, W. D. and Cowley, R. A. Plasma amino acids in normal humans and patients with shock. *Surg. Gynecol. Obstet.* 125 (1967) 516–520

Palmer, T., Rossiter, M. A., Levin, B. and Oberholzer, V. G. The effect of protein loads on plasma amino acid levels. *Clin. Sci. Mol. Med.* 45 (1973) 827–832

Romshe, C. A., Hilty, M. D., McClung, H. J., Kerzner, B. and Reiner, C. B. Amino acid pattern in Reye syndrome: Comparison with clinically similar entities. *J. Pediatr.* 98 (1981) 788–790

J. Inher. Metab. Dis. 9 *Suppl.* 2 *(1986) 257–261*

Short Communication

Treatment of Hereditary Tyrosinaemia (Fumarylacetoacetase Deficiency) by Enzyme Substitution

B. LINDBLAD[1], J. FRIDÉN[2], J. GRETER[2], E. HOLME[2], S. LINDSTEDT[2] and C. SIÖSTEEN[3]
[1]*Department of Pediatrics, Mölndal's Hospital, S-431 80 Mölndal, Sweden;* [2]*Department of Clinical Chemistry, Gothenburg University, Sahlgren's Hospital, S-413 45 Gothenburg, Sweden;* [3]*Blood Centre, Sahlgren's Hospital, S-413 45 Gothenburg, Sweden*

Dietary treatment in hereditary tyrosinaemia (McKusick 27670) has repeatedly been shown to decrease or heal the renal tubular damage, but the effect on the progressive liver disease has been variable. Despite dietary treatment about 20% of Swedish patients have died before the age of 1 year (Lindblad *et al.*, unpublished). Hepatomas develop in about 40% for those surviving the first years (Weinberg *et al.*, 1976). Even patients treated with a diet from the time of diagnosis get hepatomas. Liver transplantation is so far the only definite treatment, and today the aim of other therapeutic regimens should be to bring the patient up to an age and time when liver transplantation is possible.

The primary defect in hereditary tyrosinaemia is a deficiency of fumarylacetoacetase (EC 3.7.1.2) (Lindblad *et al.*, 1977; Fällström *et al.*, 1979). In patients, lowactivities of this enzyme have been found even in tissues not damaged by the disease process (Kvittingen *et al.*, 1983). We have recently shown that fumarylacetoacetase is present in normal erythrocytes and that patients have low activities (Holme *et al.*, 1985). We therefore suggested that enzyme substitution by erythrocyte exchange transfusion might be beneficial to patients with hereditary tyrosinaemia.

To test this hypothesis we have performed blood exchange transfusions in three cases aged 4, 10 and 12 years.

PATIENTS

Case S.J. – A boy born 1972. He has been treated with a diet since diagnosis at 6 months of age, is presently in an excellent general health and has normal values for standard liver enzymes and P-Simplastin-A® (measuring coagulation factors II, VII and X), but still has an increased S-α-fetoprotein concentration, 0.7–1.2 mg/l (ref. value <0.015 mg/l).

Case M.S. – A girl born 1980, on dietary treatment since diagnosis at 6 months of age, but still with signs of active regenerating liver disease (S-ASAT 1.0–0.8 μkat/l,

Journal of Inherited Metabolic Disease. ISSN 0141–8955.

P-Simplastin-A® 37–65% (ref. value 70–130%), S-α-fetoprotein concentration 8–18 mg/l).

Case F.P. – A boy born 1975, also on dietary treatment since diagnosis at 7 months of age. He has no signs of progressing liver disease, i.e. normal values for S-bilirubin, S-ASAT, S-ALAT, and S-α-fetoprotein. P-Simplastin-A® is only slightly subnormal (57–66%).

PROCEDURE

Donor blood was antibody-negative for hepatitis B, HTLV-III and when indicated cytomegalovirus. The donor blood contained no antigen not present in the patient's blood of the Rh (CcDEe), Kell (Kk) or Duffy (Fya) types. It was also less than 1 week old and had a comparatively high erythrocyte fumarylacetoacetase activity. Exchange transfusions corresponding to 30–50% of the estimated blood volume of the patient were performed during 2–3 days. The effect of the treatment was followed, when possible, by weekly controls of blood and 24 h urine collections.

RESULTS

The first exchange transfusion was performed in case S.J. The effect on the variables reflecting tyrosine metabolism (S-tyrosine, tU-phenolic acids, tU-succinylacetoacetate plus succinylacetone) or the factors reflecting liver damage (S-α-fetoprotein) or renal tubular damage (tU-β_2-microglobulin) was followed weekly. The values after the transfusion are compared in Figure 1 with the basal period, which was taken as all values during the preceding year. All values decreased after the transfusion with the maximal effect observed 5–10 weeks after the transfusion. During this period S-tyrosine became normal or subnormal (85–22 μmol/l) and the excretion of phenolic acids was normalized (<10 mmol/mol creatinine). Such low values had never been found during the previous 12 years of dietary treatment in this patient. There was still a small excretion of succinylacetoacetate and succinylacetone (18–29 mmol/mol creatinine) and the excretion of 5-aminolevulinate decreased only slightly. During the last 2 years there had been slight renal tubular damage, as evidenced by an elevated excretion of β_2-microglobulin, 2.8–8.6 mg/l (ref. value <0.37 mg/l). The excretion declined steadily after the transfusion and was after 8 weeks almost normalized (0.46 mg/l).

The effect on the measured variables decreased after 10 weeks and a second exchange transfusion was performed 14 weeks after the first one. No decrease of S-tyrosine concentration was seen and a third exchange transfusion was therefore done 8 weeks later. Although the effect on tyrosine metabolism from the first trial could not be repeated, the excretion of β_2-microglobulin has continued to be less than during the previous year. The S-α-fetoprotein concentration has shown a steady decline with an approximate half-life of 18 months.

Case M.S. also showed an effect on all variables, except α-fetoprotein, after the first exchange transfusion. Four of 14 values of S-tyrosine were below 100 μmol/l,

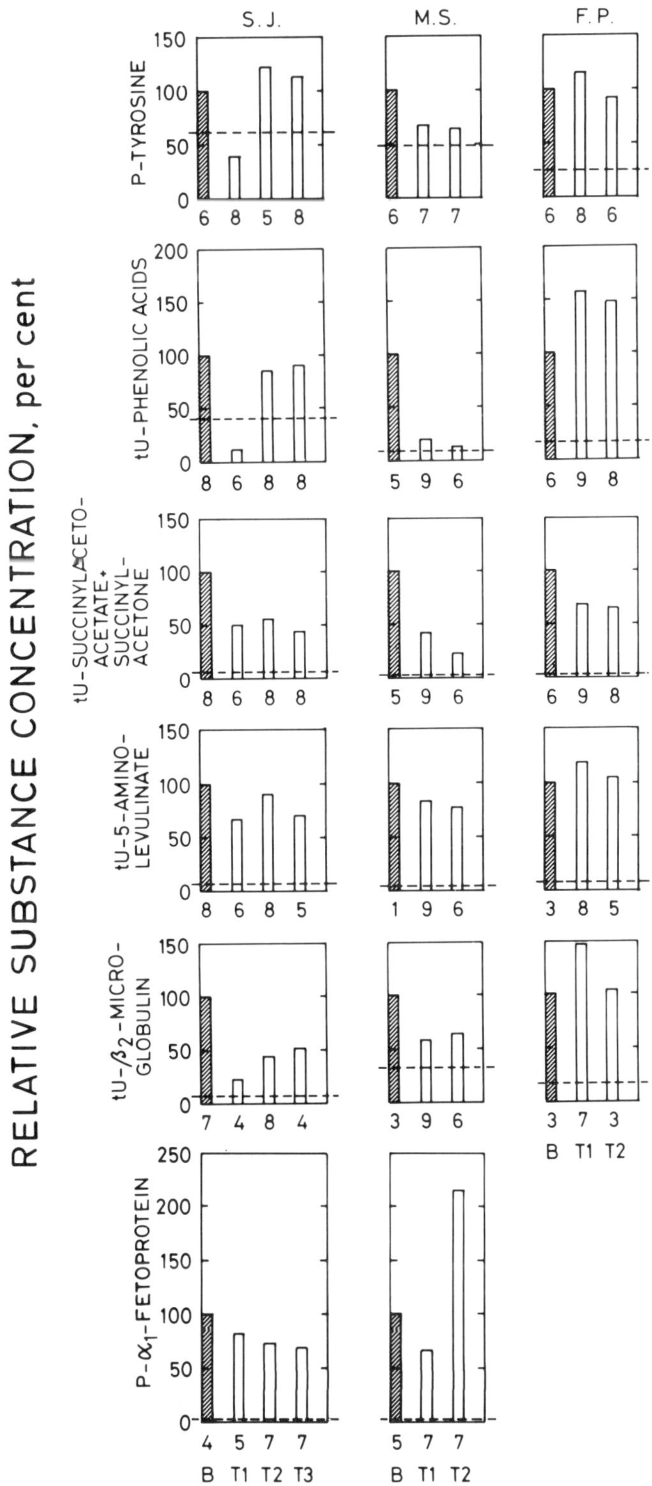

Figure 1 The excretion of tyrosine metabolites (phenolic acids, succinylacetoacetate plus succinylacetone) and of 5-aminolevulinate has been measured in relation to creatinine excretion. The bar labelled B is the basal period; T1, T2, T3, correspond to the periods after the three transfusions. The dotted line shows the upper reference limit for the different compounds. The figures below the bars show the number of samples analysed from each period. When possible, one sample per week was obtained from each patient.

and the lowest excretion of phenolic acids was around 10% of the pretreatment values. Her pretreatment renal tubular damage was less than in case S.J. (tU-β_2-microglobulin 1.1 mg/l). However, also in the case of M.S. the renal tubular damage became less marked, and a few almost normal values for β_2-microglobulin (0.39–0.50 mg/l) were obtained. The second blood transfusion was performed 5 weeks after the first. It was an ordinary blood transfusion caused by an acute large gastrointestinal bleeding. Thereafter her general condition deteriorated and increases in liver enzyme and α-fetoprotein concentrations were found to be due to a hepatocellular carcinoma. A liver transplantation was therefore performed 10 weeks after the last transfusion.

In case F.P. two exchange transfusions were performed. When the post-transfusion periods of altogether 14 weeks are compared with the preceding 10 weeks an increase in S-tyrosine concentration and in the excretion of phenolic acids was found but the excretion of succinylacetoacetate and succinylacetone decreased as in the other two patients. The renal tubular damage was unchanged with excretion of β_2-microglobulin 1.6–4.2 mg/l. It might be relevant that this boy had a varicella infection during the period between the blood transfusions.

DISCUSSION

We have suggested that maleylacetoacetate and/or fumarylacetoacetate are the toxic compounds in hereditary tyrosinaemia (Lindblad *et al.*, 1977). These compounds have, however, not been found in urine but the reduced compound succinylacetoacetate is present in both blood and urine. Intravenous injection of the precursor of maleylacetoacetate, i.e. of homogentisate, causes renal tubular damage (Fällström *et al.*, 1981).

A relationship between the excretion of succinylacetone plus succinylacetoacetate and the severity of liver and kidney involvement seems to exist in the single patient although this may not be the case between patients (Fällström *et al.*, 1981). By dietary manipulations or other forms of treatment, a reduction of S-tyrosine concentration and of the excretion of tyrosine metabolites can be achieved (Lindblad *et al.*, in preparation). However, the patients' acceptance of the diet or of the pharmacological treatment and the requirement for growth set a limit to the intensity of treatment.

It appears that enzyme substitution could reduce the toxic metabolites to an extent which had not been achieved by strict dietary control alone. The results in the patients were variable and more experience is needed to evaluate the role of enzyme substitution as supportive therapy.

ACKNOWLEDGEMENTS

This study was supported by a grant (03X-585) from the Swedish Medical Research Council.

REFERENCES

Fällström, S. P., Lindblad, B., Lindstedt, S. and Steen, G. Hereditary tyrosinaemia – fumarylacetoacetase deficiency. *Pediatr. Res.* 13 (1979) 78

Holme, E., Lindblad, B. and Lindstedt, S. Possibilities for treatment and for early prenatal diagnosis of hereditary tyrosinaemia. *Lancet* 1 (1985) 527

Kvittingen, E. A., Halvorsen, S. and Jellum, E. Deficient fumarylacetoacetate fumarylhydrolase activity in lymphocytes and fibroblasts from patients with hereditary tyrosinaemia. *Pediatr. Res.* 14 (1983) 541–544

Lindblad, B., Lindstedt, S. and Steen, G. On the enzymic defects in hereditary tyrosinaemia. *Proc. Natl. Acad. Sci. (USA)* 74 (1977) 4641–4645

Weinberg, A. G., Mize, C. E. and Worthen, H. G. The occurrence of hepatoma in the chronic form of hereditary tyrosinaemia. *J. Pediatr.* 88 (1976) 434–438

J. Inher. Metab. Dis. 9 Suppl. 2 (1986) 262–264

Short Communication

Presentation of the Data of the Italian Registry for Oculocutaneous Tyrosinaemia

A. Fois[1], P. Borgogni[1], M. Cioni[1], M. Molinelli[1], R. Frezzotti[2], A. M. Bardelli[2], G. Lasorella[2], L. Barberi[2], P. Durand[3], M. Di Rocco[3], C. Romano[4], R. Parini[5], C. Corbetta[6], M. Giovannini[7], E. Riva[7], N. Balato[8], R. Sartorio[9], F. Mollica[10], E. Zammarchi[11] and M. L. Battini[11]

[1]*Institute of Clinical Paediatrics, University of Siena, Via P.A. Mattioli 10, Siena, Italy;* [2]*Institute of Ophthalmological Sciences, University of Siena, Italy;* [3]*Department of Paediatrics 3, G. Gaslini Institute, Genoa, Italy;* [4]*Institute of Clinical Paediatrics, University of Genoa, Italy;* [5]*Institute of Clinical Paediatrics 2, University of Milan, Italy;* [6]*Department of Clinical Research, University of Milan, Italy;* [7]*Institute of Clinical Paediatrics 5, University of Milan, Italy;* [8]*Institute of Clinical Dermatology, University of Naples, Italy;* [9]*Institute of Clinical Paediatrics, University of Naples, Italy;* [10]*Institute of Clinical Paediatrics, University of Catania, Italy;*[11]*Institute of Clinical Paediatrics, University of Florence, Italy*

Hereditary type II tyrosinaemia (McKusick 27660) is an autosomal recessive disorder characterized by hypertyrosinaemia and tyrosyluria, without signs of hepatic and renal damage. The patients have a dendritic keratopathy, painful hyperkeratosis of the palms and soles and sometimes mental retardation. Hypertyrosinaemia with values ranging from 14 to 62 $mg\,dl^{-1}$, tyrosinuria and tyrosyluria are found. A defect of hepatic tyrosine aminotransferase (EC 2.6.1.5) in the cytosol is considered to be the molecular abnormality (Kennaway and Buist, 1971; Goldsmith *et al.*, 1979).

Twenty-one cases have been reported in Italy (Zammarchi *et al.*, 1974; Bardelli *et al.*, 1977; Garibaldi *et al.*, 1979). In order to evaluate all these patients together, the Italian Society for the Study of Inborn Errors of Metabolism has promoted a cumulative survey. We present the clinical and biochemical findings of the cases; the related data are given in Table 1.

CONCLUSIONS

Type II tyrosinaemia in Italy has no regional preponderance. Neuromotor retardation and/or microcephaly seem to be correlated with the higher values of tyrosine. Enzyme studies have been refused in all patients. Treatment with a low tyrosine diet has been successful when accepted: since in many patients the diagnosis was made rather late, it is not possible to evaluate the results of the diet for the prevention of neuromotor retardation.

Journal of Inherited Metabolic Disease. ISSN 0141–8955.

Table 1 Italian cases of tyrosinaemia type II

Patient	*Sex/Age*	*Region*	*Age at onset* *Keratitis*	*Age at onset* *Hyperkeratosis*	*Mental retardation*	*Neurological symptoms*	*Blood tyrosine* ($mg\,dl^{-1}$)
(1) A.C.	M/29 y	Tuscany	1 mon	Infancy	—	—	14–15
(2) L.C.	F/26 y	Tuscany	1 mon	Infancy	—	—	15–16
(3) M.M.	M/20 y	Tuscany	3 mon	Infancy	—	Convulsions	25
(4) M.V.	F/24 y	Basilicate	8 mon	Infancy	—	—	20
(5) P.G.	M/4 mon	Calabria	3 mon	—	IQ 84	—	21
(6) R.M.	F/4 y	Calabria	5 mon	5 mon	IQ 73	—	35
(7) F.M.	F/20 y	Calabria	—	—	—	—	18
(8) I.M.	F/28 y	Calabria	—	Infancy	IQ borderline	—	30
(9) M.L.B.	F/23 y	Lombardy	3–4 y	3–4 y	—	—	22
(10) R.B.	M/27 y	Lombardy	9–10 y	15 y	—	—	19
(11) G.A.	F/9y	Lombardy	3 mon	12 mon	Mild	—	33
(12) R.M.	M/6 y	Puglia	3 mon	3 mon	IQ 67	—	30
(13) L.S.	M/12 mon	Lombardy	8 mon	8 mon	Severe	Microcephaly	53
(14) A.S.	F/24 mon	Lombardy	12 mon	12 mon	Severe	Hypertonia	35
(15) P.L.	M/28 y	Campania	13 mon	14 y	—	—	21
(16) E.L.	F/33 y	Campania	3 mon	3 y	—	—	17
(17) G.R.	M/9 mon	Sicily*	3 mon	—	—	—	—
(18) L.L.	F/37 y	Tuscany	4 y	4 y	—	—	28
(19) F.B.	M/40 d	Tuscany	1 mon	1 mon	—	—	30
(20) B.G.	F/4 mon	Tuscany	1 mon	—	—	Mild neuromotor retardation	48
(21) L.R.	M/36 y	Campania	15 y	15 y	IQ borderline	—	16

* Diagnosis formulated in USA

Three children of a mentally normal mother with a mild degree of hypertyrosinaemia have a normal neuromotor development. However, two other children of a mother with 30 mg dl^{-1} of blood tyrosine have microcephaly and neuromotor retardation: one also has convulsions.

REFERENCES

Bardelli, A. M., Borgogni, P., Farnetani, M. A., Fois, A., Frezzotti, R., Mattei, R., Molinelli, M. and Sargentini, I. Familial tyrosinaemia with eye and skin lesions. Presentation of two cases. *Ophthalmologica* 175 (1977) 5–9

Garibaldi, L., Pregliasco, P., Romano, C., Siliato, F. and Durand, P. Oculocutaneous tyrosinosis. An Italian problem? *Med. Surg. Pediatr.* 1 (1979) 279–284

Goldsmith, L. A., Thorpe, J. and Roe, C. Hepatic enzymes of tyrosine metabolism in tyrosinemia II. *J. Invest. Dermatol.* 73 (1979) 530–532

Kennaway, N. G. and Buist, N. R. M. Metabolic studies in a patient with hepatic cytosol tyrosine aminotransferase deficiency. *Pediatr. Res.* 5 (1971) 287

Zammarchi, F., La Cauza, C. and Calzolari, C. Un caso di ipertirosinemia con tirosiluria. *Min. Pediatr.* 26 (1974) 203–213

J. Inher. Metab. Dis. 9 Suppl. 2 (1986) 265–267

Short Communication

A New Case of Hyperlysinaemia with Saccharopinuria

C. VIANEY-LIAUD[1], M. O. ROLLAND[1], P. DIVRY[1], G. PUTHET[2], M. T. ZABOT[1] and J. COTTE[1]
[1]*Laboratoire de Biochimie, Hôpital Debrousse, 69322 Lyon Cedex 05, France*
[2]*Service de Néonatologie, Pavillon J, Hôpital Edouard Herriot, 69374 Lyon Cedex 08, France*

The main pathway for lysine catabolism in mammalian tissues proceeds through oxidative degradation forming saccharopine as a stable intermediate. The initial reaction is catalysed by lysine α-ketoglutarate reductase and the second by saccharopine dehydrogenase. It has been demonstrated (Marcovitz *et al.*, 1984) on bovine liver that a single protein catalyses both reactions; this bifunctional enzyme has been called α-aminoadipic semialdehyde synthase by these authors. The second catabolic pathway for lysine, via pipecolic acid, although significant in some tissues (such as the central nervous system) is of less physiological importance. Familial hyperlysinaemia (McKusick 23870) was described for the first time in 1964. Until now, 13 patients in 9 families have been reported. Studies on skin fibroblasts identified the defective enzyme as lysine α-ketoglutarate reductase – but further studies in 7 of these patients revealed that saccharopine dehydrogenase activity was reduced to a similar extent (Dancis *et al.*, 1979). Moreover, three other patients have been described who excreted excessive amounts of saccharopine as well as lysine (Carson *et al.*, 1968; Simell *et al.*, 1972, 1973; Cederbaum *et al.*, 1979) and who have been reported as having saccharopinuria (McKusick 26870). The patient of Carson and colleagues exhibited a reduced activity of saccharopine dehydrogenase while lysine α-ketoglutarate reductase was only partially deficient (Fellows and Carson, 1974). Conversely, the patient of Cederbaum and colleagues (1979) had a multiple enzyme defect. Clinically, the three patients are slightly to deeply mentally retarded, with mild ataxia or small stature. We report here a new patient with hyperlysinaemia and hyperlysinuria in association with saccharopinuria.

CASE REPORT

The patient, B.S., is a 5-month-old girl. She was hospitalized at birth because of fetal distress. Slight dysmorphia and axial and peripheral hypotonia were noticed. She was rehospitalized at 9 days of life for spontaneously regressive seizures. The child always remained hypotonic. EEG and standard biological parameters, including ammonaemia, were normal. Amino acid analysis revealed hyperlysinaemia with high urinary excretion of lysine and saccharopine. The parents are Tunisian, issuing from the same village. They are in good health. The three other

Journal of Inherited Metabolic Disease. ISSN 0141–8955.

children, B.M., B.D. and B.Y., born respectively in 1974, 1976 and 1980, are also in excellent health and have developed normally until now.

MATERIALS AND METHODS

Quantitative amino acid analysis was performed by classical ion exchange chromatography on Biotronik LC 6000 and Chromakon 500 automatic analysers. Saccharopine was determined in plasma, urine and cerebrospinal fluid (CSF) after oxidation of cystine to cysteic acid, because the two amino acids cochromatographed in our system. Pipecolic acid was determined with acidic ninhydrin according to the method of Trijbels and colleagues (1979). An L-lysine oral loading test was performed with 100 mg/kg body weight. Lysine oxidation was measured in cultured skin fibroblasts according to the method of Dancis and colleagues (1979) using L-[U-^{14}C] lysine, L-[6-^{14}C] lysine and DL-α-amino-[6-^{14}C]adipic acid as substrates.

RESULTS

Plasma amino acid analysis of our patient at 20 days of life revealed a high level of lysine (665 μmol l^{-1}: normal range 220±75 μmol l^{-1}), while other amino acids including α-aminoadipic acid were normal. Urinary lysine excretion was also increased (1956 mmol mol of creatinine^{-1}: normal range 68±61 mmol mol of creatinine^{-1}). Urine analysis after oxidation of cystine revealed high levels of saccharopine (139 mmol mol of creatinine^{-1}). Plasma saccharopine was also detected but at a low level (8 μmol l^{-1}). Organic acid profile was normal, including α-ketoadipic and glutaric acids. Moreover, pipecolic acid was slightly elevated both in plasma and urine. A restricted protein diet (1.5 g kg body weight^{-1} day^{-1}) was started and the patient was reinvestigated 4 months later. The child seemed to improve as hypotonia was less marked. Staturoponderal and intellectual development were correct although weight remained always at −1 SD. The diet also resulted in an apparent decrease of lysine and saccharopine both in plasma (respectively 494 and 4 μmol l^{-1}) and urine (219 and 42 mmol mol of creatinine^{-1}). CSF amino acids were determined at that time, and demonstrated elevated values for lysine (122 μmol l^{-1}: normal range 19±6 μmol l^{-1}) and saccharopine (22 μmol l^{-1}), the latter being higher than in plasma (CSF/plasma ratio : 5.5).

Compared to a normal subject, the oral L-lysine loading test resulted in a large increase in lysine (plasma lysine concentrations reached a peak level of 2835 μmol l^{-1}). Conversely, saccharopine urinary excretion was only slightly increased while the levels in plasma remained unchanged.

Enzyme studies demonstrated a defective lysine degradation in fibroblasts of the patient (less than 15%), both with L-[U-^{14}C] lysine and L-[6-^{14}C] lysine, while DL-α-amino-[6-^{14}C]adipic acid was metabolized normally.

The parents and the three siblings of our patient were also investigated. Amino acid profiles in plasma and urine were strictly normal except for child B.Y., a 5-year-old girl, who exhibited the same profile as the propositus.

DISCUSSION

The biochemical abnormalities observed in our two patients are in agreement with the diagnosis of hyperlysinaemia with saccharopinuria. The saccharopine level in the spinal fluid was 5 times higher than in plasma, similar to levels in the patients of Carson and colleagues (1968) and of Cederbaum and colleagues (1979), suggesting significant production of saccharopine in the brain. The slightly elevated levels of pipecolic acid, in plasma and urine, have not been described in the other published cases. It can be explained as the main catabolic pathway of lysine is blocked: the secondary pathway, via pipecolic acid, may be enhanced with accumulation of this metabolic intermediate. The oral L-lysine load did not lead to elevation of saccharopine as we expected. This had not been performed in other patients and so it is difficult to give an interpretation. So far, the exact localization of the enzyme defect has not been proved (lysine α-ketoglutarate reductase and/or saccharopine dehydrogenase). However, Dancis and colleagues (1979) suggested that familial hyperlysinaemia and saccharopinuria cannot be considered as different entities, as small amounts of saccharopine can be detected in urine of patients with hyperlysinaemia (Cederbaum *et al.*, 1979). They proposed that the designation familial hyperlysinaemia type I be applied to patients with combined enzyme defect and that familial hyperlysinaemia type II be used for patients in whom significant amounts of lysine α-ketoglutarate reductase activity are retained. Besides this problem of the exact localization of the enzyme defect in hyperlysinaemia with saccharopinuria, another point should be emphasized. The occurrence of the same amino acid profile in a normal 5-year-old sibling of our index case raises the question of cause-and-effect relationship between the biochemical abnormalities and the clinical status.

REFERENCES

Carson, N. A. J., Scally, B. G., Neill, D. W. and Carre, I. J. Saccharopinuria: a new inborn error of lysine metabolism. *Nature* 218 (1968) 679

Cederbaum, S. D., Shaw, K. N. F., Dancis, J., Hutzler, J. and Blaskovics, J. C. Hyperlysinemia with saccharopinuria due to combined lysine ketoglutarate reductase and saccharopine dehydrogenase deficiencies presenting as cystinuria. *J. Pediatr.* 95 (1979) 234–238

Dancis, J., Hutzler, J. and Cox, R. P. Familial hyperlysinemia: enzyme studies, diagnostic methods, comments on terminology. *Am. J. Hum. Genet.* 31 (1979) 290–299

Fellows, F. C. I. and Carson, N. A. J. Enzyme studies in a patient with saccharopinuria: a defect of lysine metabolism. *Pediatr. Res.* 8 (1974) 42–49

Markovitz, P. J., Chuang, D. T. and Cox, R. P. Familial hyperlysinemias. Purification and characterization of the bifunctional aminoadipic semialdehyde synthase with lysine ketoglutarate reductase and saccharopine dehydrogenase activities. *J. Biol. Chem.* 259 (1984) 11643–11646

Simell, O., Johansson, T. and Aula, P. Enzyme defect in saccharopinuria *J. Pediatr.* 82 (1973) 54–57

Simell, O., Visakorpi, J. K. and Donner, M. Saccharopinuria. *Arch. Dis. Child.* 47 (1972) 52–55

Trijbels, J. M. F., Monnens, L. A. H., Bakkeren, A. J. M., Van Raay-Selten, A. H. J. and Cortiaensen, J. M. B. Biochemical studies in the cerebro-hepato-renal syndrome of Zellweger: a disturbance in the metabolism of pipecolic acid. *J. Inher. Metab. Dis.* 2 (1979) 39–42

J. Inher. Metab. Dis. 9 *Suppl.* 2 *(1986) 268–271*

Short Communication

Failure of Early Diazepam Treatment in a Neonate with Non-ketotic Hyperglycinaemia

A. AUKETT,[1] R. A. BRAITHWAITE[2] and A. GREEN[3]
[1]*Sorrento Maternity Hospital, Moseley, Birmingham 13;* [2]*Regional Toxicology Laboratory, Dudley Road Hospital, Birmingham 18;* [3]*Department of Clinical Chemistry, The Children's Hospital, Birmingham, B16 8ET, UK*

Non-ketotic hyperglycinaemia (NKH) is an inborn error of glycine metabolism (McKusick 23830). The primary defect is thought to be in the glycine cleavage enzyme system, although a reduced level of threonine dehydratase (EC 4.2.1.16) has been documented in one case (Krieger and Booth, 1984) leading to an accumulation of glycine especially in the CNS.

The presentation of non-ketotic hyperglycinaemia is variable and there appear to be three types–neonatal, infantile and late-onset. The most severe form presents in the neonatal period with rapidly progressing neurological symptoms. The majority of these children, if untreated, die within a few weeks. All survivors beyond early infancy have had severe psychomotor retardation (Carson, 1982).

Previous attempts at treatment have involved dietary restriction, conjugation or removal of glycine, supply of one-carbon units or cofactors and the use of glycine antagonists such as strychnine. These have often been used as a combination of approaches, but have not produced any real success when used in patients with the severe form of the disease. Treatment with diazepam in combination with sodium benzoate, choline, folic acid and moderate protein restriction has been used to treat two older infants with encouraging results (Matalon *et al.*, 1982). We are not aware that this regime has been tried in neonates, and we report its use in a baby with NKH who was diagnosed at age 4 days.

CASE HISTORY

After a normal pregnancy and delivery, a female baby (S.M.) presented at 40 h with lethargy, not feeding and myoclonic jerks. She was hypotonic, areflexic and unresponsive. Over the next 24 h she became virtually unrousable and developed hiccups. By 72 h the baby required ventilation. The parents were first cousins and one previous male child had died age 4 days in Pakistan with similar symptoms. There were three normal female siblings.

At age 78 h the following investigations were performed: CSF glycine 197 μmol/l, plasma glycine 1900 μmol/l, urine glycine 6700 μmol/mmol creatinine, CSF/plasma glycine ratio of 0.1. Blood ammonia and urinary organic acids were normal. There was no acidosis and no urinary ketones. There was a characteristic burst/suppression pattern on the EEG (Mises *et al.*, 1982).

Journal of Inherited Metabolic Disease. ISSN 0141–8955.

TREATMENT AND RESULTS

The treatment regime commenced on day 4 and consisted of diazepam in combination with choline, sodium benzoate and folate, all given orally. In addition protein intake was moderately reduced to approximately 2 g/kg/day. Diazepam was given,

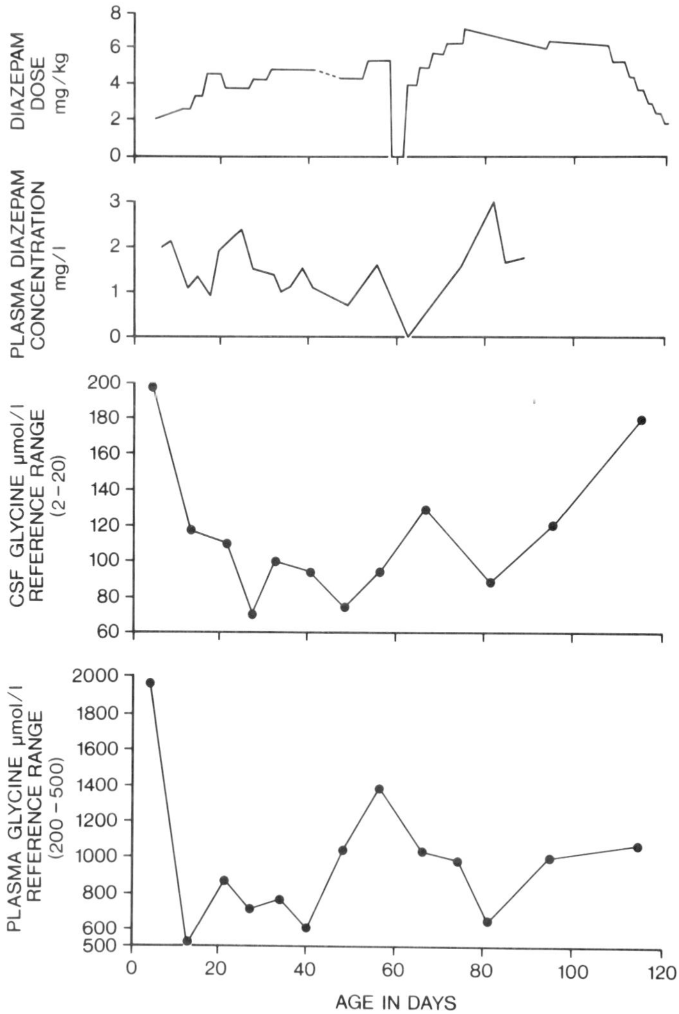

Figure 1 CSF and plasma glycine concentrations during diazepam therapy

2–7 mg/kg/day (Figure 1), in four divided doses (max. 36 mg/day). Plasma diazepam and desmethyl diazepam concentrations were measured and were maintained between 0.75 and 3.0 mg/l and 1.8 and 8.0 mg/l respectively. The ratio of desmethyl diazepam to diazepam varied between 1.8 and 4.5 with a mean of 3.1 mg/l.

Choline (0.5–1.0 g per day) was adjusted according to the presence of trimethylamine in the urine. This was judged by appearance of a fishy smell of the urine. Sodium benzoate dose was 100–200 mg/kg/day and folic acid 5 mg daily.

Progress was monitored by serial EEGs and measurement of CSF and plasma glycine concentrations. Nine days following commencement of treatment there had been a significant fall of both plasma and CSF glycine to 530 μmol/l and 70 μmol/l respectively (see Figure 1). Throughout the duration of treatment plasma glycine was between 530 μmol/l and 1393 μmol/l and CSF 74 μmol/l and 130 μmol/l.

Initially there was some clinical improvement. Over the first 2 weeks after the start of treatment, movements increased and artificial ventilation was no longer required. One month later she could bottle-feed and she was discharged home age 42 days. Over this period her EEG also improved.

However, this improvement was not maintained and at 47 days she again presented with lethargy and not feeding. Her EEG had deteriorated. There was concern that there had been non-compliance as the serum diazepam level was lower than on previous occasions. Diazepam dose was therefore increased to 4.4 mg/kg but with no effect. At this stage the possibility of diazepam toxicity was considered and therefore therapy was withheld for 3 days but there was clinical deterioration.

By 3 months, although S.M. was growing normally, there was no psychomotor development. Neurogically she remained very abnormal, with severe hypotonia and frequent myoclonic jerks. Her only response was to pain. As there was no sustained clinical improvement, treatment with diazepam was discontinued at age 3 months and she died at 13 months.

DISCUSSION AND CONCLUSIONS

Diazepam was reported to act as a specific competitor for glycine receptors in the CNS (Young *et al.*, 1974) although this has since been disputed (Hunt and Raynaud, 1977). This activity would appear to be weak and non-specific and the dose of diazepam required to exert any direct effect on the glycine receptors would be impossible to achieve therapeutically.

However, the favourable response of two older infants treated with diazepam (Matalon *et al.*, 1982) had indicated that diazepam might be effective in the treatment of NKH, although studies in the newborn were needed to determine whether this treatment regime, given early, would improve the prognosis in this condition. As the diagnosis was made early in this child we were in a position to try this.

The treatment of S.M. produced some significant biochemical and EEG changes. It would seem that, even when used from early in the neonatal period, such treatment does not result in any sustained clinical improvement as, apart from some seizure control, she remained neurologically very abnormal with no appreciable psychomotor development. This is perhaps not surprising, as there is evidence that brain damage occurs prenatally. The EEG has been demonstrated to be abnormal soon after birth (Von-Wendt *et al.*, 1981) and CSF glycine levels are also very raised at birth (De Groot *et al.*, 1977). *In utero* a raised glycine/serine ratio can be seen as early as 17–18 weeks gestation (Garcia-Castro *et al.*, 1982).

There would therefore seem to be little sound basis for post-natal treatment of this disorder, and although our experience is limited to one case, we feel that diazepam therapy is of no value in the treatment of the acute neonatal form of non-ketotic hyperglycinaemia.

REFERENCES

Carson, N. A. J. Non-ketotic hyperglycinaemia – a review of 70 patients. *J. Inher. Metab. Dis.* 5 Suppl. 1 (1982) 126–128

De Groot, C. J., Touwen, B. C., Huisjes, H. J. and Hommes, F. A. Early findings of a case of non-ketotic hyperglycinaemia. *Ann. Clin. Biochem.* 14 (1977) 140–141

Garcia-Castro, J. M., Isalas-Forsythe, C. M., Levy, H. L., Shih, V. E., Lao-Velez, C. R., Gonzalez-Rios, M. C. and Reyes de Torres, L. C. Pre-natal diagnosis of non-ketotic hyperglycinaemia. *N. Engl. J. Med.* 306 (1982) 79–81

Hunt, P. and Raynaud, J-P. Benzodiazepine activity: is interaction with the glycine receptor, as evidenced by displacement of strychnine binding, a useful criterion? *J. Pharm. Pharmacol.* 29 (1977) 442–444

Kreiger, I and Booth, F. Threonine dehydratase deficiency: a probable cause of non-ketotic hyperglycinaemia. *J. Inher. Metab. Dis.* 7 (1984) 53–56

Matalon, R., Michals, K., Naidu, S. and Hughes, J. Treatment of non-ketotic hyperglycinaemia with diazepam, choline and folic acid. *J. Inher. Metab. Dis.* 5 Suppl. 1. (1982) 3–5

Mises, J., Moussali-Salefranques, F., Laroque, M. L., Ogier, H., Coude, F. X., Charpentier, C. and Saudubray, J. M. EEG findings as an aid to the diagnosis of neonatal non-ketotic hyperglycinaemia. *J. Inher. Metab. Dis.* 5 Suppl. 2. (1982) 117–120

Von Wendt, L., Simila, S., Saukkonen, A-L., Koivisto, M. and Kouvalainen, K. Prenatal brain damage in non-ketotic hyperglycinemia. *Am. J. Dis. Child.* 135 (1981) 1072

Young, A. B., Zukin, S. R. and Snyder, S. H. Interaction of benzodiazepines with central nervous glycine receptors. Possible mechanism of action. *Proc. Natl. Acad. Sci. USA* 71 (1974) 2246–2250

J. Inher. Metab. Dis. 9 Suppl. 2 (1986) 272–274

Short Communication

Gyrate Atrophy of the Choroid and Retina: 3 Cases in one Italian Family

A. Fois[1], P. Borgogni[1], M. Cioni[1], G. M. S. Mancini[1], M. Molinelli[1], M. Pizzetti[1], A. M. Bardelli[2], L. Biagini[2], L. Barberi[2], C. Malpassi[2], E. Harms[3] and W. J. Kleijer[4]
[1] *Institute of Clinical Paediatrics, University of Siena, Via P. A. Mattioli 10, 53100 Siena, Italy;* [2]*Institute of Ophthalmological Sciences, University of Siena, Italy;* [3]*Department of Paediatrics, University of Munich, West Germany;* [4]*Department of Clinical Genetics, Erasmus University, Rotterdam, The Netherlands*

Gyrate atrophy of the choroid and retina is a tapetoretinal dystrophy in which Simell and Takki (1973) observed an increase in plasma ornithine. The disease seems to be more frequent in Finland (Sipila *et al.*, 1979) and the acronym HOGA, hyperornithinaemia-gyrate-atrophy, (McKusick 25887)has been suggested. A defect of ornithine-ketoacid aminotransferase (EC 2.6.1.13) has been demonstrated in transformed lymphocytes (Valle *et al.*, 1977), and in fibroblasts (Trijbels *et al.*, 1977), which do not convert L-ornithine to proline (O'Donnell *et al.*, 1978). The inheritance of this condition is autosomal recessive (Takki and Simel, 1974).

The first symptoms, appearing during childhood, are night blindness and increasing myopia. There is a progressive narrowing of the optical fields and by the age of 30 most patients are practically blind. Fundoscopic examination reveals patchy atrophic areas which enlarge progressively and diffusely towards the optic disk. The electroretinogram (ERG) and visual evoked potential (VEP) become extinguished (Sipila *et al.*, 1979). A posterior cataract appears at puberty.

We describe the clinical and biochemical findings in an Italian family.

PERSONAL OBSERVATIONS

The disease was discovered in a 7½-year-old child (R.P.) who was referred to the Institute of Clinical Paediatrics with language retardation. Automated plasma and urine amino acid anaylsis showed a marked increase in ornithine (Table 1). Ophthalmologic evaluation revealed gyrate atrophy of the choroid and retina and abnormalities in VEP and ERG. With systematic ophthalmological and biochemical investigations two more affected members of the family were later identified: a brother (V.P.) aged 13 years 5 months and a sister (M.P.) aged 15 years 5 months. They complained only of mild visual difficulties. In Table 1 plasma and urinary values of ornithine in all family members are reported. The father had normal fundoscopy and a slight increase in basal plasma ornithine with normal urinary values. The mother was clinically and biochemically normal.

Journal of Inherited Metabolic Disease. ISSN 0141–8955.

Table 1 Results of laboratory investigations on HOGA family members

Patients	*Ornithine*		*[^{14}C]Ornithine incorporation in proteins relative to [^{3}H] leucine incorporation*		*OKT* activity in fibroblasts (nmol mg protein^{-1} h^{-1})*
	Plasma (μmol l^{-1})	*Urine* (mol (mol creatinine)$^{-1}$)	(dpm [^{14}C]/ [^{3}H]×10^{2})	(% of control)	
M. P. father	151	4	84	74	63
G. DiB. mother	87	3	—	—	—
R. P. son (HOGA)	2095	592	5	4.7	no activity
V. P. son (HOGA)	1175	692	12	10.5	23
A. P. son	149	2	58	51	—
G. P. son	103	4	112	98	164
M. P. daughter (HOGA)	1489	133	8	6.5	11
F. P. daughter	154	15	81	71	—
M. O. nephew	66	2	60	53	169
F. O. nephew	167	1	58	51	66
Known HOGA patient			2	2.0	
Control			114	—	

*OKT: Ornithine-ketoacid aminotransferase

The incorporation of [^{14}C] ornithine into cultured fibroblasts and ornithine-ketoacid aminotransferase activity (using the method of Trijbels and colleagues, 1977) reported in Table 1.

The proband and his affected sister M.P. have accepted a low protein diet supplemented with Vitamin B_6 and L-proline (UCD 2 Milupa). There has been a reduction in the values of plasma ornithine to 217 and 287 μmol l^{-1} respectively. V.P. has refused treatment.

CONCLUSIONS

Our study reports the first comprehensive evaluation of HOGA in an Italian family, and is thus intended to alert Italian ophthalmologists and paediatricians to this potentially treatable condition in children with even apparently mild visual disturbances. The typical fundoscopic findings make diagnosis possible. Extensive epidemiological investigations could be justified to determine the incidence of this disorder in Italy.

REFERENCES

O'Donnell, J. J., Sandman, R. P. and Martin, S. R. Gyrate atrophy of the retina: Inborn error of L-ornithine: 2-oxoacid aminotransferase. *Science* 200 (1978) 200–201

Simell, O. and Takki, K. Raised plasma ornithine and gyrate atrophy of the choroid and retina. *Lancet* 1 (1973) 1031–1033

Sipila, I., Simell, O., Rapola, J., Sainio, K. and Tuuteri, L. Gyrate atrophy of the choroid and retina with hyperornithinaemia: tubular aggregates and type 2 fibre atrophy in muscle. *Neurology* 29 (1979) 996–1005

Takki, K. and Simell, O. Genetic aspects in gyrate atrophy of the choroid and retina with hyperornithinaemia. *Br. J. Ophthalmol.* 59 (1974) 907–916

Trijbels, J. M. F., Sengers, R. C. A., Bakkeren, J. A. J. M., De Kort, A. F. M. and Deutman, A. F. L-Ornithine–ketoacid- transaminase deficiency in cultured fibroblasts of a patient with hyperornithinaemia and gyrate atrophy of the choroid and retina. *Clin. Chim. Acta* 79 (1977) 371-377

Valle, D., Kaiser-Kupfer, M. I. and Del Valle, L. A. Gyrate atrophy of the choroid and retina: deficiency of ornithine aminotransferase in transformed lymphocytes. *Proc. Natl. Acad. Sci. USA* 74 (1977) 5159-5161

J. Inher. Metab. Dis. 9 Suppl. 2 (1986) 275–276

Short Communication

Methylenetetrahydrofolate Reductase and Methyltetrahydrofolate Methyltransferase in Human Fetal Tissues and Chorionic Villi

Y. S. Shin, G. Pilz and W. Endres
Children's Hospital, University of Munich, Lindwurmstrasse 4, 8 München 2, West Germany

Interconversion of reduced derivatives of folic acid such as tetrahydrofolate (THF), methyl-THF and others is mediated by several enzymes. The defects in methylene-THF reductase (EC 1.1.1.58) and methyl-THF methyltransferase (methionine synthetase, EC 2.1.1.5) lead to megaloblastic anaemia, homocystinuria and other problems, possibly due to a block in methylation of homocysteine and in methyl-THF or THF regeneration. Clinical symptoms of both defects vary from hypotonia and mental retardation to severe neurological abnormalities. Prenatal diagnosis of methylene-THF reductase deficiency (Christensen and Brandt, 1985), cobalamin C disease (Saudubray, J. M., Baumgartner, R., Bouè, M. and Shin Y. S. Unpublished data, 1984) and cobalamin E deficiency (Rosenblatt *et al.*, 1985) has been performed using cultivated amniotic fluid cells. In this report we have investigated the characteristics of both enzymes in human fetal tissues and chorionic villi in order to explore possibilities for early prenatal diagnosis using the latter.

MATERIALS AND METHODS

Two fetuses at the gestational age of 18–20 weeks were obtained from a legal abortion. Tissues were frozen at −20°C immediately until used. Chorionic villi sampling was done at 7–13 weeks of gestation and the samples were frozen at −20°C until assayed.

The activity of methylene-THF reductase was determined using the modified method of Kuntzbach and Stokstad (1971). The activity of methionine synthetase was determined by the method of Taylor and Weissbach (1967), further modified in our laboratory. The holoenzyme activity was measured without B_{12} in the reaction mixture, and the total activity with CN-cobalamin or methyl-B_{12}.

RESULTS

As shown in Table 1, the methylene-THF reductase activity in chorionic villi was similar to that in fetal intestine. The activity in fetal liver and muscle was much higher than that in the other tissues investigated. However, the apparent K_m value for methyl-THF was similar in these tissues (0.05–0.08 mmol l^{-1}). The enzyme

Journal of Inherited Metabolic Disease. ISSN 0141–8955. Printed in Great Britain by Titus Wilson & Son Ltd., Kendal.

Table 1 Methylene-THF reductase and methyl-THF methyltransferase activities (nmol h^{-1} (mg protein)$^{-1}$) in human tissues

Sample	*n*	*Reductase*	*Transferase*	
			Holoenzyme	*Total enzyme*
Fibroblasts	17	4.39±1.88* (1.80–7.40)**	0.59±0.28 (0.20–1.10)	2.53±1.89 (0.82–8.70)
Amniotic fluid cells	11	3.70±0.92 (1.70–6.62)	0.58±0.16 (0.30–0.76)	2.69±1.46 (0.48–5.00)
Fetal liver	2§	8.7, 11.5	0.75, 1.45	3.45, 5.90
Fetal muscle	2	9.5, 13.2	1.30, 1.65	1.98, 2.85
Fetal intestine	2	2.70, 3.75	1.65, 1.85	2.27, 2.93
Chorionic villi	17#	2.79±0.78 (1.70–4.70)	0.85±0.14 (0.40–0.85)	2.29±1.12 (1.25–5.40)

* mean ± SD
** rangc
§ 18–20th week of gestation
\# 7–13th week of gestation

activity in chorionic villi was comparable to that in cultivated fibroblasts and amniotic fluid cells.

The methionine synthetase activity in chorionic villi was almost the same as that in fetal tissues (Table 1). The activity values were also similar to those in cultured fibroblasts and amniotic fluid cells. The K_m value for methyl-THF was also similar, at about 0.10–0.15 mmol l^{-1}.

DISCUSSION

These results for the methylene-THF reductase activity and the methionine synthetase activity indicate that early prenatal diagnosis may be possible with the application of uncultured chorionic villi samples. It may also be feasible to perform the diagnosis of defects of vitamin B_{12} such as cobalamin C, cobalamin D and cobalamin E deficiencies.

REFERENCES

Christensen, E. and Brandt, N. J. Prenatal diagnosis of 5,10–methylenetetrahydrofolate reductase deficiency. *N. Engl. J. Med.* 313 (1985) 50–51

Kutzbach, C. and Stokstad, E. L. R. Mammalian methylenetetrahydrofolate reductase. Partial purification, properties, and inhibition by *S*-adenosylmethionine. *Biochim. Biophys. Acta* 250 (1971) 459–477

Rosenblatt, D. S., Cooper, B. A., Schmutz, S. M., Zaleski, W. A. and Casey, R. E. Prenatal vitamin B_{12} therapy of a fetus with methylcobalamin deficiency (cobalamine E disease). *Lancet* 1 (1985) 1127–1129

Taylor, R. T. and Weissbach, H. N^5-methyltetrahydrofolatehomocysteine transmethylase. *J. Biol. Chem.* 242 (1967) 1502–1508

J. Inher. Metab. Dis. 9 Suppl. 2 (1986) 277–279

Short Communication

Kinetic Studies on the Glucose-6-phosphate Transport System in Rat Hepatic Microsomal Membrane

Y. IGARASHI, S. KATO and K. TADA
Department of Pediatrics, Tohoku University School of Medicine, 1–1 Seiryo-machi, Sendai 980, Japan

It has been demonstrated that glycogen storage disease type Ib is the congenital disorder due to a defect of glucose-6-phosphate (G6P) transport system in hepatic microsomal membrane (Igarashi *et al.*, 1979, 1984). The kinetics of the G6P transport system in rat hepatic microsomal membrane have been studied (Igarashi *et al.*, 1985). In this paper the effects of sugars, sugar-phosphates and some other chemicals on G6P uptake into rat hepatic microsomes are described.

MATERIALS AND METHODS

Preparation of rat hepatic microsomal fraction and the experimental procedure of G6P uptake studies were described in the previous paper (Igarashi *et al.*, 1985). The chemicals used to study the inhibitory effect on G6P uptake were galactose, fructose, deoxy-D-glucose-6-phosphate (deoxy-G6P), glucose-1-phosphate (G1P), glucose-6-sulphate, (G6-sulphate), galactose-6-phosphate (Gal-6P), fructose-6-phosphate (F6P), fructose-1, 6-diphosphate (FDP), carbamyl phosphate, pyrophosphate, ATP and benzenesulphonic acids. From the Lineweaver-Burk type plot and Dixon's plot of data, the inhibition constant K_i of each inhibitor on G6P transport was estimated.

RESULTS

In this series of studies on the G6P transport system, the kinetic parameters of G6P uptake into rat hepatic microsome were 20.3 nmol (mg prot)$^{-1}$ (30 s)$^{-1}$ for the maximum rate (J_{max}) and 0.84 mmol/l for the half saturation concentration (Michaelis constant, K_t), respectively. A high concentration of D-galactose or D-fructose (100 mmol/l each) did not have any effect on the kinetic parameters of G6P uptake, as with 100 mmol/l D-glucose (Igarashi *et al.*, 1985). 50 mmol/l ATP slightly changed the J_{max} and K_t to 28.7 nmol (mg prot)$^{-1}$ (30 s)$^{-1}$ and 1.64 mmol/l respectively. When 100 mmol/l pyrophosphate was added to the incubation mixture, J_{max} of G6P uptake was unchanged but the K_t was 1.5 mmol/l. On the other hand, phosphoric acid and carbamyl phosphate showed competitive inhibition with K_i for G6P uptake of 31 and 32 mmol/l respectively. The inhibitory effects of sugar-

Journal of Inherited Metabolic Disease. ISSN 0141–8955.

Table 1 Effects of inhibitors on G6P uptake into rat hepatic microsomes

Inhibitors[1]	*Concentration*	*Type of inhibition*	K_i
Mannose-6-P	25–100 mM	competitive	62 mM
2–Deoxy-D-glucose-6-P	25–100 mM	competitive	22 mM
Glucose-1-P	25–100 mM	competitive	77 mM
Glucose-6-sulphate	25–100 mM	competitive	147 mM
Galactose-6-P	25– 50 mM	competitive	12 mM
Fructose-6-P	25–100 mM	competitive	39 mM
Fructose-1-P	25–100 mM	competitive	44 mM
Fructose-1, 6-diP	25–100 mM	competitive	74 mM
Phosphoric acid	25–100 mM	competitive	31 mM
Carbamyl phosphate	10– 50 mM	competitive	32 mM
DIDS	10– 50 μM	competitive	7.5 μM
SITS	10– 50 μM	competitive	12.6 μM
Benzenesulphonic acid	10– 50 mM	competitive	12 μM
Phlorizin	1– 4 mM	mixed	–

[1]The abbreviations used are: DIDS, 4,4′-diisothiocyanostilbenene-2,2′-disulphonic acid; SITS, 4-acetamido-4′-isothiocyanostilbene-2,2′-disulphonic acid

phosphates were investigated as shown in Table 1. All of those investigated in this study had weak inhibitory effects and the pattern of inhibition was competitive. The values of K_i were Gal-6-P<deoxy-G6P<F6P<M6P<FDP<G1P<G-6-sulphate. The K_i value of benzenesulphonic acid was 12 mmol/l. Phlorizin, known as a competitive inhibitor of active sugar transport, showed a mixed type inhibition on G6P uptake.

DISCUSSION

In this study the effects of some sugars, phosphate, sugar-phosphate and other chemicals on G6P uptake into rat hepatic microsome were investigated to elucidate the kinetic properties of the G6P transport system in hepatic microsomal membrane. Glucose, galactose, and fructose were without influence on G6P uptake, showing that these sugars themselves do not bind to the G6P transport system. In contrast DIDS and SITS, known as potent anion-exchange transport inhibitors in human erythrocytes, strongly inhibited G6P uptake (Igarashi *et al.*, 1985) and phosphoric acid, carbamyl phosphate and benzenesulphonic acid also inhibited competitively. Therefore the anion (phosphate) moiety seems to be very important in the binding to the G6P transport system. However, high concentrations of pyrophosphate (PPi) and ATP showed only very weak inhibitory effects. It had been demonstrated in the studies on glycogen storage disease type Ib that PPi is transported by a specific transport system separate from the G6P transport system (Arion *et al.*, 1980; Narisawa *et al.*, 1983).

The different effects of sugar-phosphates and G-6-sulphate on G6P uptake were investigated. All of them showed weak but significant inhibitory effects on the G6P uptake. Gal-6-P was the most potent (K_i 12 mmol/l). Of the sugar-6-Ps, M6P was the weakest inhibitor.

The structure of the sugar moiety, especially the location of OH and H at C-2, seems to affect the affinity for the G6P transport system. The change of the phosphate residue on glucose from G6P to G1P and the substitution of the phosphate moiety by sulphate (G6P to G-6-sulphate) significantly decreased the affinity of substrates for the G6P transport system.

REFERENCES

Arion, W. J., Lange, A. J., Walls, H. E. and Balls, L. M. Evidence for the participation of independent translocases for phosphate and glucose-6-phosphate in the microsomal glucose-6-phosphatase system. *J. Biol. Chem.* 255 (1980) 10396–10406

Igarashi, Y., Kato, S., Narisawa, K. and Tada, K. A direct evidence for defect in glucose-6-phosphate transport system in hepatic microsomal membrane of glycogen storage disease type Ib. *Biochem. Biophys. Res. Commun.* 119 (1984) 593–597

Igarashi, Y., Kato, S. and Tada, K. Kinetic properties of the glucose-6-phosphate transport system in rat hepatic microsomal membranes. *J. Inher. Metab. Dis.* 8 (1985) 153–154

Igarashi, Y., Otomo, H., Narisawa, K. and Tada, K. A new variant of glycogen storage disease type I: probably due to a defect in the glucose-6-phosphate transport system. *J. Inher. Metab. Dis.* 2 (1979) 45–49

Narisawa, K., Otomo, H., Igarashi, Y., Arai, N., Otake, M., Tada. K. and Kuzuya, T. Glycogen storage disease type Ib: microsomal glucose-6-phosphatase system in two patients with different clinical findings. *Pediatr. Res.* 17 (1983) 545–549

J. Inher. Metab. Dis. 9 Suppl. 2 (1986) 280–283

Short Communication

Long-term Cornstarch Therapy in Glycogen Storage Disease Types I, Ib and III

R. Gatti[1], G. Lamedica[2], M. Di Rocco[1], D. Massocco[1], N. Marchese[2] and C. Borrone[1]

[1]*III Divisione di Pediatria and* [2]*Labaratorio di Chimica Clinica, Istituto 'G. Gaslini', Via V Maggio 39, 16148 Genoa, Italy*

The purpose of treatment of hepatic glycogen storage disease (GSD) is to prevent fasting hypoglycaemia and its clinical and metabolic consequences: growth retardation, hepatomegaly, metabolic acidosis, hyperuricaemia and hyperlipidaemia. This problem is particularly severe for patients with GSD type I (McKusick 23220) and for young patients with GSD type III (McKusick 23240). In recent years frequent day feedings associated with continuous intragastric infusion have been proposed as the treatment of choice (Burr *et al.*, 1979; Fernandes *et al.*, 1984b; Greene *et al.*, 1980). Gastric drip night feeding is effective, but serious complications such as symptomatic hypoglycaemia and acidosis resulting from acute gastroenteritis, vomiting and delays in feeding are reported (Greene *et al.*, 1980). The regimen requires monitoring by infusion pump and specific training for parents; furthermore, some patients have psychological problems in accepting it.

Recently the use of uncooked cornstarch has been proposed as an alternative therapy for patients with GSD I when continuous intragastric feeding is impracticable (Chen *et al.*, 1984; Sloan and Zipt, 1983; Smit *et al.*, 1984), but long-term experiences are still not available. In this paper we report the results in 10 children with GSD I, Ib and III after one year of cornstarch therapy.

METHODS AND RESULTS

Informed consent was obtained from parents and from children able to understand. We studied 10 patients (5 with GSD I, 2 with GSD Ib and 3 with GSD III), 5 males and 5 females, whose ages were between 3 and 12 years. In none of them had nocturnal intragastric feeding been tried.

At first admission we measured weight, height and liver size and evaluated skeletal age. Serum triglycerides, lactic acid, bicarbonate, uric acid and transaminases were assayed and a 24 h blood glucose profile was obtained. In patients with GSD Ib, a leukocyte count was also performed. The optimal dose of cornstarch to maintain normoglycaemia for 6–8 h was determined for each patient by testing blood glucose level every 2 h after uncooked cornstarch administration. When individual dosages had been determined, patients started treatment: cornstarch was administered every 6 h (20 min after a meal) and the diet consisted of 6 meals, the

Journal of Inherited Metabolic Disease. ISSN 0141–8955.

last at midnight and the first at 6 a.m. GSD I patients received 50–70% of calories as carbohydrates, 10–15% as proteins and 10–30% as fats; galactose and fructose were reduced. GSD III patients had 40–50% of calories as carbohydrates, 15–20% as proteins and 40% as fats (polyunsaturated and MCT). After 3 days of treatment a 24 h glycaemic profile was checked and the dose of cornstarch adjusted as necessary. The dosage of cornstarch ranged from 1.5 to $2\,g\,kg^{-1}$. After 6 months and after 1 year the patients were readmitted to hospital and submitted to the same protocol.

Long-term cornstarch regimen induced biochemical improvement in all the patients as well as accelerated growth rate. The only complication was a transient diarrhoea at the beginning of treatment, easily controlled by loperamide or spontaneously resolved within a few days. No patients had problems in accepting this regimen. Clinical and biochemical findings for the patients are reported in Table 1.

DISCUSSION

Cornstarch has proved to be the most slowly absorbed carbohydrate. In fact, oral uncooked cornstarch produces a relatively constant normal blood glucose level (>70 mg%) for almost 6 h; uncooked rice starch results in initially higher glucose levels followed by a rapid fall; uncooked potato starch has no effect on glycaemia; glucose, polycose or cooked starches maintain blood glucose level over 70 mg% for less than 3 h (Chen *et al.*, 1984).

Chen reported the response of 7 GSD I patients (4 children and 3 adults) treated for 4 to 20 months: all of them had clinical and biochemical improvements except for an eight-month-old child who had never taken foods containing starch before and who had a poor activity of amylase. Sloan and Zipt (1983) had positive results but these were limited to a 14-week treatment in 3 GSD I patients, and to a 2-week treatment in 2 GSD Ib patients. Smit *et al.* (1984) studied the effect of uncooked cornstarch on 8 patients with GSD I and on one patient with GSD Ib, but did not report long-term experience.

We tried the cornstarch regimen in 5 patients with GSD I, 2 with GSD Ib and 3 with GSD III. One year after the beginning of treatment all patients showed an improvement in glycaemia, triglyceridaemia and uricaemia. Lactic acidaemia was not completely corrected. However, this abnormality appears difficult to control even with intragastric nocturnal feeding; furthermore, Fernandes and colleagues (1984a) mean a moderate hyperlacticacidaemia to be maintained as lactate is a fuel for the brain. An accelerated growth rate was seen in all patients, up to 1 cm every month.

The treatment did not improve haematological parameters in our 2 patients with GSD Ib, which seems to support the hypothesis that neutropenia is related to the basic defect and not to secondary metabolic derangement.

Collateral effects were insignificant and all patients and their families had no problems in accepting this treatment. In conclusion, our study, carried out for 1 year, confirms the first encouraging results of short-term cornstarch regimen and

Table 1 Effects of cornstarch treatment

Case	*Sex*	*Age at diagnosis*	*Age at beginning of treatment*	*Dose of cornstarch* ($g\ kg^{-1}$)	*Minimal level of glycaemia* ($mg\ dl^{-1}$)	*Triglycerides* ($mg\ dl^{-1}$)	*Lactic acid* ($mg\ dl^{-1}$)	*Uric acid* ($mg\ dl^{-1}$)	*Linear growth* ($cm\ y^{-1}$)
GSD I									
I.F.	F	3 y	7 y	2	40[b]	933	79	6.2	6.0
					55[a]	414	77	4.5	7.0
A.P.	M	3 y	4 y	1.5	45[b]	121	16	5.0	3.5
					60[a]	97	27	3.9	12.0
A.S.	M	3 y	4 y	1.5	43[b]	126	49	6.1	4.0
					52[a]	85	51	4.4	11.0
A.F.	M	3 y	4 y	1.5	41[b]	210	15	5.5	5.0
					58[a]	77	22	3.8	11.0
G.F.	M	3 y	4 y	2	29[b]	1116	95	6.8	6.0
					54[a]	239	98	5.6	7.5
GSD Ib									
O.R.	F	8 y	12 y	1.5	20[b]	675	52	5.3	2.0
					68[a]	132	35	3.0	6.0
L.P.	F	5 mon	4 y	2	13[b]	389	45	7.2	4.0
					52[a]	280	49	4.1	9.0
GSD III									
S.A.	F	4 y	10 y	1.5	35[b]	279	—	5.6	6.0
					59[a]	213		3.9	9.0
Z.M.	F	1 y	6½ y	1.5	40[b]	412	—	4.4	5.0
					65[a]	202		3.5	8.0
S.G.	M	4 y	4 y	2	36[b]	380	—	5.5	5.0
					61[a]	226		3.7	6.5

[b]: before cornstarch treatment
[a]: after 1 y of cornstarch treatment

indicates that cornstarch is effective, safe and cheap and that it can replace nocturnal intragastric feeding.

REFERENCES

Burr, I. N., O'Neall, T. A., Karson, D. B., Howard, L. J. and Green, H. L. Comparison of the effect of total enteral nutrition, continuous intragastric feeding and portocaval shunt on a patient with type I glycogen storage disease. *J. Pediatr*. 85 (1979) 792

Chen, Y. T., Cornblath, M. and Sidbury, T. B. Cornstarch therapy in type I glycogen storage disease. *N. Engl. J. Med*. 310 (1984) 171

Fernandes, J., Berger, R. and Smit, G. P. A. Lactate as a cerebral metabolic fuel for glucose-6-phosphatase deficient children. *Pediatr. Res*. 18 (1984a) 335

Fernandes, J., Smit, G. P. A. and Berger, R. Dietary treatment of children with liver glycogenosis. In Benson, P. F. (ed.) *Screening and Management of Potentially Treatable Genetic Metabolic Disorders*. MTP Press, Lancaster, 1984b, pp. 161–176

Greene, H. L., Slonin, A. E., Burr, J. M. and Moran, R. Type I glycogen storage disease: five years of management with nocturnal intragastric feeding. *J. Pediatr*. 96 (1980) 590

Sloan, H. R. and Zipt, W. B. Cornstarch therapy of glycogen storage disease type I (GSD I). *Pediatr. Res*. 17 (1983) 220A

Smit, G. P. A., Boyer, R., Potasmick, R., Morel, S. W and Fernandes, J. The dietary treatment of children with type I glycogen storage disease with slow release carbohydrate. *Pediatr. Res*. 18 (1984) 879

J. Inher. Metab. Dis. 9 *Suppl.* 2 *(1986) 284–286*

Short Communication

Galactose-1-Phosphate-Uridyl Transferase Activity in Chorionic Villi: A First Trimester Prenatal Diagnosis of Galactosaemia

M. O. ROLLAND[1], G. MANDON[1], J. P. FARRIAUX[2] and C. DORCHE[1]
[1]*Laboratoire de Biochimie, Hôpital Debrousse, 69005 Lyon, France;*
[2]*Service de Génétique, CHU, 59000 Lille, France*

Antenatal diagnosis of galactosaemia was until now based on galactitol detection in amniotic fluid and enzymatic measurement in cultured amniotic cells from second trimester pregnancy (Jakobs *et al.*, 1984; Fensom *et al.*, 1974).

The use of chorionic villi for early prenatal diagnosis is rapidly gaining practical importance. Its main advantage is that fetal tissue can be obtained early, without any penetration of the fetal membrane (Gosden *et al.*, (1982).

We report the determination of galactose-1-phosphate-uridyl transferase activity (Gal-transferase) (EC 2.7.7.12) in a first-trimester fetus suspected of galactosaemia through a direct assay on chorionic villus material.

METHODS

Erythrocyte Gal-transferase activity was measured by the UDPG-consumption method (Beutler and Baluda, 1966). The Gal-transferase activity in other tissues was determined by the method of Ng *et al.* (1964), using [^{14}C] galactose-1-phosphate as a substrate but with separation of product and substrate on DEAE cellulose microcolumns. Genotype determination was carried out by starch gel electrophoresis according to Sparkes *et al.* (1977). The protein content of lysates was measured by the method of Lowry.

Chorionic villi were obtained by ultrasound-directed aspiration. Pure chorionic villi were selected under a microscope by separation from maternal decidua. Fetal tissue was homogenized in forty parts of buffer, sonicated twice for 10 seconds, and Gal-transferase activity determined using the radioisotopic method.

CASE REPORT

The index case was the first child of unrelated parents. He developed early severe neonatal disorders ending with coma and death 12 days after birth. The biological diagnosis was performed *a posteriori*, on a screening card revealing a mild hyper-phenylalaninaemia (Guthrie test at 5 days of life) and a Beutler's spot test positive for galactosaemia. Subsequently, Gal-transferase activity in erythrocytes and

Journal of Inherited Metabolic Disease. ISSN 0141–8955.

fibroblasts of the parents confirmed the risk of galactosaemia for their future offspring.

When the mother became pregnant once again, it was decided to perform a trophoblast biopsy in the first trimester, followed, in the case of a result indicating a non-affected fetus, by an amniocentesis during the 17th week of gestation for a direct analysis of galactitol combined with enzymatic activity measurement in cultivated cells.

Chorionic villi obtained in Lille, were sent in NaCl (0.9% solution) to Lyon. At the same time controls were obtained from elective pregnancy terminations and sent in the same conditions (20 h at room temperature).

RESULTS

Gal-transferase of the parents was shown to be lowered when compared to controls, both in red blood cells (mother 38%, father 54% of controls) and in fibroblasts (mother 36%, father 64% of controls). The enzymatic mobility on starch gel electrophoresis showed that while the mother had a normal electrophoretic pattern, the father, on the contrary, had an enzyme with bands moving faster than controls. The decreased activity associated with fast mobility indicated a genotype of Los Angeles galactosaemia compound heterozygote for the father. The decreased activity associated with a normal migration led to a genotype of a classical galactosaemia carrier for the mother.

The results obtained on trophoblastic tissue for the fetus at risk are shown in Table 1. Three controls gave activities between 12.5 and 21.3 units. The propositus had an activity at 11. This indicated the occurrence of a non-affected child.

Table 1 Gal-transferase activity in trophoblasts and cultured amniotic cells and trophoblastic cells measured as μkat/kg protein

	Trophoblast	*Cultured amniotic cells*	*Cultured trophoblastic cells*
Propositus	11	8.5	8.4
Range in controls (n = 3)	12.5–21.3	7.1–10.8	6.3–9.3

The amniocentesis was carried out later: Dr Jakobs in Amsterdam did not find a pathological level of galactitol in the amniotic fluid. The Gal-transferase activity determined in cultivated trophoblastic and amniotic cells was found in the same range as controls (Table 1).

To help determine the genotype of the fetus, a starch gel electrophoresis was performed directly on chorionic villi and on cultivated trophoblasts. A faster mobility for the propositus than for controls was obtained. The pattern for controls was the same as in skin fibroblasts showing three bands of different intensities; for the propositus the anodic bands were more intense indicating that the Los Angeles variant was present.

DISCUSSION AND CONCLUSION

The availability of chorionic villi biopsy opens up new perspectives for antenatal diagnosis, allowing direct enzyme analysis. This study has shown that Gal-transferase is easily measured in as little as 15 mg of tissue and furthermore that rare variants can be detected with usual electrophoretic methods. Thus we can conclude that chorionic villi represents an adequate material on which to perform early antenatal diagnosis of galactosaemia.

REFERENCES

Beutler, E. and Baluda, M. Improved method for measuring galactose-1-phosphate uridyl transferase activity of erythrocytes. *Clin. Chim. Acta* 13 (1966) 369–379

Fensom, A., Benson, P. and Blunt, S. Prenatal diagnosis of galactosaemia. *Br. Med. J.* 4 (1974) 386

Gosden, J., Mitchell, A., Gosden, C., Rodeck, C. and Morsman J. Direct vision chorion biopsy and chromosome specific DNA probes for determination of fetal sex in first trimester prenatal diagnosis. *Lancet* 2 (1982) 1416

Jakobs, C., Warner, T., Sweetman, L. and Nyhan W. Stable isotope dilution analysis of galactitol in amniotic fluid an accurate approach to the prenatal diagnosis of galactosaemia. *Pediatr. Res.* 18 (1984) 714

Ng, W., Bergren, W. and Donell, G. Galactose 1 Ph uridyltransferase assay by use of radioactive galactose-1-phosphate. *Clin. Chim. Acta* 10 (1964) 337–343

Sparkes, M., Crist, M. and Sparkes R. Improved technique for electrophoresis of human galactose-1-phosphate uridyl transferase. *Hum. Genet.* 40 (1977) 93

J. Inher. Metab. Dis. 9 Suppl. 2 (1986) 287–290

Short Communication

Molecular Heterogeneity of McArdle Disease

D. Daegelen, S. Gautron, F. Mennecier, J.-C. Dreyfus and A. Kahn
Laboratoire de Recherches en Génétique et Pathologie Moléculaires, Unité 129 de L'INSERM, 24 rue du Fg St Jacques, 75674 Paris Cedex 14, France

McArdle disease (McKusick 23260) is a rare form of metabolic myopathy due to the lack of glycogen phosphorylase activity in muscle. This disease, genetically transmitted as an autosomal recessive character, is clinically characterized by weakness, cramps and attacks of myoglobinuria. Glycogen phosphorylase isoenzymes (muscle, liver and brain types) show a specific tissue distribution, so that the defect is limited to skeletal muscle.

Research on the molecular mechanism of the disease has long been confined to the search for altered or inactive proteins: immunological and/or electrophoretic methods (Daegelen-Proux *et al.*, 1981) have led to the differentiation of two kinds of aetiology: in most cases no protein was present while in a few other cases inactive protein could be detected (Feit and Brooke, 1976).

To gain more insight into the molecular defect in the case of patients with no cross-reacting material (CRM$^-$), the presence of muscle phosphorylase translational activity in muscle mRNAs of patients was investigated in our laboratory (Daegelen *et al.*, 1983). In the two cases studied no functional messenger could be detected. Nevertheless our experiments could not distinguish between absence of mRNA and presence of non-translatable mRNA.

To investigate further the molecular defect responsible for absence of CRM in most cases of McArdle disease we developed a specific human glycogen phosphorylase probe. We present in this paper the results obtained with this probe in 'Northern' blot and 'Southern' blot analysis of five unrelated cases of McArdle disease.

MATERIAL AND METHODS

Muscle biopsies (30–50 mg) were obtained from five patients with McArdle disease. The absence of phosphorylase activity was ascertained by both histoenzymological and biochemical methods. All cases have been checked for the presence of any detectable altered protein (Daegelen-Proux *et al.*, 1981) and were shown to be CRM$^-$. Human control muscle was obtained from a leg amputation.

Phosphorylase and aldolase A probes – Specific phosphorylase cDNA clones were isolated from a muscle human cDNA library in *E. coli* plasmid pBR 322 (Hanauer *et al.*, 1983). This was achieved by hybridization with a rabbit muscle phosphorylase cDNA, a gift from Dr Putney (Boston). Specific human aldolase A clones were isolated from the same library by using cross-hybridization with a human aldolase

B cDNA (Simon *et al.*, 1983). Subcloning of these cDNA was performed in M-13 bacteriophage (Messing, 1983).

RNA studies – The method of mRNA purification was scaled down to be compatible with the size of clinical muscle biopsies (Munnich *et al.*, 1982). Detection and characterization of mRNA for normal and McArdle muscle was realized by 'Northern blot' analysis (Simon *et al.*, 1983). Blots were hybridized with both phosphorylase and aldolase A probes and submitted to autoradiography. The autoradiograms were scanned on a 'Shimadzu' densitometer. The signal given by aldolase A probe was used as an internal reference for standardization of the amount of phosphorylase mRNA.

DNA studies – Blood samples from patients and controls were kept frozen until purification of DNA from the white blood cells. DNA studies were performed by Southern blot analysis (Southern, 1975).

RESULTS AND DISCUSSION

By heterologous hybridization with a rabbit muscle glycogen phosphorylase labelled cDNA probe, three cDNA clones corresponding to human muscular glycogen phosphorylase were isolated by screening about 8000 clones from an adult muscle cDNA library. Characterization of these clones was achieved by restriction mapping and partial sequencing according to Maxam and Gilbert, and after subcloning in the M-13 vector according to Sanger. Comparison of the deduced amino acid sequence with the known rabbit protein sequence showed an about 90% homology (Gautron *et al.*, in preparation). The most interesting clone covered 1300 bases; it overlaps half of the C-terminal coding region of the protein.

Studies of the RNA of several human tissues by 'Northern blot' revealed complementarity with a specific mRNA of 3400 bases (3.4 kb) and this only in tissues expressing muscle glycogen phosphorylase (at the protein level).

Five McArdle patients with no detectable inactive protein were investigated by Northern blot analysis for the presence or absence of phosphorylase mRNA. For this purpose we used the 1300 bases cDNA subcloned in M-13, in order to obtain highly labelled monostrand (improved) probes.

In three cases no specific phosphorylase mRNA could be detected while in two other cases normal size mRNA was present although in lowered amount: about 20% of normal as quantified with an internal constant mRNA (aldolase A mRNA). Typical results are shown in Figure 1. These results demonstrate that different molecular mechanisms can be responsible for the absence of cross-reacting material; even in the case where mRNA is present no detectable protein is translated. Therefore it cannot be excluded that these patients are compound heterozygotes carrying a mutation leading to no mRNA on one allele and on the other allele, another type of lesion leading to no translatable RNA.

Comparative studies of DNA from four patients and control white blood cells by Southern blot analysis showed no detectable deletion or rearrangement in the 20 kb region scanned by our probe. One of the cases studied corresponded to a

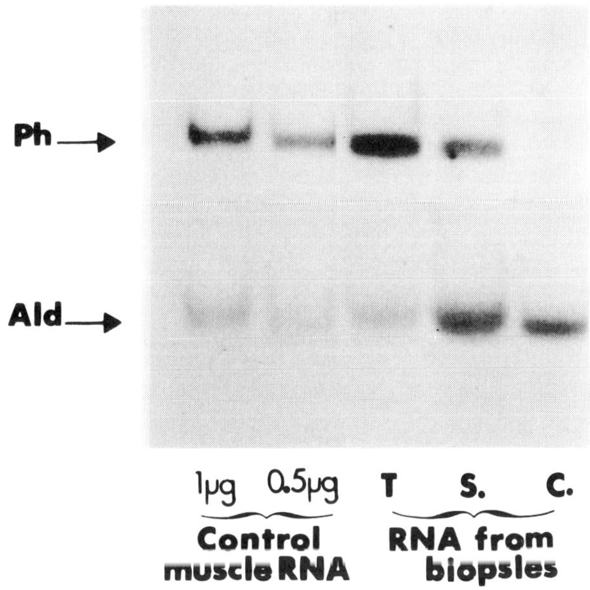

Figure 1 Northern blot analysis of RNA from a control (T) and two McArdle's patient biopsies (S. and C.), hybridized with both human muscle phosphorylase and aldolase A probes. About one-quarter of the total RNA purified from each biopsy was deposited in the corresponding slot. The intensities of the phosphorylase and aldolase A signals given by known amounts (0.5 and 1 μg) of human muscle RNA, and those obtained for the control biopsy were used to determine the normal phosphorylase/aldolase A signal intensity ratio.

patient with no mRNA and another with lowered amount. Our observations seem to favour small or point mutations leading to absent or unstable mRNA. For example non-sense mutations are known to lead to lowered amount of RNA.

REFERENCES

Daegelen-Proux, D., Kahn, A., Marie, J. and Dreyfus, J. C. Research on molecular mechanisms of McArdle's disease – Use of new protein mapping and immunological techniques. *Ann. Hum. Genet.* 45 (1981) 113–120

Daegelen, D., Munnich, A., Levin, M. J., Girault, A., Gosguen, J., Kahn, A. and Dreyfus, J. C. Absence of functional messenger RNA for glycogen phosphorylase in the muscle of two patients with McArdle's disease. *Ann. Hum. Genet.* 47 (1983) 107–115

Feit, H. and Brooke, M. H. Myophosphorylase deficiency: two molecular etiologies. *Neurology* 26 (1976) 963–967

Hanauer, A., Levin, M., Hielig, R., Daegelen, D., Kahn, A. and Mandel, J. L. Isolation and characterization of cDNA clones for human skeletal muscle actin. *Nucleic Acids Res.* 11 (1983) 3503–3516

Messing, J. New M13 vectors for cloning. *Methods Enzymol.* 101 (1983), 20–78

Munnich, A., Daegelen, D., Besmond, C., Marie, J., Dreyfus, J. C. and Kahn, A. Cell-free translation of mRNAs from human muscle biopsies: a miniaturized tool for investigation of neuromuscular diseases. *Pediatr. Res.* 16 (1982) 335–339

Simon, M. P., Besmond, C., Cottreau, D., Weber, A., Dreyfus, J. C., Sala-Trepat, J.,

Marie, J. and Kahn, A. Molecular cloning of cDNA for rat L-type pyruvate kinase and aldolase B. *J. Biol. Chem.* 258 (1983) 14576–14584

Southern, E. M. Detection of specific sequences among DNA fragments separated by gel electrophoresis. *J. Mol. Biol.* 98 (1975) 503–517

J. Inher. Metab. Dis. 9 Suppl. 2 (1986) 291–292

Short Communication

Decreased Affinity of Phosphorylase *a* for Glucose-1-phosphate in Polymorphonuclear Leukocytes of a Patient with Glycogenosis Type VI

D. PIENIĄŻEK and E. PRONICKA
Memorial Hospital Child Health Centre, Al. Dzieci Polskich 20, 04-736 Warsaw, Poland

Polymorphonuclear leukocytes are normally used for the diagnosis of glycogen storage disease (GSD) type VI (McKusick 23270), caused by the inherited deficiency of glycogen phosphorylase. Although the tissue for the investigation is readily available, little is known about the enzymatic defect(s). The deficiency of glycogen phosphorylase may be due to the reduced number of normal molecules of phosphorylase or to a structural change or changes in this protein.

The purpose of the present study was to determine the affinity of phosphorylase *a* and *b* for glucose-1-phosphate in polymorphonuclear leukocytes of a patient with GSD type VI.

PATIENT AND METHODS

J.P., a boy, was born in 1971. The parents are unrelated and have 3 healthy children. In the first years of life hepatomegaly and retarded growth were observed. At the age of 13 GSD type VI was recognized on the basis of the selective deficiency of phosphorylase *a* in leukocytes and liver tissue. The activities of other enzymes involved in glycogen degradation (phosphorylase *b* kinase, amylo-1, 6-glucosidase, glucose-6-phosphatase) were normal. At that time the physical and mental development of the patient was normal. The routine analysis of blood revealed a decreased concentration of glucose (50 mg dl^{-1}, control 70–140), increased lactate (28 mg dl^{-1}, control 7–18) and increased activities of aspartate and alanine aminotransferase (64 and 84 IU l^{-1}, control 4–32). The concentrations of total lipids, triglycerides and uric acid were similar to the control values. More details on the clinical and biochemical picture were presented in an earlier paper (Pieniążek *et al.*, 1985).

Phosphorylase *a* activity was determined by measuring the production of inorganic phosphate (P_i) from glucose-1-phosphate in the presence of 0.5 mmol l^{-1} caffeine by the method of Hers (1964). Phosphorylase *b* activity was estimated by the same method, except that caffeine was omitted and 1.0 mmol l^{-1} 5-AMP was added to the incubation mixture. The estimation of this enzyme was performed after the specific elimination of phosphorylase *a* from the homogenate. For this reason, an

Journal of Inherited Metabolic Disease. ISSN 0141–8955.

earlier 30 min preincubation of polymorphonuclear leukocytes in 0.125 mmol l^{-1} glycyl-glycine buffer, pH 7.4 at 25°C, was carried out. The affinities of phosphorylase *a* and *b* for glucose-1-phosphate as a substrate were determined at concentrations of 3.5–235 mmol l^{-1}. Protein in the tissue homogenate was estimated by the method of Lowry and colleagues (1951). Leukocytes from the whole blood were isolated by the method of Young and Patrick (1970).

RESULTS AND COMMENTS

The specific activities of phosphorylase *a* and *b* and the affinities of both forms of the enzyme for glucose-1-phosphate in polymorphonuclear leukocytes of the patient are presented in Table 1.

Table 1 The activities and affinities of phosphorylase *a* and *b* with glucose-1-phosphate in polymorphonuclear leukocytes of a patient with GSD type VI

	Activities (μmol P_i (mg protein)$^{-1}$ h^{-1})		K_m (mmol l^{-1})	
	Phosphorylase a	*Phosphorylase b*	*a*	*b*
Patient	0.17	1.10	35	10
Control ($n = 7$)	1.17±0.54	1.40±0.90	12±3	16±6

Phosphorylase *a* activity was significantly decreased in comparison with the control value, whereas the activity of phosphorylase *b* was similar to the control value. This indicated that the deficiency of phosphorylase *a* was not caused by a decreased rate of synthesis of the proenzyme, phosphorylase *b*. The affinity of phosphorylase *b* for glucose-1-phosphate was similar to the control value but the K_m of phosphorylase *a* was about 3 times higher than normal. This suggests that the low activity of phosphorylase *a* could be due to a structural change in the enzyme.

The analysis of the kinetic properties of phosphorylase *a* and *b* in leukocytes of other patients with this type of glycogenosis would be interesting.

REFERENCES

Hers, H. G. Glycogen storage disease. *Adv. Metab. Disord.* 1 (1964) 4–44

Lowry, O. H., Rosenbrough, N. J., Farr, A. L. and Randall, R. J. Protein measurements with the Folin phenol reagent. *J. Biol. Chem.* 193 (1951) 265–275

Pieniążek, D., Pronicka, E., Cabalska, B., Borowska, B., Maciejko, D., Miłoszewska. E., Kulczycka, H. and Prokopowicz, K. Glycogenosis type VI and VIa - biochemical and clinical documentation. *Pediatria Polska* 60 (1985) 489–496

Young, E. P. and Patrick, A. D. Deficiency of acid esterase activity in Wolman's disease. *Arch. Dis. Child.* 45 (1970) 664–668

J. Inher. Metab. Dis. 9 Suppl. 2 (1986) 293–296

Short Communication

The Diagnosis and Treatment of a Patient with Medium-chain Acyl-CoA Dehydrogenase Deficiency: Overnight Fasting Does Not Result in the Expected Urinary Metabolite Profile

A. H. VAN GENNIP[1], H. D. BAKKER[1], M. DURAN[2] and L. J. VAN OUDHEUSDEN[3]

[1]*Children's Hospital 'Het Emma Kinderziekenhuis', Spinozastraat 51, 1018 HJ Amsterdam;* [2]*University Children's Hospital 'Het Wilhelmina Kinderziekenhuis', Nieuwegracht 137, 3512 LK Utrecht;* [3]*Westfries Gasthuis, Wabenstraat 19, 1624 GM Hoorn, The Netherlands*

A patient with medium-chain acyl-CoA dehydrogenase (MCAD, EC 1.3.99.3) deficiency was subjected to a fasting experiment in order to test her ability to produce ketone bodies and maintain her blood glucose level within acceptable limits. Moreover, the organic acid excretion profile in relation to fasting was investigated in order to evaluate the necessity and risk of prolonged fasting experiments for the diagnosis of MCAD-deficiency. Finally, the effect of treatment with carnitine and riboflavin in preventing hypoketotic hypoglycaemia and dicarboxylic aciduria was studied in a second fasting experiment.

CASE REPORT

Patient S.K., a girl, is the first child born to healthy unrelated parents after an uneventful full-term pregnancy and normal delivery. At the age of 16 months she was found in her bed in a semi-comatose condition and she was slightly vomiting. Shortly thereafter she was admitted to a local hospital. During preceding days she had had a moderate slimy diarrhoea and a cold. Physical examination revealed no abnormalities. Routine laboratory tests showed a metabolic alkalosis and a severe hypoglycaemia, which was corrected by glucose infusion. A 24 h urine collected after recovery was referred to our laboratory for metabolic investigation.

GLC-analysis of organic acids revealed dicarboxylic aciduria without ketonuria, and considerable amounts of 5-hydroxyhexanoic and hexanoic acids, a pattern indicating MCAD deficiency. Plasma free carnitine was at the lower limit of the normal range. The excretion of free carnitine was decreased, but that of acylcarnitine was increased.

The patient was subjected to a fasting experiment under constant medical observa-

Journal of Inherited Metabolic Disease. ISSN 0141–8955. Queen Square, Lancaster, UK. Printed in Great Britain by Titus Wilson & Son Ltd., Kendal.

tion. After treatment with frequent feedings rich in carbohydrates, 3×1 g D,L-carnitine daily and riboflavin 2×50 mg daily for 10 weeks, a second fasting experiment was carried out in order to evaluate the effect of the treatment.

METHODS

Organic acids were extracted with ethyl acetate. Gas chromatography of the trimethylsilyl derivatives was performed on a capillary fused silica WCOT column (25 m×0.22 mm I.D.) coated with CP^{tm} Sil 19 CB (film thickness 0.2 μm). Identification of the compounds was performed by GC-MS (Kamerling *et al.*, 1979).

Free fatty acids were extracted from plasma or urine with a mixture of chloroform/*n*-heptane/methanol (28 : 21 : 1, v/v) according to the method described by Samson and Hensley (1975). The organic phase was evaporated to dryness under reduced pressure. After trimethylsilylation, the compounds were analysed by GLC as described above.

For the analysis of conjugated acids 5 ml 10N NaOH was added to an equal amount of urine. In a screw-capped vial this mixture was heated at 100°C for 1 h. After cooling below 5°C the sample was adjusted to pH 1.5 and then processed as for unhydrolysed urine.

Carnitine measurements in plasma and urine were done enzymatically according to Pearson *et al.* (1969). Urinary acylcarnitines were separated and determined according to Duran *et al.* (1983).

RESULTS

After a 12 h overnight fast during the first fasting experiment blood glucose was still 4.6 mmol/l and a urine sample collected at that time showed virtually no abnormalities. After alkaline hydrolysis of the urine only small amounts of suberic acid and of octanoic acid could be detected. Even in a urine sample collected after 18 h of fasting only slightly increased amounts of adipic acid, 5-hydroxyhexanoic acid and 7-hydroxyoctanoic acid were found; alkaline hydrolysis of the urine sample revealed the presence of conjugated hexanoic, octanoic and suberic acids. At this time blood glucose was 4.2 mmol/l. It was not until 24 h of fasting that the glucose concentration had dropped to 3.2 mmol/l and at 32 h of fasting it was still 3.1 mmol/l. Within the next 2 h clinical symptoms of hypoglycaemia appeared and blood glucose level decreased to 2.1 mmol/l. At that time there was a tremendous increase in the excretion of free and conjugated dicarboxylic acids and other medium-chain acids (Table 1).

During the second fasting test performed after 10 weeks of treatment, the blood glucose level decreased from 5.0 mmol/l to 2.9 mmol/l within 24 h. After 30 h of fasting the level was still 2.6 mmol/l, but within 2 h the level dropped to 0.5 mmol/l. This time the urinary metabolite profile after 18 h of fasting was even more pronounced than during the first experiment (Table 1). Urine samples collected later on during the test showed the full-blown metabolite pattern.

Table 1 Urinary metabolite profile in relation to fasting (excretion values in μmol/g creat.)

		First fasting test on 7 March 1985			*Second fasting test on 14 May 1985*				
Metabolite	*24 h sample*	*0-12 h*	*12-18 h*	*18-35 h*	*0-12 h*	*12-18 h*	*18-27 h*	*27-28½ h*	*28½-37½ h*
decanoic	–	–	trace	16	trace	18	31	35	39
decan. conj.	trace	–	19	591	[illegible]2	29	55	n.a.	43
sebacic	694	56	trace	350	trace	168	1619	1739	1959
uns. sebacic.	1103	–	–	1664	–	137	1363	1423	1779
sebacic. conj.	–	–	–	105	–	trace	164	101	289
3-OH-sebacic	365	–	–	630	–	167	1044	1319	2315
octanoic	trace	–	trace	568	trace	35	766	1224	2472
octan. conj.	391	84	174	1912	5[illegible]1	1464	3246	608	1580
octan. carnitine	n.a.	n.a.	n.a.	n.a.	–	n.a.	n.a.	n.a.	+
7-OH-octan.	–	–	64	trace	–	–	–	–	+
suberic	1150	31	129	1991	trace	204	[illegible]106	1157	1553
uns. suberic	731	trace	trace	932	–	trace	511	546	828
sub. conj.	1532	80	485	1666	177	979	3324	3878	3476
sub. glycine	–	–	+	+	n.a.	n.a.	n.a.	n.a.	+
hexanoic	75	–	51	326	trace	trace	+	+	98
hexan. conj.	326	+	243	416	43[illegible]	796	944	n.a.	732
hex. glycine	+	–	–	–	–	+	+	+	+
hex. carnitine	n.a.	n.a.	n.a.	n.a.	+	n.a.	n.a.	n.a.	+
5-OH-hexan.	729	36	72	2443	5[illegible]	135	465	423	1202
adipic	3218	91	113	4641	5[illegible]	122	2109	2099	4964
ß-OH-but.	<4904	trace	trace	1240	–	295	1295	1340	1451
ß-keto-but.	trace	–	–	624	–	528	1847	1887	1943

n.a. = not analysed.

DISCUSSION

Routine GLC analysis of urine collected after an overnight fast showed virtually no abnormalities. However, after alkaline hydrolysis of the urine small amounts of suberic, hexanoic and octanoic acids could be detected, a pattern indicating MCAD deficiency (Gregersen *et al.*, 1983). Therefore, GLC of hydrolysed urine should be included in the analysis programme when MCAD deficiency is suspected. Prolonged fasting by a patient is recommended for diagnostic evaluation, but has the risk of life-threatening hypoglycaemia. However, in our patient 18 h fasting appeared to be adequate for the purpose of diagnosis whereas blood glucose remained within the normal range.

Treatment with carnitine and riboflavin did not improve the capacity of β-oxidation and could not prevent hypoketotic hypoglycaemia and dicarboxylic aciduria in a second fasting experiment. In our opinion this treatment can be omitted. A dietary protocol of frequent feedings rich in carbohydrates seems to be the only substantiated method to prevent hypoglycaemic attacks.

REFERENCES

Duran, M., De Klerk, J. B. C., Van Pelt, J., Wadman, S. K., Scholte, H. R., Beekman, R. P. and Jennekens, F.G.I. The analysis of plasma and urinary organic acids during prolonged fasting differentiates between systemic carnitine deficiency and a defect of fatty acid oxidation. *J. Inher. Metab. Dis.* 6 Suppl. 2 (1983) 121–122

Gregersen, N., Kølvraa, S., Rasmussen, K., Mortensen, P. B., Divry, P., David, M. and Hobolth, N. General (medium-chain) acyl-CoA dehydrogenase deficiency (non-ketotic dicarboxylic aciduria): quantitative urinary excretion pattern of 23 biologically significant organic acids in three cases. *Clin. Chim. Acta* 132 (1983) 181–191

Kamerling, J. P., Brouwer, M., Ketting, D. and Wadman, S. K. Gas chromatography of urinary *N*-phenylacetylglutamine. *J. Chromatogr.* 164 (1979) 217–221

Pearson, D. J., Tubbs, P. K. and Chase, J. F. A. Carnitine and acylcarnitines. *Methods Enzymol.* 14 (1969) 1758–1771

Samson, D. and Hensley, W. J. A rapid gas chromatographic method for the quantitation of underivatised individual free fatty acids in plasma. *Clin. Chim. Acta* 61 (1975) 1–8

J. Inher. Metab. Dis. 9 *Suppl.* 2 *(1986) 297–299*

Short Communication

A New Case of C_6–C_{14} Dicarboxylic Aciduria with Favourable Evolution

E. RIUDOR[1], A. RIBES[2], M. BORONAT[1], C. SABADO[1], C. DOMINGUEZ[1] and A. BALLABRIGA[1]
[1]*Children's Hospital, Ciutat Sanitaria Vall d'Hebron, Barcelona, Spain*
[2]*Institut de Bioquimica Clinica, Diputacio de Barcelona, Cerdanyola, Spain*

Acyl-CoA dehydrogenation deficiencies and carnitine deficiencies result in several biochemical disturbances with no specific organic acid profile and similar symptoms (Duran *et al.*, 1984). We present here a case of C_6–C_{14}dicarboxylic aciduria with an unusual major peak, eluting just before adipic acid, which is currently under investigation. The patient responded to treatment with carnitine, riboflavin and a high carbohydrate, low fat diet with frequent intakes.

CASE REPORT

The patient was a boy aged 3 years and 3 months, the fourth child of unrelated parents, who has been admitted on two occasions due to vomiting, obnubilation and metabolic acidosis. His family history included two sisters who died at 4 months and 25 months respectively. The first died following cardiorespiratory failure during a slight episode of diarrhoea, and the second died following an attack of severe dehydration with vomiting and hepatomegaly. Fatty infiltration of the liver, cerebral oedema, fatty myocardiac vacuoles and fatty renal tubular cell vacuoles were observed at necropsy. The third child is a normal girl.

The patient was first referred to the hospital in November 1984 with a 4–5 day history of vomiting, hypotonia and hepatomegaly coinciding with a cold. He had non-ketotic hypoglycaemia ($50\,mg\,dl^{-1}$) with metabolic acidosis; NH_3 $211\,\mu mol\,l^{-1}$; serum free carnitine $17\,\mu mol\,l^{-1}$. Plasma and urine amino acids were normal except for low glutamine and alanine plasma values. Echocardiographic studies showed dilation of the left ventricle. Myopathy was revealed by EMG and pigmentous retinitis was confirmed by electroretinography. Histopathology showed fatty vacuoles in liver, as in Reye's syndrome, and alterations in muscle ratio of type I and II fibres. Carnitine therapy ($100\,mg\,kg^{-1}$) and frequent high carbohydrate, low fat intakes were instituted.

Two months later he was readmitted, with a clinical picture similar to the previous one which improved in a few days. Since then the patient has presented with two similar but less serious episodes: one coincided with a slight infection and the other with no known triggering factor. In addition to the other therapy, he began treatment with riboflavin (50 mg every 12 hours). At present he has a normal lifestyle without clinical disturbances.

Journal of Inherited Metabolic Disease. ISSN 0141–8955.

RESULTS AND DISCUSSION

Organic acids of urine were analysed by GC–MS of their trimethylsilyl (TMS) derivatives after overnight extraction with diethyl ether.

Table 1 Urinary organic acids (μmol (g creatinine)$^{-1}$). The response factor of the corresponding saturated dicarboxylic acid has been applied to the other compounds

	First crisis	*Second crisis*	*24 h post-second crisis*	*Fasting test*			
				Basal	*8 h*	*16 h*	*24 h*
3-Hydroxybutyric acid	2032	1452	512	298	246	156	1029
Unidentified peak (given as adipic acid)	1402	1009	1095	496	681	879	1159
Adipic acid	2173	6027	1641	108	193	229	1882
Octenedioic acid	377	682	158	101	47	80	396
Suberic acid	530	1937	369	88	92	99	513
Decenedioic acid I	—	1311	335	Tr	Tr.	Tr.	682
Decenedioic acid II	749	1601	576	215	267	138	692
Hydroxydecenedioic acid	315	651	139	69	34	43	284
Hydroxysebacic acid	735	1756	588	125	162	176	899
Hydroxydodecenedioic acid	276	660	219	Tr.	Tr.	Tr.	420
Hydroxydodecanedioic acid	211	1211	381	31	64	50	649
Hydroxytetradecenedioic acid	Tr.	505	91	Tr.	Tr.	Tr.	306

On the first admission (Table 1), C_6–C_{14}dicarboxylic aciduria with increased 3-hydroxybutyric acid was found along with the presence of a peak eluting just before adipic acid. This is under investigation: base peak *m/z* 75 by electron impact MS, molecular weight of TMS derivative 216 by chemical ionization with ammonia gas, parent molecular weight 144; hypothetical structure 2-hydroxyadipic acid lactone.

On the second admission, a urine sample taken during the crisis fully repeated the profile described above. Analysis was repeated 24 h after the crisis and showed a notable decrease in pathologic metabolites. A 24 h fasting test was performed which showed the organic acid profile previously described, without hypoglycaemia or clinical decompensation (Tables 1 and 2).

In none of the urine samples was the presence of acylglycines detected by GC–MS of methylated derivatives, nor has an increase of dicarboxylic acids been found on hydrolysis of these acylglycines. Similarly, no octanoic acid has been observed in urine, or in hydrolysed urine (search for octanoylcarnitine). The absence of acylglycines and octanoic acid suggests that medium chain acyl-CoA dehydrogenase activity was normal. No pipecolic acid was found. The history of the patient suggests a long chain acyl-CoA dehydrogenase deficiency (Gregersen, 1985) or a possible carnitine deficiency (Engel and Rebouche, 1984).

Pathological metabolites in minor concentration were observed in the father's urine. Though this could clarify the possible deficiency, it is difficult to choose one therapeutic factor as determinant of clinical improvement. The high concentration of an unidentified endogenous peak adds a new question: is it secondary to dicarboxylic acid accumulation or is it a primary metabolite in an unknown pathway?

Table 2 Plasma metabolites during fasting test

	Basal: on remission	*24 h*
Glucose (mg dl^{-1})	132	89
3-Hydroxybutyric acid (mmol l^{-1})	0.25	0.54
Glycerol (mg dl^{-1})	1.61	4.91
Free fatty acids (μmol l^{-1})	696	2310
Octanoic acid (μmol l^{-1})	22.6	21.6
Decanoic acid (μmol l^{-1})	4.3	4.6
Free carnitine (nmol ml^{-1})	16.7	17.3
FFA/3-Hydroxybutyrate	2.78	4.28

REFERENCES

Duran, M., de Klerk, J. B. C., Wadman, S. K., Bruinvis, L. and Ketting, D. The differential diagnosis of dicarboxylic acidurias. *J. Inher. Metab. Dis.* 7 Suppl. 1 (1984) 48–51

Engel, A. G. and Rebouche, C. J. Carnitine metabolism and inborn errors. *J. Inher. Metab. Dis.* 7 Suppl. 1 (1984) 38–44

Gregersen, N. The acylCoA dehydrogenation deficiencies. *Scand. J. Clin. Lab. Invest.* 45 Suppl. 174 (1985)

J. Inher. Metab. Dis. 9 *Suppl.* 2 *(1986)* 300–302

Short Communication

Pyruvate Carboxylase Responsive to Ketosis in a Multiple Carboxylase Deficiency Patient

A. VELÁZQUEZ[1], D. VON RAESFELD[2], A. GONZÁLEZ-NORIEGA[1], L. GONZÁLEZ[1], C. GARAY[1], R. ORTIZ[1] and V. DEL CASTILLO[2].
[1]*Instituto de Investigaciones Biomédicas, Universidad Nacional Autónoma de México Apdo. Postal 70228, C.P. 04510 Ciudad Universitaria, D.F., México*
[2]*Instituto Nacional de Pediatría, Servicio de Genética Insurgentes Sur 3700-C, 3er piso Col. Insurgentes Cuicuilco CP 04530 México, D.F.*

Pyruvate carboxylase (PC; EC 6.4.1.1) is a key enzyme for carbohydrate and lipid metabolism. Deficient patients have been described, the deficiency being either isolated (McKusick 26615) or combined with other carboxylase deficiencies (McKusick 25327) (Bartlett *et al.*, 1984). The effects of ketosis are quite different depending on whether it occurs in a normal or in a deficient individual. In the former it is associated with enhanced gluconeogenesis (Newsholme and Leech, 1983); in the latter, ketosis may cause severe acidosis (DeVivo *et al.*, 1977). We have studied a multiple carboxylase deficient (MCD) child with a phenotype resembling PC deficiency (Velázquez *et al.*, in preparation), who did not present an acidotic response to ketosis but instead improved clinically and biochemically when this metabolic state was induced in her.

CASE HISTORY

The patient was a female whose fetal movements were weak and of late onset. There was severe psychomotor and somatic retardation, intractable seizures and spastic paraparesia, but no ketoacidotic episodes. Alanine, pyruvate and lactate were elevated and were further increased after a glucose load. High doses of biotin diminished their blood concentration to the normal range but no clinical improvement was observed. There was also a small urinary excretion of methylcitrate and 3-hydroxypropionate but no metabolites related to 3-methylcrotonyl-CoA carboxylase could be detected. The patient died at 6 years of age: there was severe cerebral atrophy. All three mitochondrial carboxylases were approximately 20% of normal in cultured fibroblasts and increased only 1.5 to 2-fold after growth in medium containing 4000 nmol biotin per litre. When biotin-depleted cells were transferred to a biotin-enriched medium (820 nmol/l), reactivation of the patient's carboxylases was slower for PC than for PCC. Holocarboxylase synthetase activity, using endogenous apoPCC as a substrate, was 15% of the control values; when assayed at varying concentrations of biotin, the V_{max} was decreased but the apparent K_m was normal.

CLINICAL STUDIES

Ketosis was induced in the patient on four occasions (Table 1), initially during the course of diagnostic evaluation, and later as an attempt to control the seizures, which did not respond to the conventional anticonvulsant therapy. Blood pyruvate and lactate reached near-normal levels during a 24 h fast, while glucose remained normal and 3-hydroxybutyrate increased moderately. Similar results were observed, and seizures disappeared, when the patient was given a fat-rich diet containing medium-chain triglycerides (MCT) during 1 week.

Table 1 **Effect of ketogenic interventions on blood pyruvate and 3-hydroxybutyrate (3-HB) levels and on lymphocyte carboxylases***

Interventions	*Pyruvate*		*3-HB*		*PC*		*PCC*	
	B	*A*	*B*	*A*	*B*	*A*	*B*	*A*
24 h fast	389	140	45	1014	ND	ND	ND	ND
Medium-chain triglycerides	225	71	37	354	ND	ND	ND	ND
72 h fast	173	48	241	1395	ND	ND	ND	ND
2.75 F:C+P diet	—	76	—	622	2.4	8.3	3.8	4.2

* Pyruvate and 3-hydroxybutyrate in μmol/l; carboxylase activities in nmol CO_2 fixed h^{-1} (mg protein)$^{-1}$. B: before, and, A: after intervention. ND: not determined. F:C+P: fat to carbohydrate plus protein ratio.

The patient was again subjected to a fast, this time of 72 h duration, followed by a fat-rich diet with coconut oil as source of MCT. Ketosis was produced during the fast and when the ratio of fat to carbohydrate plus protein (F:C+P) was 2.75. On these two occasions, blood pyruvate reached normal concentrations, seizures disappeared and anticonvulsant therapy could be discontinued. However, seizures reappeared when a normal diet was readministered. During this last intervention PC and PCC activities were measured simultaneously in lymphocytes from the patient and from a control eating a normal diet. PC increased to near-normal levels in the patient while PCC (and both carboxylases from the control cells) did not vary significantly (Table 1).

DISCUSSION

Other patients deficient in PC have responded with hypoglycaemia to fasting (Van Biervliet *et al*., 1977) and with severe acidosis to a ketogenic diet (DeVivo *et al*., 1977). However, compared to those other patients, ours had substantial residual enzyme activity, which might have been further activated by an enlarged pool of acetyl-CoA during the ketotic episodes. However PC activity in the patient fibroblasts remained at 20% that of control cells in spite of the addition of increasing amounts of acetyl-CoA to the reaction mixture, up to a concentration of 1000 μmol/l (PC is usually assayed with 300 μmol/l acetyl-CoA; Atkin *et al*., 1979). Therefore, it seems that the *in vivo* effect was not the result of direct activation of residual PC but a consequence of ketosis-induced *in vivo* regulatory events, including hormone-mediated changes and perhaps stabilization of the enzyme by acetyl-CoA.

Another possible mechanism might be an activation of holocarboxylase synthetase by acetyl-CoA, as has been described in yeast (Cazzulo *et al.*, 1968) and in *B. stearonthermophilus* (Cazzulo *et al.*, 1970). However, this is an unlikely explanation for our observations since it has not been observed in chick liver (Madappalli and Mistry, 1970) nor in mouse cultured cells (Chang and Cohen, 1983).

Finally, it is noteworthy that in our patient ketosis had an effect greater than that of biotin, on PC activity and on the control of seizures.

ACKNOWLEDGEMENTS

The financial support from Consejo Nacional de Ciencia y Tecnología, Programa Universitario de Investigación Clínica and Fondo Ricardo J. Zevada is gratefully acknowledged.

REFERENCES

Atkin, B. M., Utter, M. F. and Weinberg, M. B. Pyruvate carboxylase and phosphoenolpyruvate carboxykinase activity in leukocytes and fibroblasts from a patient with pyruvate carboxylase deficiency. *Pediatr. Res.* 13 (1979) 38–43

Bartlett, K., Ghneim, H. K., Stirk, J. H., Dale, G. and Alberti, G. M. M. Pyruvate carboxylase deficiency. *J. Inher. Metab. Dis.* 7, Suppl. 1 (1984) 74–78

Cazzulo, J. J., Claisse, L. M. and Stoppani, O. M. Carboxylase levels and carbon dioxide fixation in bakers' yeast. *J. Bact.* 96 (1968) 623–628

Cazzulo, J. J., Sundaram, T. K. and Kornberg, H. L. Properties and regulation of pyruvate carboxylase from *Bacillus stearonthermophilus. Proc. Roy. Soc. London B* 176 (1970) 1–19

Chang, H. I. and Cohen, N. D. Regulation and intracellular localization of the biotin holocarboxylase synthetase of 3T3-L1 cells *Arch. Biochem. Biophys.* 225 (1983) 237–247

DeVivo, D. C., Haymond, M. W., Leckie, M. P., Bussman, Y. L., McDougal, D. B. and Pagliara, A. S. The clinical and biochemical implications of pyruvate carboxylase deficiency. *J. Clin. Endocrinol. Metab.* 45 (1977) 1281–1296

Madappalli, M. M. and Mistry, S. P. Synthesis of chicken liver holocarboxylase *in vivo* and *in vitro. Biochim. Biophys. Acta* 215 (1970) 316–322

Newsholme, E. A. and Leech, A. R. *Biochemistry for the Medical Sciences,* John Wiley & Sons, Chichester, 1983, p. 452

Van Biervliet, J. P. G. M., Bruinvis, L., van der Heiden, C., Ketting, D., Wadman, S. K., Willemse, J. L. and Monnens, L. A. H. Report of a patient with severe, chronic lactic acidaemia and pyruvate carboxylase deficiency. *Develop. Med. Child Neurol.* 19 (1977) 392–401

J. Inher. Metab. Dis. 9 Suppl. 2 (1986) 303–306

Short Communication

Neonatal Screening for Biotinidase Deficiency: An Update

B. Wolf[1,2], G. S. Heard[1], L. G. Jefferson[1], K. A. Weissbecker[1], J. R. Secor McVoy[1], W. E. Nance[1,2], P. L. Mitchell[3], F. W. Lambert[3] and A. S. Linyear[4]

[1]*Department of Human Genetics and* [2]*Department of Pediatrics, Children's Medical Center, Medical College of Virginia, Richmond, Virginia 23298, USA;* [3]*Department of General Services, Division of Consolidated Laboratory Services, Bureau of Microbiological Science, Richmond, Virginia 23219, USA and* [4]*Bureau of Maternal and Child Health, Commonwealth of Virginia, Richmond, Virginia 23219, USA*

Biotinidase (EC 3.5.1.12) hydrolyses biotin from small biotinyl peptides and biocytin that result from the proteolytic degradation of biotin-dependent holocarboxylases (Pispa, 1965; Craft *et al.*, 1985). The released biotin can then be reutilized by the body. Biotinidase also appears to play an important role in the processing of biotin from dietary protein-bound sources (Wolf *et al.*, 1984). We have shown that most individuals with late-onset multiple carboxylase deficiency have a primary defect in biotinidase activity (Wolf *et al.*, 1983a). Children with this autosomal recessively inherited disorder may exhibit seizures, hypotonia, ataxia, alopecia, skin rashes, hearing loss and developmental delay, which may ultimately result in coma or death (Wolf *et al.*, 1983b). Although most affected individuals have had metabolic ketoacidosis and organic aciduria, some have not. All children who have been diagnosed early have improved markedly after treatment with pharmacologic doses of biotin. Others who are diagnosed late often sustain neurologic abnormalities even after biotin therapy. Therefore, biotinidase deficiency qualifies for inclusion in a newborn screening programme for inherited metabolic disorders by satisfying three major criteria. First, symptoms of the disease do not appear at birth but usually occur at several months of age. Second, affected individuals may manifest serious physical and mental disability. Third, the disorder can be treated easily and effectively with vitamin supplementation. In order to determine the feasibility of screening and the incidence of biotinidase deficiency, we have conducted a pilot neonatal screening programme in the Commonwealth of Virginia.

METHODS

We developed a semi-quantitative colorimetric assay for biotinidase activity which employs the same samples of blood-soaked filter paper that are used in most neonatal screening programmes (Heard *et al.*, 1984). An artificial substrate, *N*-

Journal of Inherited Metabolic Disease. ISSN 0141–8955.

biotinyl-*p*-aminobenzoate, an analogue of biocytin, is used in the assay. During incubation of blood spots with this substrate, biotinidase liberates *p*-aminobenzoate. The *p*-aminobenzoate reacts with several colour developing reagents, including a diazonium compound, to produce a distinctive purple colour. Blood spots lacking activity (less than 10% normal activity) remain straw-coloured. Each individual diagnosed previously has had less than 5% normal activity based on quantitative determination (Wolf *et al.*, 1983a). Biotinidase remains active in the paper filters for up to 18 months. We use sample trays that hold disposable wells for the incubations, but a 'dimple' tray such as that used in the Beutler test is satisfactory.

RESULTS AND DISCUSSION

During the 18 months since the programme commenced 115 262 newborn infants were screened for biotinidase deficiency in Virginia. We detected two newborns with the disorder (Wolf *et al.*, 1985). These infants, a 4-month-old female and a 2-month-old male, were not noted previously to have any medical problems. Closer examination of both children revealed the presence of increased deep-tendon reflexes and mild hypertonia. Both were developing normally and neither had cutaneous or biochemical abnormalities. Biotin treatment was begun, and at 1 year of age the hypertonia has resolved and both infants are doing well.

The parents and several other relatives were shown to be heterozygous for this disorder. Unexpectedly, two siblings of the second infant, a 2-year-old male and a 3-year-old female, were also found to have biotinidase deficiency. They had slight facial skin rashes, some neurologic abnormalities, but no acidosis or organic aciduria. Both are now being treated with biotin.

The diagnosis in the affected infants was confirmed at several months of age. Because the screening was conducted in a separate laboratory we did not have access to the efficient follow-up procedures that are available in the state's metabolic screening programme. More rapid confirmation is anticipated when the test becomes incorporated into the state programme.

A summary of the results of the screening programme is shown in Table 1. The overall rate of false positive tests (based on requests for second filter cards, not repeated tests of the initial card) is 0.12% of the total newborns screened. This compares favourably to that for the other screening tests currently being conducted. The highest percentage of false positive results occurs in infants born prematurely. Serum biotinidase activity increases from about 25% of normal in children born at 26 weeks of gestation to 50–75% of normal in infants born at term. Infants with hepatic damage may also have low enzyme activity.

There are five important advantages of screening for biotinidase deficiency. First, the screening assay measures enzyme activity rather than elevated concentrations of a metabolite. A sample without activity must be retested, whereas a sample with activity almost certainly represents an unaffected child. Although the presence of sulphonamides in a blood sample may cause the development of purple colour, these antibiotics are not usually used in the treatment of newborns. However, all tests performed on samples from second cards are tested for the presence of

Table 1 Results of neonatal screening for biotinidase deficiency in Virginia

Age of newborns from whom the initial sample was obtained	*Number of infants screened*	*Second card requested and tested* (percentage of infants screened in the age category)*	*Number of infants with biotinidase deficiency*
Premature	2387	28 (1.17%)	0
Less than 1 day	2646	2 (0.08%)	0
1 to 10 days	89 711	110 (0.12%)	1
Older than 10 days	20 518	2 (<0.01%)	1
Total	115 262	142 (0.12%)	2

* Does not include seven children from whom a second card was requested but is still pending, one child lost to follow-up and four premature infants who died before a second card could be requested.

chromogenic substances unrelated to biotinidase activity by incubating and developing the filter disc in the absence of substrate. Second, the diagnosis of biotinidase deficiency can be confirmed easily in affected infants and heterozygotes can be reliably identified using the quantitative colorimetric test. Therefore, the genotype of other members of the family of an affected infant, particularly siblings, can be determined and this information can be used for genetic counselling. Third, all biotinidase-deficient patients have responded to biotin therapy, and since treatment circumvents the enzyme defect, we would expect all affected individuals detected subsequently to respond to vitamin supplementation. Fourth, the cost of 24 cents per test is about one quarter that of the least expensive test currently performed in the Virginia metabolic screening programme. Fifth, it is anticipated that maternal biotinidase deficiency will not be a problem.

From the results of this screening programme, we estimate the incidence of biotinidase deficiency at between 1 in 17 500 and 1 in 340 000 births (95% confidence limits), which places the disorder within the range of frequencies of other disorders currently screened for in most programmes. Furthermore, our findings indicate that biotinidase deficiency should be strongly considered among the metabolic disorders which are screened for in the neonatal period.

REFERENCES

Craft, D. V., Cross, N. H., Chandramouli, N. and Wood, H. G. Purification of biotinidase from human plasma and its activity on biotinyl peptides. *Biochemistry* 24 (1985) 2471–2476

Heard, G. S., Secor McVoy, J. R. and Wolf, B. A screening method for biotinidase deficiency in newborns. *Clin. Chem.* 30 (1984) 125–127

Pispa, J. Animal biotinidase. *Ann. Med. Exp. Biol. Fenn.* 43 Suppl. 5 (1965) 5–39

Wolf, B., Grier, R. E., Allen, R. J., Goodman, S. I. and Kien, C. L. Biotinidase deficiency: the enzymatic defect in late-onset multiple carboxylase deficiency. *Clin. Chim. Acta* 131 (1983a) 272–281

Wolf, B., Grier, R. E., Allen, R. J., Goodman, S. I., Kien, C. L., Parker, W. D., Howell,

D. M. and Hurst, D. L. Phenotypic variation in biotinidase deficiency. *J. Pediatr.* 103 (1983b) 233–237

Wolf, B., Heard, G. S., Jefferson, L. G., Proud, V. K., Nance, W. E. and Weissbecker, K. A. Clinical findings in four children with biotinidase deficiency detected through a statewide neonatal screening program. *N. Engl. J. Med.* 313 (1985) 16–19

Wolf, B., Heard, G. S., McVoy, J. S. and Raetz, H. M. Biotinidase deficiency: the possible rôle of biotinidase in the processing of dietary protein-bound biotin. *J. Inher. Metab. Dis.* 7, Suppl. 2 (1984) 121–122

J. Inher. Metab. Dis. 9 Suppl. 2 (1986) 307–310

Short Communication

GM$_2$ Gangliosidosis with Hexosaminidase A and B Defect: Report of a Family with Motor Neuron Disease-like Phenotype

A. FEDERICO[1], G. CIACCI[1], I. D'AMORE[1], R. PALLINI[1], S. PALMERI[1], A. ROSSI[1], N. RIZZUTO[2] and G. C. GUAZZI[1]
[1]*Istituto di Scienze Neurologiche e Centro per lo studio delle Encefalo-neuromiopatie genetiche dell'Università di Siena, 53100 Siena, Italy*
[2]*Cattedra di Neuropatologia, Università di Verona, Italy*

GM$_2$ Gangliosidosis is an inherited dysmetabolic disease, characterized by accumulation of GM$_2$ and GA$_2$ gangliosides in neuronal as well as in non-neuronal tissues. Biochemically the disorder can be due either to a deficiency of hexosaminidase isoenzyme A (Tay–Sachs form) or isoenzymes A and B (Sandhoff variant) or to absence of the activator protein of the enzyme (Sandhoff and Christomanov, 1979). Infantile, juvenile and adult phenotypes are known. Recently patients with late-onset disease with amyotrophic lateral sclerosis-like or Kugebelg–Welander phenotypes or spinocerebellar ataxia have been described, and a large heterogeneity is increasingly being discovered (Johnson, 1981; Federico, in press).

In this report we describe two brothers, now 49 and 44 years old, presenting a slowly progressive ataxia, fasciculations, peripheral neuropathy and autonomic nervous system involvement, and biochemically, severe deficiency of both hexosaminidase (Hex) A and B isoenzymes. A preliminary report on these patients has been previously communicated (Guazzi *et al*., 1983).

CASE REPORTS

The family derived from Piancastagnaio, a small village in the Amiata region in Tuscany, where few familial names are present. No consanguinity was present in the family. The father of our propositi at 40 years of age developed gait difficulties and died at 59 years of age. He had seven children; two of them are our patients.

Case 1 – San . . . Francesco, 49 years old, miner, was in good health until the age of 37, when fatigue and cramps in his legs with pain appeared. He was first hospitalized at 40 years of age in a department of neurology where examination showed hypotrophy of quadriceps muscles and fasciculations. At that time EMG showed a bilateral neurogenic peripherial lesion at quadriceps muscles.

At 44 years, neurovegetative troubles appeared as diffuse high perspiration at right hemithorax and left leg, pili at legs and libido loss.

At 47 years of age he was first examined by us. Neurologic examination showed a moderately ataxic gait, atrophy of the distal part of the legs, hypotrophy of

Journal of Inherited Metabolic Disease. ISSN 0141–8955.

quadriceps and of the distal part of the arms, moderate hypertonus, normal deep tendon reflexes at upper limbs and hypoactive reflexes at lower limbs, slight dysmetria and moderate nystagmus, and fasciculations at lower limbs. Psychic examination was normal. EMG showed moderate increase of potential duration and amplitude, increase of incidence of polyphasic potentials, fasciculations. Sural sensory nerve conduction velocity was slightly reduced (35 m/s) while peroneal motor and median sensory and motor nerve conduction velocities were normal. CT head scan showed a bilateral basal nuclear calcification.

Leukocyte lysosomal enzymes showed normal activity for α-mannosidase, β-galactosidase, β-glucosidase, and arylsulphatase A, while total Hex activity was present at 10% (Table 1).

Table 1 Leukocyte lysosmal enzyme activities (mU (mg protein)$^{-1}$ min^{-1})

Enzyme	*Case 1*	*Case 2*	*Controls*
α-Fucosidase	0.38	0.48	0.14–0.90
α-Mannosidase	2.39	3.55	0.50 3.94
β-Glucosidase	0.61	0.88	0.20–0.90
β-Glucuronidase	1.68	1.22	0.68–1.35
Arylsulphatase A	0.42	0.37	0.30–3.28
Arylsulphatase B	1.03	1.39	0.90–3.93
Hexosaminidase (tot.)	1.82	1.49	5–24
Hexosaminidase A (%)	78	79	50–80
β-Galactosidase	0.37	0.50	0.32–3.69

Case 2 – San . . . Gino, 43 years old, miner, was in good health until the age of 20, when he presented with fasciculations. At the age of 32 he experienced gait troubles, cramps in the lower limbs and paraesthesias in the feet. At the age of 34 there was a decrease of libido. At the age of 40 he was hospitalized in the Institute of Neurological Sciences of the University of Siena, where neurological examination showed a moderately ataxic gait, moderate pyramidal hypertonus, hypotrophy of the scapular girdle and of the lower limbs, brisk deep tendon reflexes at upper limbs and moderately hypoactive reflexes at lower limbs, tremor at hands and fasciculations of quadriceps. Psychic examination showed anxiety and depression. All routine blood and urine examinations, including analysis of urinary mucopolysaccharides and oligosaccharides, CT head scan and echography of liver, pancreas and spleen were normal. EEG showed non-specific diffuse electric abnormalities. Auditory evoked potentials were bilaterally abnormal in morphology and latency. On a cervical spynogram there was bilateral increase of latency in S11–S13 complexes. EMG showed loss of motor units, severely increased potential duration and amplitude, severe increase of incidence of polyphasic potentials, and fasciculations. Motor nerve conduction velocities at sural, peroneal and median nerve were normal with a slight decrease of sensory nerve conduction velocity at the median nerve.

Skin biopsy examined by electron microscopy was normal. Nerve biopsy (superficial peroneus nerve) showed severe myelin fibre loss (2800 mm^2, n.v. 7000–11 000) without signs of recent demyelination, few clusters of axonal regeneration, short internodes and decreased numbers of amyelinic fibres with an increase of endoneural collagen. The perinevrium was enlarged with hyalinization and enlargement of the wall of endo- and peri-neuronal vessels. Amyloid deposits were absent.

Leukocyte lysosomal enzyme determination showed a 10% activity of total Hex isoenzymes (Table 1).

DISCUSSION

The number of phenotypes of GM_2 gangliosidosis with Hex deficiency has increased in recent years. Cases have been reported with atypical spinocerebellar ataxia, amyotrophic lateral sclerosis or Kugebelg–Welander phenotypes, due to α-locus mutation and Hex A deficiency. β-Locus mutation and total Hex deficiency have been reported in cases with juvenile cerebellar ataxia and adult onset spinocerebellar ataxia (Johnson, 1981, 1983). More recently Barbeau *et al.* (1984) reported two adult brothers with the clinical phenotype of atypical Kugebelg–Welander disease, in one case associated with dystonia and ataxia, and total hexosaminidase deficiency. In both cases onset of symptoms was in infancy.

If we consider the father of our patients as probably affected by the same disease, the hereditary transmission in our family would be of dominant type. Clinical and genetic findings were suggestive of a familial amyloidosis, but nerve and skin biopsies were not able to show any amyloid storage. Enzymatic analysis of leukocytes showed a decreased activity of total hexosaminidase (10%) for a β-locus mutation. This family thus is an example of an adult motor neurone like phenotype of GM_2 gangliosidosis with autonomic nervous system involvement, due to β-locus mutation and both Hex A and B deficiency.

Clinically our patients are closely similar to five cases reported by Argov and Navon (1984), all with Hex A defect only. In this family also a pseudodominant transmission has been found. Dominant hereditary transmission is not typical of lysosomal disorders. Such 'pseudodominant' inheritance could be secondary to a marriage of an affected subject with a carrier of the same disorder.

The molecular pathogenesis of the adult forms of GM_2 gangliosidosis is still under discussion. Different allelic mutations in one gene locus may lead to extremely variable clinical forms of the same biochemical variant. The different clinical forms, therefore, e.g. infantile, juvenile and adult forms, must result from allelic mutations yielding gene products with different residual activities against their natural substrates *in vivo* (Conzelman and Sandhoff, 1984). The 10% residual activity of the enzyme present in our case could influence the very slow clinical course of the syndrome.

ACKNOWLEDGEMENTS

This research has been in part supported by a grant of Ministero della Pubblica Istruzione and CNR (Proggetto finalizzato Ingegneria Genetica e basi molecolari delle malattie ereditarie).

REFERENCES

Argov, Z. and Navon, R. Clinical and genetic variations in the syndrome of adult GM_2 gangliosidosis resulting from hexosaminidase A deficiency. *Ann. Neurol.* 16 (1984) 14–20

Barbeau, A., Plasse, L., Cloutier, T., Paris, S. and Roy, M. Lysosomal enzymes in ataxia: discovery of two cases of late-onset hexosaminidase A and B deficiency (adult Sandoff disease) in French Canadians. *Canad. J. Neurol. Sci.* 11 (1984) 601–606

Conzelman, E. and Sandhoff, K. Partial enzyme deficiencies: residual activities and the development of neurologic disorders. *Dev. Neurosci.* 6 (1984) 58–71

Federico, A. GM_2 gangliosidosis with motor neuron disease phenotype: clinical heterogeneity of hexosaminidase deficiency disease. In Kato, A., Cosi V., Parlette W., Pinelli, P. and Poloni, M. (eds.) *Therapeutic, Psychologic and Research Aspects of ALS,* Plenum Press, London, in press

Guazzi, G. C., Rizzuto, N., Ciacci, G., D'Amore, I. and Rossi, A. Polyneuritiform spinocerebellar ataxia with dominant autosomic transmission. *Neuropath. Acta Neurol.* 5 (1983) 303–304

Johnson, W. G. The clinical spectrum of hexosaminidase deficiency diseases. *Neurology* 31 (1981) 1453–1456

Johnson, W. G. Genetic heterogeneity of the hexosaminidase deficiency diseases. In Kety, S., Rowland, L. P., Sidman, R. L. and Matthysse, S. W. (eds.) *Genetics of Neurological and Psychiatric Disorders,* Raven Press, New York, 1983, pp. 215–237

Sandhoff, K. and Christomanov, H. Biochemistry and genetics of gangliosidoses. *Hum. Genet.* 50 (1979) 107–147

J. Inher. Metab. Dis. 9 Suppl. 2 (1986) 311–313

Short Communication

A Comparison between Hepatocytes and Macrophages of Sphingomyelin, Cholesterol and Acid Lipase in Various Types of Niemann-Pick Disease

A. LAGERON
INSERM U9, 184 rue du Faubourg, Saint Antoine 75012, Paris, France

Niemann-Pick disease (NPD) represents a group of inborn errors of metabolism with (McKusick 25720) or without (McKusick 25725) sphingomyelinase (s'ase) deficiency. Although the clinical classification proposed by Crocker (1961) has been extended, the dividing line between type A and C is not clear. Studying the sphingomyelin and cholesterol storage, and the degree of s'ase deficiency may help to clarify this problem. We attempted to determine which material was stored, its amount and the cells involved. Is there a relation between s'ase activity and sphingomyelin storage? Is there a relation between cholesterol storage and acid lipase activity?

MATERIALS AND METHODS

Seventeen biopsies from patients with NPD (15 livers (L), one spleen (S), one bone marrow (BM)) were studied in our laboratory by histoenzymological techniques: sphingomyelin was assessed with Baker and OTAN reactions after alkaline hydrolysis; cholesterol revealed with Schultz reaction and differentiation between esterified and free forms carried out using digitonin and oil red staining; acid lipase activity (EC 3.1.1.1) was evaluated according to the method described by Lake and Patrick (1970). The sphingomyelinase activity (EC 3.1.4.1.2) was measured by a biochemical technique (Kanfer *et al.*, 1966) in leukocytes or in fibroblasts in culture. Among these patients, aged from 3 months to 27 years, three belonged to type A, eight to type B and six to type C.

RESULTS AND DISCUSSION

The main results are summed up in Table 1 and the following points warrant emphasis.

Often in NPD, the storage involves not only macrophages but also hepatocytes whereas only macrophages are laden in Gaucher disease.

The group of the three patients belonging to type A is relatively homogeneous and seems to be different from types B and C in that hepatocytes are not involved

Journal of Inherited Metabolic Disease. ISSN 0141–8955. Queen Square, Lancaster, UK. Printed in Great Britain by Titus Wilson & Son Ltd., Kendal.

in the storage of sphingomyelin or cholesterol, macrophages contain both cholesterol and sphingomyelin but there is less of the former than of the latter, and acid lipase exhibits a normal or increased activity.

Table 1 Sphingomyelin and cholesterol amounts and acid lipase activity in hepatocytes (H) and macrophages (M) from 17 cases of Niemann-Pick disease. SBH indicates the presence of sea blue histiocytes

Type	*Cases (tissue)*	*S'ase (% control)*	*Sphingomyelin*		*Free cholesterol*		*Acid lipase activity*	
			H	*M*	*H*	*M*	*H*	*M*
A	J. (L)	5	+±	+++	−	++±	+	++
	Cha. (L)		±	++	−	+	+++	++
	R. (L)		+,+±	++±	−	+±	+++	−,++
B	Ber. (L)	5	±	++	+++	+	−	+
	S. (L)		++	++++	±	++	−	+,+++ SBH
	M. (L)	18	++	+++	±	−,+±	−	−,+±
	Z. (S)	1		+,++++		+		+,+++ SBH
	D. (L)	15	−	−,++	+,++±	−,+±	−	−,++ SBH
	Chi. (BM)			+++		+		−
	L.A. (L)	5	−	+++	++±	−,±		−
	L.B. (L)	5	−	+++	+±	−,±	−	−
C	G. (L)	100	+	++	−	++	−	+ SBH
	F. (L)	100	++	−	+±	+++	−	−,+±
	Bel. (L)	45	+	−	++	+++	−	−
	Lav. (L)		+	+++	+±	+++	−	−
	Br. (L)		+++±	++++	+±	++±	−	−
	E. (L)		++±	+++±	+±	+	−	−

The group of type B (eight cases) includes four Tunisians, Z., Chi., L.A. and L.B. (uncle and nephew), whose livers react similarly. In all eight patients the macrophages from the liver, spleen and bone marrow contain more sphingomyelin than cholesterol. More often, however, the hepatocytes contain little sphingomyelin except for the two adult cases (S., M.) where it is slightly increased. Its distribution in the cell was homogeneous except in the liver of patient S. where sphingomyelin is stored in the peribiliary area. This pattern seems more obvious in the cases reported by Elleder *et al.* (1980). In hepatocytes cholesterol storage is greater than sphingomyelin storage and higher than macrophage cholesterol storage. In this group the epithelial cells (hepatocytes and sometimes, tubule kidney cells (Lageron *et al.*, 1977)) are involved in the storage process. Acid lipase is negative in hepatocytes, negative or slightly positive in macrophages, but when some of them become sea blue histiocytes (SBH), they recover this enzymatic activity. Elleder did not find any acid lipase activity in hepatocytes in type A or B, whereas in our series type A and B give opposite results.

In type C, macrophages store more cholesterol than hepatocytes but the latter always store cholesterol. In both cells acid lipase is nearly negative. Perhaps this deficiency plays a part in type C. Curiously this activity seems closely dependent on cholesterol storage: in the liver from patient M. periportal macrophages, without cholesterol overload, demonstrate acid lipase activity whereas those lining sinusoids with cholesterol overload, have no acid lipase activity.

Sphingomyelin storage and s'ase deficiency do not always occur together. This therefore opens the possibility that an activating factor may be present.

REFERENCES

Crocker, A. C. The cerebral defect in Tay Sachs disease and Niemann-Pick disease. *J. Neurochem.* 7 (1961) 69–80

Elleder, M., Smid, F., Harzer, K. and Cihula, J. Niemann-Pick disease. Analysis of liver tissue in sphingomyelinase-deficient patients. *Virchows Arch. A Path. Anat. Histol.* 385 (1980) 215–231

Kanfer, J. N., Young, O. M., Shapiro, D. and Brady, R. O. The metabolism of sphingomyelin. I Purification and properties of a sphingomyelin cleaving enzyme from rat liver tissue. *J. Biol. Chem.* 240 (1966) 1081–1084

Lageron, A., Brière, J., Calman, F., Hinglais, N. and Emerit, J. Etude clinique histoenzymologique, ultrastructurale, biochimique d'un cas de forme B de Niemann-Pick. *Acta Histochem.* 59 (1977) 106–121

Lake, B. D. and Patrick, A. D. Wolman's disease deficiency of E600 resistant acid esterase activity with storage of lipids in lysosomes. *J. Pediatr.* 76 (1970) 262–266

J. Inher. Metab. Dis. 9 Suppl. 2 (1986) 314–316

Short Communication

Juvenile Dystonia without Vertical Gaze Paralysis: Niemann–Pick Type C Disease

A. FEDERICO[1], S. PALMERI[1], O. VAN DIGGELEN[2], E. FERRARI[3] and G. C. GUAZZI[1]

[1]*Istituto di Scienze Neurologiche e Centro per lo studio delle Encefalo-Neuro-Miopatie genetiche dell'Università di Siena, Italy;* [2]*Department of Cell Biology and Genetics, University of Rotterdam, The Netherlands;* [3]*Istituto di Clinica Neurologica dell'Università di Bari, Italy*

Niemann–Pick disease (NPD, McKusick 25720) is a group of inherited disorders of widely different clinical phenotypes, pathologically characterized by sphingomyelin storage. Crocker and Farber (1958) classified it into four groups: type A is the acute neuronopathic infantile form; type B is the chronic non-neuronopathic form; type C is the juvenile chronic neuronopathic form. Patients with a slower course, all of Nova Scotia extraction and of French ancestry, constituted group D. Brady *et al.* (1966) showed that in the tissue from type A and type B patients a profound deficiency of sphingomyelinase was present; sphingomyelinase activity was either normal or partially deficient (10–60%) in NPD-types C and D. Crocker's classification has been slightly modified into types A to F by Brady (1983) to include a few particular adult cases. Of all the groups, NPD-type C is the most complex due to clinical and biochemical heterogeneity of the reported cases. It is not even established whether or not NPD-type C is a single disease, as the nature of the primary biochemical lesion is unknown: the hypothesis of a defect of a specific sphingomyelinase isoenzyme (Callahan *et al.*, 1974) or of an activator protein (Christomanou, 1980) is yet under discussion.

We here report a new case of NPD-type C in which the clinical signs were characterized only by slight gait difficulties with choreo-athetoid movements, without vertical gaze paralysis that is one of the typical clinical findings at onset of this disorder (Vanier and Roussou, 1984).

CASE REPORT

Cam . . . Nicoletta has been observed at the age of 11 years. She was born of healthy unrelated parents after a normal delivery and did not show the neonatal icterus usually reported in such cases (Vanier and Roussou, 1984). No other cases were reported in the family. She appeared normal until 10 years old when she presented slowly progressive gait difficulties, dystonic movements of left foot and tremor of hands during intentional movements.

Neurological examination showed dystonic movement during gait, at rest pre-

Journal of Inherited Metabolic Disease. ISSN 0141–8955.

sence of myoclonus at feet, generalized hypotonus, brisk deep tendon reflexes at legs (normal at arms) and dysgraphia. Neuropsychologic and ophthalmologic examinations were normal. Within normal limits were all the routine blood and urine examinations including urinary mucopolysaccharides, Reuma test, Waaler Rose test, serum ceruloplasmin and urinary copper excretion. Urinary oligosaccharides examined by thin-layer chromatography showed abnormal presence of oligosaccharides with mobilities of 0.2, 0.4 and 0.6 cm. EEG was normal, as was X-ray of skeleton and CT head scan. An examination of bone marrow showed foamy histiocytes with presence of intracytoplasmic PAS-positive material. Leukocyte (α-mannosidase, β-galactosidase, β-glucosidase, β-hexosaminidase arylsulphatase A and B) and cultured skin fibroblast (hexosaminidase, β-galactosidase, β-glucosidase, arylsuphatase A, α-neuraminidase) lysosomal enzymes were normal. Sphingomyelinase activity was normal in leukocytes, while it was decreased (50%) in cultured skin fibroblasts either by using HNP substrate or methyl [^{14}C]sphingomyelin, according to Vanier *et al.* (1980) (Table 1).

Table 1 Lysosomal enzyme activities in leukocytes and fibroblasts. Values are expressed as nmol (mg protein)$^{-1}$ h^{-1} except for hexosaminidase A which is expressed as a percentage of total β-hexosaminidase

Enzyme	*Leukocytes*		*Fibroblasts*	
	NPD-C	*N.V.*	*NPD-C*	*N.V.*
α-Mannosidase	128	110–325	–	–
β-Galactosidase	98	90–200	480	450–1200
β-Glucosidase	4.4	5–13	181	90–350
β-Hexosaminidase (total)	1093	1100–3200	6140	4000–15 000
Hexosaminidase A	79%	50–80%	76%	40–80%
Arylsulphatase A	50	35–100	354	300–800
Arylsulphatase B	188	105–240	–	–
α-Neuraminidase	–	–	20	25–80
Sphingomyelinase (HNP-substrate)	24	10–36	57/43/58	100–400
Sphingomyelinase (methyl[^{14}C]sphingomyelin)	–	–	11	21–38

NPD-C = Niemann–Pick disease type C; N.V. = normal value.

DISCUSSION

The reported case, clinically characterized by moderate gait difficulties with choreoathetoid movements and rare myoclonus without vertical supranuclear ophthalmoplegia and without hepatomegaly, with presence of foamy histiocytes in bone marrow, represents an example of NPD-type C in an early stage.

Clinical diagnosis has been confirmed by sphingomyelinase assay that showed normal activity in leukocytes and decreased (50%) activity in cultured skin fibroblasts.

In NPD-type C sphingomyelinase activity has been reported normal in leukocytes, liver (Vanier *et al.*, 1980), spleen and brain (Brady, 1983), but in 80% of the cases a partial deficiency was found in cultured skin fibroblasts (Vanier and Rousson, 1984).

The nature of the molecular defect in NPD-type C remains unknown. After the postulation of a defect of a specific sphingomyelinase isoenzyme (Callahan *et al.*, 1974) or of a natural activator of the enzyme (Christomanou, 1980), Poulos *et al.*, (1983) suggested that the heterogeneity observed in fibroblast extracts may reflect an interaction of the enzyme either with itself or with other hydrophobic components present in the cellular extracts. Vanier and Rousson (1984), considering the complexity of the lipid profile in NPD-type C, doubted that in this disorder sphingomyelin represents the basic storage material and that the observed sphingomyelinase alterations are of primary origin.

In conclusion, our case, without the vertical gaze paralysis that is usually reported as an early symptom in NPD-type C, suggests that a dysmetabolic disorder such as NPD has to be suspected in subjects presenting only with mild dystonia and with other minor neurological signs.

ACKNOWLEDGEMENTS

This research has been supported in part by a grant from the Ministero della Pubblica Istruzione (Roma) and by a grant from the Consiglio Nazionale delle Ricerche (Progetto Finalizzato Ingegneria Genetica e Basi Molecolari delle Malattie Ereditarie). The authors acknowledge Prof. Dispensa (Div. Haematology, Siena), for bone marrow examination. The technical assistance of Dr. C. Salvadori and of Mrs. B. Cinelli is gratefully acknowledged.

REFERENCES

Brady, R. O. Sphingomyelin lipidoses: Niemann–Pick disease. In Stanbury, J. B., Wyngaarden, J. B., Fredrickson, D. S., Goldstein, J. L., Brown, M. S. (eds.), *The Metabolic Basis of Inherited Diseases* 5th Edn., McGraw-Hill, New York, 1983, pp. 831–841

Brady, R. O., Kanfer, J. N., Mock, M. B. and Fredrickson, D. S. The metabolism of sphingomyelin. II – Evidence of an enzymatic deficiency in Niemann–Pick disease. *Proc. Nat. Acad. Sci. USA* 55 (1966) 366–369

Callahan, J. W., Khalil, M. and Gerrie, J. Isoenzymes of sphingomyelinase and the genetic defect of Niemann–Pick disease type C. *Biochem. Biophys. Res. Commun.* 58 (1974) 384–390

Christomanou, H. Niemann–Pick disease type C: evidence for the deficiency of an activating factor stimulating sphingomyelin and glucocerebroside degradation. *Hoppe Seyler's Z Phys. Chem.* 361 (1980) 1489–1502

Crocker, A. C. and Farber, S. Niemann–Pick disease: a review of 18 patients. *Medicine* 37 (1958) 1–98

Poulos, A., Hudson, N. and Ranieri, E. Sphingomyelinase in cultured skin fibroblasts from normal and Niemann–Pick type C patients. *Clin. Genet.* 24 (1983) 225–233

Vanier, M. T., Revol, A. and Fichet, M. Sphingomyelinase activities of various human tissues in control subjects and in Niemann–Pick disease. Development and evaluation of a microprocedure. *Clin. Chim. Acta* 106 (1980) 257–267

Vanier, M. T. and Rousson, R. Niemann–Pick disease: a clinical and biochemical study. In Vanier, M. T. (ed.) *Recent Progress in Neurolipidoses and Allied Disorders*. Collection Fond. M. Merieux, Lyon, 1984, pp. 183–201

J. Inher. Metab. Dis. 9 Suppl. 2 (1986) 317–320

Short Communication – Noel Raine Award

Pre- and Postnatal Diagnosis of the Cerebro-hepato-renal (Zellweger) Syndrome via a Simple Method Directly Demonstrating the Presence or Absence of Peroxisomes in Cultured Skin Fibroblasts, Amniocytes or Chorionic Villi Fibroblasts

R. J. A. WANDERS[1], G. SCHRAKAMP[2], H. VAN DEN BOSCH[2], J. M. TAGER[3], H. W. MOSER[4], A. E. MOSER[4], P. AUBOURG[5], W. J. KLEIJER[6] and R. B. H. SCHUTGENS[1]

[1]*Department of Paediatrics, University Hospital Amsterdam, Meibergdreef 9, 1105 AZ Amsterdam, The Netherlands;* [2]*Laboratory of Biochemistry, State University Utrecht, Padualaan 8, 3584 CH Utrecht, The Netherlands;* [3]*Laboratory of Biochemistry, Meibergdreef 15, 1105 AZ Amsterdam, The Netherlands;* [4]*The John F. Kennedy Institute, Baltimore, Maryland, USA;* [5]*Hôpital Saint-Vincent de Paul, Paris, France;* [6]*Department of Clinical Genetics, University Hospital, Rotterdam, The Netherlands*

The cerebro-hepato-renal (Zellweger, McKusick 21410) syndrome is an autosomal recessive disease characterized clinically by severe hypotonia, typical cranio-facial dysmorphism, hepatomegaly, disturbances in liver function, renal cysts, failure to thrive and severe psychomotor and sensorial retardation (see Kelley, 1983 and Heymans, 1984). Most patients usually die within the first year of life. Biochemical abnormalities associated with this disease include a deficiency of plasmalogens in tissues and an accumulation of very long chain fatty acids, pipecolic acid and di- and trihydroxycoprostanoic acid in tissues and/or body fluids. The absence of morphologically distinct peroxisomes in liver and kidney of Zellweger patients as described by Goldfischer and colleagues in 1973 has generally been held responsible for this multitude of biochemical aberrations.

We recently described a simple method which directly demonstrates whether peroxisomes are present or deficient in cultured skin fibroblasts (Wanders *et al.*, 1984). Here we report that this method can also be used in cultured amniotic fluid cells and chorionic villi fibroblasts, thus allowing unequivocal prenatal diagnosis of Zellweger syndrome.

Journal of Inherited Metabolic Disease. ISSN 0141–8955.

MATERIALS AND METHODS

Enzyme activity measurements

The activities of dihydroxyacetone phosphate acyltransferase (EC 2.3.1.42) and catalase (EC 1.11.1.6) are measured as described previously (Schutgens *et al.*, 1984; Wanders *et al.*, 1984).

Latency measurements

Intact cultured skin fibroblasts or amniotic fluid cells were incubated in isotonic sucrose media containing different concentrations of digitonin. The free activities of catalase and lactate dehydrogenase were measured as described previously (Wanders *et al.*, 1984).

RESULTS

We have previously reported that acylCoA-dihydroxyacetonephosphate acyltransferase, a peroxisomal membrane-bound enzyme, is deficient in tissues, cultured skin fibroblasts and thrombocytes from Zellweger patients (Schutgens *et al.*, 1984; Wanders *et al.*, 1985). However, catalase, a soluble peroxisomal matrix enzyme, was found to be present in normal amounts (Wanders *et al.*, 1984; see also Table 1).

The results in Table 1 illustrate the same pattern in cultured amniotic fluid cells: whereas acylCoA-dihydroxyacetonephosphate acyltransferase was found to be deficient in homogenates of amniotic fluid cells from two fetuses affected by Zellweger syndrome as reported recently (Schutgens *et al.*, 1984), catalase was found not to be deficient.

The results obtained raise the question of the intracellular localization of catalase in control and Zellweger amniocytes respectively. We have previously shown that

Table 1 Activity of catalase and acylCoA-dihydroxyacetonephosphate acyltransferase in cultured skin fibroblasts and cultured amniocytes from controls and Zellweger patients and the minimal amount of digitonin required to release the latency of catalase in these cells

	Dihydroxyacetone-phosphate acyltransferase activity (nmol (2 h)$^{-1}$ (mg protein)$^{-1}$)*	*Catalase activity* (μmol O_2 min^{-1} (mg protein)$^{-1}$)*	*Minimal amount of digitonin required to release the latency of catalase* (μg ml^{-1})*
Cultured skin fibroblasts			
Controls	9.80±2.10 (*n*=27)	14.1±4.8 (*n*=21)	240±12 (*n*=18)
Zellweger patients	0.66±0.50 (*n*= 9)	26.7±9.1 (*n*=17)	8± 1 (*n*= 8)
Cultured amniocytes			
Controls	8.52±2.52 (*n*= 7)	2.74±0.83 (*n*= 7)	230±20 (*n*= 4)
Zellweger fetus 1	0.14	4.2	7
Zellweger fetus 2	0.04	3.4	8

* Results are mean±SD

the intracellular localization of enzymes within a cell can be determined in a relatively simple way. The method we used makes use of digitonin to permeabilize selectively the different intracellular compartments, and is based on the fact that the activity of an enzyme within a cell is latent due to the presence of an impermeable membrane preventing free interaction between the enzyme and its substrates present in the incubation medium (Wanders *et al.*, 1984).

The results in Table 1 indicate that, as in control fibroblasts, high levels of digitonin (about 230 μg ml^{-1}) were required to abolish the latency of catalase in control amniocytes. This indicates that catalase-containing particles (peroxisomes) are present in control amniocytes, a conclusion supported by the presence of the peroxisomal membrane-bound enzyme acylCoA-dihydroxyacetonephosphate acyltransferase in these cells. The data in Table 1 show that very low levels of digitonin (about 8 μg ml^{-1}) were required to abolish the latency of catalase in cultured amniocytes from two Zellweger fetuses. Identical amounts of digitonin were required to abolish the latency of lactate dehydrogenase, a cytosolic marker enzyme. Hence catalase is a cytosolic enzyme in Zellweger amniocytes.

Digitonin titration experiments revealed that catalase-containing particles (peroxisomes) are also present in chorionic villi fibroblasts

In one pregnancy at risk for Zellweger syndrome we recently found a deficiency of peroxisomes with this method. Furthermore, dihydroxyacetonephosphate acyltransferase was found to be deficient (0.55 nmol (2 h)$^{-1}$ mg^{-1}). From these results it was concluded that the fetus was affected by Zellweger syndrome and the pregnancy was terminated in the 13th week of gestation. Subsequent biochemical studies confirmed the diagnosis.

DISCUSSION

The absence of catalase-positive particles (peroxisomes) in liver and kidney from Zellweger patients was first documented by Goldfischer and colleagues in 1973. We have recently described a method which directly demonstrates whether peroxisomes are present or deficient in cultured skin fibroblasts (Wanders *et al.*, 1984). With the aid of this technique peroxisomes were shown to be deficient in fibroblasts from Zellweger patients. The present results indicate that this method, which makes use of digitonin to determine the subcellular localization of catalase, can also be used in cultured amniocytes and cultured chorionic villi fibroblasts. Use of the digitonin titration technique together with determination of dihydroxyacetonephosphate acyltransferase activity in cultured amniocytes or chorionic villi (fibroblasts) has so far resulted in the detection of four Zellweger fetuses.

This study was supported by grants from the Netherlands Foundation for Pure Scientific Research (ZWO) under the auspices of the Netherlands Foundation for Fundamental Medical Research (FUNGO) and from the Princess Beatrix Fund (The Hague, The Netherlands).

REFERENCES

Goldfischer, S., Moore, C. L., Johnson, A. B., Spiro, A. J., Valsamis, M. P., Wisniewski, H. K., Ritch, R. H., Norton, W. T., Rapin, I. and Gartner, L. M. Peroxisomal and mitochondrial defects in the cerebro-hepato-renal syndrome. *Science* 182 (1973) 62–64

Heymans, H. S. A. Cerebro-hepato-renal (Zellweger) syndrome: clinical and biochemical consequences of peroxisomal dysfunction. *PhD Thesis* (1984), University of Amsterdam

Kelley, R. I. The cerebro-hepato-renal syndrome of Zellweger: morphological and metabolic aspects. *Am. J. Med. Genet.* 16 (1983) 503–517

Schutgens, R. B. H., Heymans, H. S. A., Wanders, R. J. A., van den Bosch, H. and Schrakamp, G. Prenatal detection of Zellweger syndrome. *Lancet* 2 (1984) 1339–1340

Schutgens, R. B. H., Romeyn, G. J., Wanders, R. J. A., van den Bosch, H., Schrakamp, G. and Heymans, H. S. A. Deficiency of acylCoA-dihydroxyacetonephosphate acyltransferase in patients with Zellweger (cerebro-hepato-renal) syndrome. *Biochem. Biophys. Res. Commun.* 120 (1984) 179–184

Wanders, R. J. A., Kos, M., Roest, B., Meijer, A. J., Schrakamp, G., Heymans, H. S. A., Tegelaers, W. H. H., van den Bosch, H., Schutgens, R. B. H. and Tager, J. M. Activity of peroxisomal enzymes and intracellular distribution of catalase in Zellweger syndrome. *Biochem. Biophys. Res. Commun.* 123 (1984) 1054–1061

Wanders, R. J. A., van Weringh, G., Schrakamp, G., Tager, J. M., van den Bosch, H. and Schutgens, R. B. H. Deficiency of acylCoA-dihydroxyacetonephosphate acyltransferase in thrombocytes from Zellweger patients: a simple postnatal diagnostic test. *Clin. Chim. Acta* 151 (1985) 217–221

J. Inher. Metab. Dis. 9 *Suppl.* 2 *(1986) 321–324*

Short Communication

Impaired Cholesterol Side Chain Cleavage Activity in Liver from Patients with the Cerebro-Hepato-Renal (Zellweger) Syndrome in Relation to the Accumulation of Di- and Trihydroxycoprostanoic Acid in Serum

R. J. A. WANDERS[1], H. S. A. HEYMANS[1], R. B. H. SCHUTGENS[1], J. VAN ELDERE[2] and H. J. EYSSEN[2]
[1]*Department of Pediatrics, University Hospital Amsterdam, Meibergdreef 9, 1105 AZ Amsterdam, The Netherlands;* [2]*Rega Institute, Katholieke Universiteit van Leuven, B-3000, Leuven, Belgium*

The cerebro-hepato-renal (Zellweger, McKusick 21410) syndrome can be considered to be the prototype of a newly recognized group of diseases in which one or more peroxisomal functions are impaired. In 1973 Goldfischer *et al.* described the absence of morphologically distinguishable peroxisomes in liver and kidney of Zellweger patients. Biochemical abnormalities associated with this disease include the accumulation of abnormal C_{27}-bile acids. Indeed, there are several reports on the accumulation of di- and trihydroxycoprostanoic acid in plasma, urine and bile of Zellweger patients (for reviews see Kelley, 1983 and Heymans, 1984).

According to current concepts on bile acid synthesis from cholesterol, changes in the sterol nucleus precede degradation of the sterol side chain (see Salen and Shefer, 1983). Furthermore, it is generally believed that C_{27}-sterol side chain cleavage starts with 26-hydroxylation followed by oxidation of the C_{26}-hydroxyl group and subsequent conversion to C_{24}-bile acids via a sequence of reactions resembling the β-oxidation process. Studies in the early 1960s showed that isolated rat-liver mitochondrial preparations catalyse the oxidative cleavage of the side chain of cholesterol with formation of different bile acids and propionic acid. The mitochondrial fractions used in these studies, however, were highly contaminated with other organelles. For this reason, Hagey and Krisans (1982) reinvestigated the subcellular distribution of the cholesterol side chain cleavage activity in rat liver. They found that peroxisomes possess the complete enzymic armamentum to cleave the cholesterol side chain.

Since peroxisomes are absent in liver from Zellweger patients, we studied cholesterol side chain cleavage in liver from controls and Zellweger patients in order to elucidate the metabolic block in bile acid synthesis in Zellweger patients. The results obtained are described here.

Journal of Inherited Metabolic Disease. ISSN 0141–8955.

MATERIALS AND METHODS

Bile acid levels in serum from controls and Zellweger patients are determined according to published procedures (Parmentier *et al.*, 1979).

Fresh liver biopsy samples were obtained from three patients with the Zellweger syndrome and, as controls, three patients with unrelated disorders. Postnuclear supernatant fractions were prepared as described before (Wanders *et al.*, 1985). Incubations were carried out essentially as described by Mitropoulos and Myant (1967) and Hagey and Krisans (1982) using a medium with the following standard components: 100 mmol/l Tris-HCl pH = 8.50, 2.3 mmol/l ATP, 0.4 mmol/l NAD^+, 2.2 mmol/l $MgCl_2$, 4.0 mmol/l Na-citrate, 5.0 mmol/l propionate, 3.0 mmol/l reduced glutathione, 0.1 mmol/l coenzyme A, 10 μmol/l [26,27-^{14}C]cholesterol in bovine serum albumin and an aliquot of human liver homogenate. Cholesterol side chain cleavage activity was determined according to the procedure of Hagey and Krisans (1982) by measuring the amount of [^{14}C]propionic acid generated.

RESULTS

In serum from the three patients used in this study large amounts of di- and trihydroxycoprostanoic acid were found, whereas the levels of the normally occurring major bile acids, cholic acid and chenodeoxycholic acid, were low (see Table 1). Normal serum contains mainly C_{24}-bile acids with only trace amounts of the C_{27}-bile acids di- and trihydroxycoprostanoic acid.

Table 1 Cholesterol side chain cleavage activity and serum bile acid levels in Zellweger patients and controls

	Patient 1	*Patient 2*	*Patient 3*	*Controls*
Cholesterol side chain cleavage activity (percentage of mean of three controls)	11	9	14	100 (66–119)
Serum bile acids				
C_{27}-bile acids (percentage of total)				
trihydroxy coprostanoic acid	22.1	45.5	42.0	0
dihydroxy coprostanoic acid	16	26.2	8.8	0
C_{24}-bile acids (percentage of total)				
cholic acid	11.5	0.5	4.9	41–67
chenodeoxycholic acid	6.1	6.6	4.4	27–59

In order to obtain information on the metabolic block in bile acid synthesis in Zellweger patients, human-liver postnuclear supernatants were incubated with [26,27-^{14}C]cholesterol (see Materials and Methods) and cholesterol side chain cleavage measured. It was found that postnuclear supernatants prepared from fresh human-liver biopsies efficiently catalyse the oxidative cleavage of cholesterol as in rat-liver. Cholesterol side chain cleavage activity was maximal at pH = 8.5; omission of NAD^+ or ATP from the standard reaction medium (see Materials and Methods) resulted in an almost complete loss in activity. Cholesterol side chain cleavage activity was measured in liver from three controls and three Zellweger patients. The results (see Table 1) indicate a strongly impaired cholesterol side chain cleavage activity in liver from the three patients with Zellweger syndrome.

DISCUSSION

Bile acid synthesis from cholesterol involves the complicated interaction between a variety of enzymes in different subcellular compartments. Di- and trihydroxycoprostanoic acid are considered to be normal intermediates in the biosynthesis of cholic acid and chenodeoxycholic acid from cholesterol. The finding of an impaired cholesterol side chain cleavage activity in liver from Zellweger patients, as described here, provides an explanation for the accumulation of these compounds in serum from Zellweger patients.

It has been suggested that the accumulation of abnormal bile acids results from mitochondrial abnormalities which have been described in some Zellweger patients (see e.g. Goldfischer *et al*., 1973). Since the demonstration (Kase *et al.*, 1983) that peroxisomes catalyse the conversion of trihydroxycoprostanoic acid to cholic acid, it is more likely that the absence of peroxisomes in Zellweger patients is directly responsible for their apparent incapability to cleave off the terminal C_3-unit. It remains to be elucidated whether the small amounts of C_{24}-bile acids found in Zellweger patients (see Table 1) are formed via a separate pathway involving initial 25-hydroxylation rather than 26-hydroxylation (see Salen and Shefer, 1983) or are synthesized via the residual cholesterol side chain cleavage activity as found in our patients.

ACKNOWLEDGEMENTS

This study was supported by grants from the Netherlands Foundation for Pure Scientific Research (ZWO) under auspices of the Netherlands Foundation for Fundamental Medical Research (FUNGO) and from the Princess Beatrix Fund (The Hague, The Netherlands).

REFERENCES

Goldfischer, S., Moore, C. L., Johnson, A. B., Spiro, A. J., Valsamis, M. P., Wisniewski, H. K., Ritch, R. H., Norton, W. T., Rapin, I. and Gartner, L. M. Peroxisomal and mitochondrial defects in the cerebro-hepato-renal syndrome. *Science* 182 (1973) 62–64

Hagey, L. R. and Krisans, S. K. Degradation of cholesterol to propionic acid by rat liver peroxisomes. *Biochem. Biophys. Res. Commun.* 107 (1982) 834–841

Heymans, H. S. A. Cerebro-hepato-renal (Zellweger) syndrome: clinical and biochemical consequences of peroxisomal dysfunction. *Ph.D. thesis* (1984), University of Amsterdam.

Kase, F., Björkhem, I. and Pedersen, J. I. Formation of cholic acid from 3α,7α,12α-trihydroxy-5β-cholestanoic acid by rat liver peroxisomes. *J. Lipid Res.* 24 (1983) 1560–1567

Kelley, R. I. The cerebro-hepato-renal syndrome of Zellweger: morphological and metabolic aspects. *Am. J. Med. Genet.* 16 (1983) 503–517

Mitropoulos, K. A. and Myant, N. B. The formation of lithocholic acid, chenodeoxycholic acid, and α- and β-muricholic acids from cholesterol incubated with rat-liver mitochondria. *Biochem. J.* 103 (1967) 472–479

Parmentier, G. G., Janssen, G. A., Eggermont, E. A. and Eyssen, H. J. C_{27} Bile acids in infants with coprostanoic acidemia and occurrence of a 3α,7α,12α-trihydroxy-5β-C_{29}dicarboxylic bile acid as a major component in their serum. *Eur. J. Biochem.* 102 (1979) 173–183

Salen, G. and Shefer, S. Bile acid synthesis. *Ann. Rev. Biochem.* 45 (1983) 679–685

Wanders, R. J. A., Schutgens, R. B. H. and Tager, J. M. Peroxisomal matrix enzymes in Zellweger syndrome: activity and subcellular localization in liver. *J. Inher. Metab. Dis.* 8 Suppl. 2 (1985) 151–152

J. Inher. Metab. Dis. 9 Suppl. 2 (1986) 325–328

Short Communication

Deficiency of Dihydroxyacetonephosphate Acyltransferase and Catalase-containing Particles in Patients with Infantile Refsum's Disease

R. J. A. WANDERS[1], R. B. H. SCHUTGENS[1], G. SCHRAKAMP[2], H. VAN DEN BOSCH[2], J. M. TAGER[3], B. T. POLL-THÉ[4] and J. M. SAUDUBRAY[4]
[1]*Department of Paediatrics, University Hospital of Amsterdam, Meibergdreef 9, 1105 AZ Amsterdam, The Netherlands;* [2]*Laboratory of Biochemistry, State University Utrecht, Padualaan 8, 3584 CH Utrecht, The Netherlands;* [3]*Laboratory of Biochemistry, Meibergdreef 15, 1105 AZ Amsterdam, The Netherlands;* [4]*Clinique de Génétique et INSERM U 12, Hôpital des Enfants Malades, 75015 Paris, France*

Cerebellar ataxia, retinitis pigmentosa and peripheral neuropathy are the primary clinical features in patients with the classical form of Refsum's disease (McKusick 26650). The age of onset may vary from early childhood to adulthood. A characteristic finding in these patients is the accumulation of phytanic acid in plasma and tissues due to a phytanic acid oxidase deficiency.

In recent years several patients have been described presenting in the first year of life with a variety of clinical aberrations including hepatomegaly, facial dysmorphism, mental retardation, and retinitis pigmentosa. The finding of elevated plasma phytanic acid levels led to the diagnosis of an infantile form of Refsum's disease (Scotto *et al.*, 1982). Recent data, however, indicate that apart from phytanic acid, pipecolic acid, very long chain fatty acids and trihydroxycoprostanoic acid are also elevated in plasma from these patients (Stokke *et al.*, 1984; Poulos and Sharp, 1984; Poulos and Whiting, 1985). These abnormalities have also been described in patients with the cerebro-hepato-renal (Zellweger, McKusick 21410) syndrome. The multitude of biochemical abnormalities in patients with Zellweger syndrome has generally been ascribed to the known absence of peroxisomes (Goldfischer *et al.*, 1973).

Since the same set of biochemical abnormalities has been described in infantile Refsum and Zellweger patients, we decided to investigate whether the multitude of biochemical aberrations in infantile Refsum patients results from a generalized loss of peroxisome functions due to a deficiency of peroxisomes. The results of this collaborative study are described here.

Journal of Inherited Metabolic Disease. ISSN 0141–8955. Queen Square, Lancaster, UK. Printed in Great Britain by Titus Wilson & Son Ltd., Kendal.

MATERIALS AND METHODS

Enzyme activity measurements

The activities of dihydroxyacetonephosphate acyltransferase (EC 2.3.1.42) and catalase (EC 1.11.1.6.) were measured as described previously (Schutgens *et al.*, 1984; Wanders *et al.*, 1984.)

Latency measurements

Intact cultured skin fibroblasts from controls, Zellweger patients and infantile Refsum patients were incubated in isotonic sucrose media containing different concentrations of digitonin. The free activities of catalase and lactate dehydrogenase were measured as described previously (Wanders *et al.*, 1984).

RESULTS

We have previously reported that the membrane-bound peroxisomal enzymes dihydroxyacetonephosphate acyltransferase and alkyldihydroxyacetonephosphate synthase are deficient in tissues and cultured skin fibroblasts from Zellweger patients (Schutgens *et al.*, 1984; Schrakamp *et al.*, 1985), whereas several soluble peroxisomal matrix enzymes were not deficient (Wanders *et al.*, 1984). Indeed, catalase was found to be present in near normal amounts in liver and cultured skin fibroblasts from Zellweger patients (Wanders *et al.*, 1984).

Table 1 Activity of dihydroxyacetonephosphate acyltransferase and catalase in cultured skin fibroblasts from controls, Zellweger patients and infantile Refsum patients and the intracellular localization of catalase in these fibroblasts

Parameter measured	*Subjects*			
	Infantile Refsum Patient 1	*Infantile Refsum Patient 2*	*Controls*	*Zellweger patients*
Dihydroxyacetonephosphate acyltransferase activity (nmol $(2\,h)^{-1}$ (mg protein)$^{-1}$)	1.08	0.32	9.8±2.1 (n = 27)*	0.66 ± 0.50 (n = 9)*
Catalase activity (μmol O_2 min^{-1} (mg protein)$^{-1}$)	23.6	22.1	14.1±4.8 (n = 21)*	26.7±9.1 (n = 17)*
Catalase-containing particles in cultured skin fibroblasts	deficient	deficient	present	deficient

*Results are mean ± SD

The results in Table 1 indicate that dihydroxyacetonephosphate acyltransferase is also deficient in fibroblasts from patients with the infantile form of Refsum's disease. As in Zellweger fibroblasts, catalase is not deficient in fibroblasts from infantile Refsum patients. This finding led us to investigate whether catalase in fibroblasts from infantile Refsum patients is present in a subcellular organelle (peroxisome) as in control fibroblasts, or whether it is present in the cytosolic compartment in these fibroblasts as in Zellweger fibroblasts (Wanders *et al.*, 1984). The method used to investigate this makes use of digitonin to permeabilize the cell selectively and is based on the fact that the activity of an enzyme within an intact cell is latent due to the presence of an impermeable membrane preventing free interaction between the enzyme and its substrates present in the incubation medium. The digitonin titration experiments revealed that in fibroblasts from patients wth infantile Refsum's disease, catalase is present in the same compartment as lactate dehydrogenase, a cytosolic marker enzyme. These results indicate a strong deficiency of peroxisomes in fibroblasts from patients with the infantile form of Refsum's disease.

DISCUSSION

Recent results from different laboratories have indicated that biochemical abnormalities associated with infantile Refsum's disease include elevated levels not only of phytanic acid but also of trihydroxycoprostanoic acid, very long chain fatty acids and pipecolic acid (see introduction). The results described in this communication indicate that this multitude of biochemical abnormalities results from a deficiency of peroxisomes as found in Zellweger syndrome, leading to the generalized loss of peroxisomal functions. Since peroxisomes are involved in the conversion of trihydroxycoprostanoic acid to cholic acid, in the β-oxidation of very long chain fatty acids and in the catabolism of pipecolic acid, the accumulation of trihydroxycoprostanoic acid, very long chain fatty acids and pipecolic acid in plasma from Zellweger patients and infantile Refsum patients is immediately explained.

A consequence of the present findings is that the methods developed to diagnose Zellweger syndrome both postnatally and prenatally can in principle also be used in the diagnosis of infantile Refsum's disease. These methods include measurement of dihydroxyacetonephosphate acyltransferase in thrombocytes, cultured skin fibroblasts, cultured amniotic fluid cells or chorionic villi and/or the direct demonstration of the presence or absence of peroxisomes in cultured fibroblasts, amniocytes and chorionic villi fibroblasts using the digitonin titration procedure.

ACKNOWLEDGEMENTS

This study was supported by grants from the Netherlands Foundation for Pure Scientific Research (ZWO) under the auspices of the Netherlands Foundation for Fundamental Medical Research (FUNGO) and from the Princess Beatrix Fund (The Hague, The Netherlands).

REFERENCES

Goldfischer, S., Moore, C. L., Johnson, A. B., Spiro, A. J., Valsamis, M. P., Wisniewski, H. K., Ritch, R. H., Norton, W. T., Rapin. I. and Gartner, L. M. Peroxisomal and mitochondrial defects in the cerebro-hepato-renal syndrome. *Science* 182 (1973) 62–64

Poulos, A. and Sharp, P. Plasma and skin fibroblasts C_{26} fatty acids in infantile Refsum's disease. *Neurology* 34 (1984) 1606–1609

Poulos, A, and Whiting, M. J. Identification of 3α, 7α, 12α-trihydroxy-5β-cholestan-26-oic acid, an intermediate in cholic acid synthesis, in the plasma of patients with Refsum's disease. *J. Inher. Metab. Dis.* 8 (1985) 13–17

Schrakamp, G., Roosenboom, C. F. P., Schutgens, R. B. H., Wanders, R. J. A., Heymans, H. S. A., Tager, J. M. and van den Bosch, H. Alkyldihydroxyacetonephosphate synthase in human fibroblasts and its deficiency in Zellweger syndrome. *J. Lipid Res.* 26 (1985) 867–873

Schutgens, R. B. H., Romeyn, G. F., Wanders, R. J. A., van den Bosch, H., Schrakamp, G. and Heymans, H. S. A. Deficiency of acylCoA-dihydroxyacetonephosphate acyltransferase in patients with Zellweger (cerebro-hepato-renal) syndrome. *Biochem. Biophys. Res. Commun.* 120 (1984) 179–184

Scotto, H. M., Hadchouel, M., Odièvre, M., Laudat, M. H., Saudubray, J. M., Dulac, C., Beucler, I. and Beaune, P. Infantile phytanic acid storage disease, a possible variant of Refsum's disease: three cases, including ultrastructural studies of the liver. *J. Inher. Metab. Dis.* 5 (1982) 83–90

Stokke, O., Skrede, S., Ek, J. and Björkhem, I. Refsum's disease, adrenoleukodystrophy and the Zellweger syndrome. *Scand. J. Clin. Lab. Invest.* 44 (1984) 463–464

Wanders, R. J. A., Kos, M., Roest, B., Meijer, A. J., Schrakamp, G., Heymans, H. S. A., Tegelaers, W. H. H., van den Bosch, H., Schutgens, R. B. H. and Tager, J. M. Activity of peroxisomal enzymes and intracellular distribution of catalase in Zellweger syndrome. *Biochem. Biophys. Res. Commun.* 123 (1984) 1054–1061

J. Inher. Metab. Dis. 9 Suppl. 2 (1986) 329–331

Short Communication

Peroxisomal Abnormalities in Rhizomelic Chondrodysplasia Punctata

H. S. A. Heymans[1], J. W. E. Oorthuys[1], G. Nelck[1], R. J. A. Wanders[1], K. P. Dingemans[2] and R. B. H. Schutgens[1]
[1]*Department of Paediatrics and* [2]*Department of Pathology, University Hospital Amsterdam, Meibergdreef 9, 1105 AZ Amsterdam, The Netherlands*

The rhizomelic type of chondrodysplasia punctata (RCDP), an autosomal recessive disorder, is clinically characterized by a disproportionally short stature affecting primarily the proximal parts of the extremities, typical facial appearance, congenital cataracts, joint contractures, characteristic ocular involvement and severe mental retardation (Spranger *et al.*, 1971). Radiological studies reveal shortening, metaphyseal cupping and disturbed ossification of humeri and/or femora, together with epiphyseal and extraepiphyseal calcifications (Spranger *et al.*, 1971). No biochemical abnormalities have been described so far.

According to the literature, clinical similarities between RCDP and Zellweger's syndrome (ZS), including stippled calcifications of the bones, have caused some confusion in the diagnosis of those two entities (Spranger *et al.*, 1971; Heymans, 1984). Kretzner and colleagues (1981) described a striking resemblance between ocular features in RCDP and ZS, suggesting a related underlying biochemical abnormality. As ZS is biochemically characterized by a generalized peroxisomal dysfunction (Heymans, 1984; Tager *et al.*, 1985) we decided to study peroxisomal functions in patients with RCDP.

We report here the outcome of our investigations of plasmalogen content of erythrocytes, acylCoA-dihydroxyacetonephosphate acyltransferase activity (DHAP-AT) in thrombocytes and fibroblasts, phytanic acid concentration in plasma and intracellular distribution of catalase in fibroblasts of patients with RCDP and ZS respectively and of controls, together with the results of an ultrastructural study of the liver of one patient with RCDP.

PATIENTS AND METHODS

Patients

We investigated 5 patients with RCDP, 4 boys and 1 girl, varying in age from 6 months to 16 years. In all cases weight, height and head circumference were below the 3rd percentile. All patients showed cataracts, rhizomelia, contractures and roentgenological abnormalities typical of RCDP. After parental consent blood samples were obtained in all cases, skin biopsies for fibroblast cultures were taken in 3 cases and a liver needle biopsy was performed on one patient.

Journal of Inherited Metabolic Disease. ISSN 0141–8955.

Methods

Plasmalogen content of erythrocytes was measured as described by Heymans and colleagues (1983). DHAP-AT was measured according to the method of Schutgens and colleagues (1984). Phytanic acid was measured as described by Poulos and Whiting (1984). The intracellular distribution of catalase was studied according to the method of Wanders and colleagues (1984). Fibroblasts were cultured according to standard procedures.

RESULTS AND DISCUSSION

The results of our investigations are summarized in Table 1. Patients with RCDP showed a severe deficiency in plasmalogens in phospholipids from erythrocytes and a deficient activity of the peroxisomal enzyme DHAP-AT both in thrombocytes and fibroblasts, as described in ZS (Heymans *et al.*, 1983; Schutgens *et al.*, 1984). Plasma phytanic acid levels were elevated, comparable to those of ZS (Poulos and Whiting, 1984). However, digitonin titration experiments revealed a normal intracellular distribution of catalase in contrast to our previous findings in ZS (Wanders *et al.*, 1984).

Ultrastructural studies of the liver of one patient showed an absence of peroxisomes in some hepatocytes, whilst other liver cells displayed an increased number of exceptionally large and irregularly shaped peroxisomes.

From these findings we conclude that RCDP is an inborn disorder clinically as well as biochemically closely related to Zellweger's syndrome. The biochemical abnormalities in RCDP, which have not been described before, will prove important

Table 1 Plasmalogen content of erythrocytes, DHAP-AT activity in thrombocytes and fibroblasts, plasma phytanic acid concentration and intracellular distribution of catalase in fibroblasts of patients with RCDP and ZS respectively and of controls

	RCDP		*ZS*		*Controls*	
Plasmalogen content of erythrocytes pPE/pPE+PE×100%[1]	2.5–11.4	(5)*	6.5–24.6	(6)	39.7±1.6§	(10)
DHAP-AT activity						
Thrombocytes[2]	0.01–1.19	(5)	0.03–1.13	(4)	2.69±0.39§	(8)
Fibroblasts[3]	0.90–2.58	(3)	0.02–1.62	(9)	9.80±2.10§	(30)
Phytanic acid[4]	49–196	(4)	0–88	(11)	<9	(15)
Catalase positive particles[5]	Present	(4)	Absent	(4)	Present	(4)

*Numbers of subjects in parentheses

§Mean ± standard deviation

[1]PE = diacylphosphatidylethanolamine; pPE = plasmalogen phosphatidylethanolamine

[2]Units are nmol $(30\,\text{min})^{-1}$ $(\text{mg protein})^{-1}$

[3]Units are nmol $(2\,\text{h})^{-1}$ $(\text{mg protein})^{-1}$

[4]Units are mg $(1\,\text{plasma})^{-1}$

[5]Intracellular distribution of catalase by digitonin titration according to the method of Wanders and colleagues (1984)

in the (prenatal) diagnosis of this serious inherited disorder. Although ultrastructural and biochemical studies show that peroxisomes are present, we consider, based on our biochemical findings suggesting the involvement of more than one peroxisomal enzyme, that RCDP is a peroxisomal disorder of which the underlying defect has still to be elucidated.

REFERENCES

Heymans, H. S. A. Cerebro-hepato-renal (Zellweger) syndrome. Clinical and biochemical consequences of peroxisomal dysfunction. *Thesis*, University of Amsterdam, 1984

Heymans, H. S. A., Schutgens, R. B. H., Tan, R., van den Bosch, H. and Borst, P. Severe plasmalogen deficiency in tissues of infants without peroxisomes (Zellweger syndrome). *Nature (London)* 306 (1983) 69–70

Kretzner, F. L., Hittner, H. M. and Mehta, R. Ocular manifestations of Conradi and Zellweger syndromes. *Metab. Pediatr. Ophthalmol.* 5 (1981) 1–11

Poulos, A. and Whiting, M. Infantile Refsum's disease (phytanic acid storage disease): a variant of Zellwegers's syndrome? *Clin. Genet.* 26 (1984) 579–586

Schutgens, R. B. H., Romeyn, G. J., Wanders, R. J. A., van den Bosch, H., Schrakamp, G. and Heymans, H. S. A. Deficiency of acylCoA:dihydroxyacetonephosphate acyltransferase in fibroblasts from patients with Zellweger (cerebro-hepato-renal) syndrome. *Biochem. Biophys. Res. Commun.* 120 (1984) 179–184

Spranger, J. W., Opitz, J. M. and Bidder, U. Heterogeneity of chondrodysplasia punctata. *Humangenetik* 11 (1971) 190–212

Tager, J. M., Ten Harmsen van der Beek, W. A., Wanders, R. J. A., Hashimoto, T., Heymans, H. S. A., van den Bosch, H., Schutgens, R. B. H. and Schram, A. W. Peroxisomal β-oxidation enzyme proteins in the Zellweger syndrome. *Biochem. Biophys. Res. Commun.* 126 (1985) 1269–1275

Wanders, R. J. A., Kos, M., Roest, B., Meijer, A. J., Schrakamp, G., Heymans, H. S. A., Tegelaers, W. H. H., van den Bosch, H., Schutgens, R. B. H. and Tager, J. M. Activity of peroxisomal enzymes and intracellular distribution of catalase in Zellweger syndrome. *Biochem. Biophys. Res. Commun.* 123 (1984) 1054–1061

J. Inher. Metab. Dis. 9 Suppl. 2 (1986) 332–335

Short Communication

Cytogenetic Studies of Three Families with Ataxia-telangiectasia (Louis–Bar Syndrome)

L. Chessa[1], A. Federico[2], S. Raimondi[2], G. C. Guazzi[2] and E. Gandini[1]

[1]*I Cattedra di Genetica Medica, Università La Sapienza, Rome, Italy*

[2]*Istituto di Scienze Neurologiche e Centro per lo studio delle Encefalo-Neuro-Miopatie Genetiche dell'Università di Siena, 53100 Siena, Italy*

Ataxia–telangiectasia (AT, McKusick 20890) is an autosomal recessive disorder characterized by progressive cerebellar ataxia starting in early infancy and leading to complete disability by the age of 10 years, and oculocutaneous telangiectasias, appearing at 3–5 years of age. The disease is clinically and genetically heterogeneous (Balbi *et al.*, 1972). The basic molecular defect is unknown. AT patients show low levels or complete absence of IgA, are highly prone to lympho-reticular proliferative disorders and show hypersensitivity to ionizing radiations (Swift *et al.*, 1976; Paterson *et al.*, 1979; Painter *et al.*, 1980; Gatti, 1984). Life expectancy can be shortened because patients may succumb to pulmonary infections or malignancies.

AT is generally considered to be in the group of DNA-repair syndromes: affected individuals show increased rates of spontaneous and induced chromosomal aberrations (Oxford *et al.*, 1975). A similar trend has also been described in obligate heterozygotes but not at significant levels with respect to normal individuals. Chromosomal instability is characterized by random chromatid and chromosome breaks, at a lower level than in the other DNA-repair diseases like Fanconi's anaemia and Bloom's syndrome. Pseudodiploid clones are common: the most frequent rearrangements involve breakpoints in the long arm of chromosome 14 at bands q12 or q3.

In order to identify the mechanisms underlying a high tendency to malignancy in subjects with mendelian diseases and to obtain a suitable cytogenetic test for the carriers, we chose to study AT, encouraged also by the results obtained by our group in Fanconi's anaemia (Dallapiccola *et al.*, 1983).

MATERIAL AND METHODS

Our methodological approach was as follows:

(a) Identification of new familial groups with one or more affected individuals.

(b) Short-term cultivation of peripheral blood lymphocytes of patients, their parents (obligate heterozygotes) and their relatives (at risk subjects) in order to define the cytogenetic pattern of all the examined individuals, the rates and types of spontaneous chromosomal aberration and the effect of various clastogenic

substances. Peripheral blood lymphocytes were cultivated for 72 h in TC 199 with 10% of fetal calf serum (FCS) at 37°C; during the last 2 h colcemid (5 μg ml^{-1}) was added. Sodium citrate (0.9%) at 37°C for 20 min was used as the hypotonic solution. Slides were stained with Giemsa 5% for 10 min; one slide for each experiment was banded with GAG banding technique. To study the ratio of chromosomal aberrations 100 mitoses were examined.
(c) Stabilization of fibroblastoid cell lines, which constitute a long-term cell population very similar to T lymphocytes in their response to clastogenic tests. The medium used was MEM with 10% FCS added.
(d) Stabilization of lymphoblastoid cell lines by cocultivation with Epstein–Barr virus; we obtained a cell population virtually immortal, very easy to cultivate and store and previously used in AT studies (Littlefield *et al.*, 1981).

Controls were chosen on the basis of negative family history for lymphoreticular, immunological and neuroiogical diseases. Results of experiments were analysed by a double blind method.

RESULTS AND COMMENT

To date we have studied four AT homozygotes (AT/AT) from three different families, six obligate heterozygotes (AT/+) (their parents) and three at risk relatives (?/+).

Cytogenetic analyses showed a normal karyotype in T lymphocytes of all subjects except two homozygotes, the first with a 7/14 translocation in 1 cell of 15, the second with a dicentric 14 and a rearranged chromosome 7 in 2 cells of 12 in the first culture, and a more complex rearrangement 46, XY,−7, −8, −9, −14, der (8) t (8;14) (qter; qll), +marl, +mar2, +mar3 in 1 cell of 5 in the second culture.

Lymphoblastoid cells were also cytogenetically normal except for an obligate heterozygote showing a 47, XY, der(12)t(12;?)(p11;?), +mar|t(12;?)(p11;?)|line in 50% of the examined mitoses. It is of interest that 50% of lymphoblastoid cells of an affected individual are lacking the Y chromosome.

The rates of spontaneous aberration in short- and-long-term cultures are peculiar to each family and appear to be significantly higher in homozygotes and slightly increased in heterozygotes with respect to controls (Table 1).

To date we have used two clastogens to try to differentiate at a significant level the cytogenetic response of heterozygotes versus homozygotes, both normal and affected. The first clastogen was tritiated thymidine, for the last 48 and 24 h of culture at final concentrations of 0.01 and 0.02 μCi ml^{-1}; the second was a radiomimetic, bleomycin, at a final concentration of 1 μmol ml^{-1} for the last 48 and 24 h of culture. These substances were chosen for the well known hypersensitivity *in vivo* and *in vitro* of AT patients, and to a lesser extent of AT carriers, to ionizing radiations. Results are reported in Table 1.

Our data, even though preliminary, suggest the following two considerations. Firstly, we did not find in peripheral lymphocytes and especially in lymphoblastoid cells as many rearrangements involving chromosome 14 as we might have expected. Secondly, we have failed to obtain a significant difference between heterozygotes

Table 1 **Distribution of spontaneous and induced chromosomal aberrations (gaps, breaks, dicentrics, rings, acentrics, triradials) in peripheral blood cultures from three families with AT and the controls. The data are calculated on 100 cells; percentages indicate the number of cells with aberrations. Data in brackets refer to lymphoblastoid cell lines.**

	Standard cultures	*[³H]TdR* 0.01 μCi ml^{-1}	*[³H]TdR* 0.02 μCi ml^{-1}	*BLM I* *24 h*	*BLM I* *48 h*	*SCE*	*Lympho-blastoid lines*	*Fibroblast lines*
Family 1								
AT/AT	–	–	–	–	–	–	NA	A
AT/+	0.13 (0.19)	0.17 (0.32)	0.27 (0.30)	0.27 (0.56)	0.34 (—)	+	A	A
AT/+	0.21 (0.12)	0.31 (0.27)	0.30 (0.24)	0.38 (0.34)	0.57 (0.38)	+	A	A
?/+	0.21 (0.23)	0.33 (0.32)	0.26 (0.38)	0.42 (0.30)	0.58 (0.40)	+	A	A
+/+	0.10 (0.15)	0.13 (0.21)	0.25 (0.17)	0.45 (0.22)	0.48 (0.23)	+	A	NA
Family 2								
AT/AT	0.32* (0.31)	0.15* (0.18)	0.25* (0.19)	1.00* (0.42)	0.50* (0.20)	–	A	NA
AT/+	0.15 (0.07)	0.18 (0.10)	0.28 (0.14)	0.53 (0.28)	0.54 (0.40)*	+	A	A
AT/+	0.14 (0.23)	0.21 (0.32)	0.24 (0.48)	0.44 (0.36)	0.52 (–)	+	A	A
?/+	0.09	0.12	0.25	0.42	0.49	+	A	A
+/+	0.08	0.11	0.19	0.40	0.46	+	A	NA
Family 3								
AT/AT	0.13	0.18	0.22	0.55	0.50	+	A	NA
AT/AT	0.16*	–	–	0.60*	0.66*	–	A	NA
AT/+	0.09	0.17	0.13	0.38	0.51	+	A	NA
AT/+	0.10	0.18	0.22	0.30	0.40	+	A	NA
+/+	0.07	0.12	0.18	0.35	0.48	+	A	NA

— : failed culture
* : these values are calculated on less than 100 mitoses
A : available ; NA : not available
AT/AT : affected individuals, homozygous for AT gene
AT/+ : normal subjects, heterozygous for AT gene
?/+ : normal subjects, at risk of being heterozygous for AT gene
+/+ : controls
SCE : sister chromatidid exchanges
[³H]TdR : tritiated thymidine
BLM : bleomycin (1 μmol ml^{-1})

and homozygotes, both in lymphocytes and lymphoblasts. Each family shows a characteristic pattern of response, but variations within the family are not significant.

In conclusion, [^{3}H]thymidine and bleomycin used as clastogens do not indicate significant differences between heterozygotes and homozygotes, both in lymphocytes and lymphoblasts of AT patients. Further experiments will be performed using other clastogens such as alkylating agents (diepoxybutane), gamma radioisotopes ([^{14}C]thymidine) and oxidants (hydrogen peroxide).

The rates of spontaneous aberration differ between families but they appear to be significantly higher in homozygotes and slightly but not significantly increased in heterozygotes with respect to controls.

This work was supported in part by grant CNR no. 84.00596.44. EB virus was kindly provided by Dr P. Ragona, Clinica Medica Generale e Terapia Medica III, Università 'La Sapienza', Rome, Italy.

REFERENCES

Balbi, R., Abbate, G., Carlomagno, S., Del Vecchio, M., Fusco, G., Malagoli, T., Ventruto, V. and Guazzi, G. C. L'Atassia-telangectasia di Louis–Bar in un isolato genetico del mezzogiorno d'Italia. *Acta Neurol.* 27 (1972) 458–478

Dallapiccola, B., Porfirio, B., Mokini, V., Alimena, G., Mandelli, F. and Gandini, E. Detection of Fanconi's anemia heterozygotes by different cytogenetic approaches. *Clin. Genet.* 24 (1983) 293–298

Gatti, R. Ataxia-telangiectasia. Immune dysfunction is one of many defects. *Immunol. Today* 5 (1984) 121–123

Littlefield, L. G., Colyer, S. P., Joinier, E. E., Du Frain, R. J., Frome, E. and Cohen, M. M. Chromosomal radiation sensitivity in ataxia telangiectasia long-term lymphoblastoid cell lines. *Cytogenet. Cell Genet.* 31 (1981) 203–213

Oxford, G. M., Harnden, D. H., Parrington, J. M. and Delhantoy, J. D. A. Specific chromosome aberrations in ataxia-telangiectasia. *J. Med. Genet.* 12 (1975) 251–262

Painter, R. B. and Young, B. R. Radiosensitivity in ataxia-telangiectasia: a new explanation. *Proc. Natl. Acad. Sci. USA* 77 (1980) 7315–7317

Paterson, M. C. and Smith, P. J. Ataxia-telangiectasia: an inherited human disorder involving hypersensitivity to ionizing radiation and related DNA-damaging chemicals. *Ann. Rev. Genet.* 13 (1979) 291–318

Swift, M., Sholman, L., Perry, M. and Chase, C. Malignant neoplasms in the families of patients with ataxia-telangectasia. *Cancer Res.* 36 (1976) 209–215